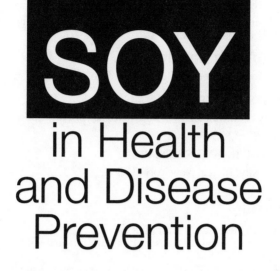

# SOY
## in Health
## and Disease
## Prevention

# NUTRITION AND DISEASE PREVENTION

## Published Titles

**Genomics and Proteomics in Nutrition**
*Carolyn D. Berdanier*, Ph.D., Professor Emerita, University of Georgia, Athens,
    Watkinsville, Georgia
*Naima Moustaid-Moussa*, Ph.D., University of Tennessee, Knoxville, Tennessee

**Perinatal Nutrition: Optimizing Infant Health and Development**
*Jatinder Bhatia*, M.B.B.S., Medical College of Georgia, Augusta, Georgia

**Soy in Health and Disease Prevention**
*Michihiro Sugano*, Ph.D., Professor Emeritus at Kyushu University, Japan

**Nutrition and Cancer Prevention**
*Atif B. Awad*, Ph.D., Department of Exercise and Nutrition Science, State University
    of New York, Buffalo, New York
*Peter G. Bradford*, Ph.D., Department of Pharmacology and Toxicology,
    School of Medicine and Biomedical Science, State University of New York,
    Buffalo, New York

# SOY

## in Health
## and Disease
## Prevention

Edited by
## Michihiro Sugano

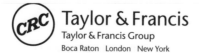

Taylor & Francis
Taylor & Francis Group
Boca Raton London New York

A CRC title, part of the Taylor & Francis imprint, a member of the
Taylor & Francis Group, the academic division of T&F Informa plc.

Published in 2006 by
CRC Press
Taylor & Francis Group
6000 Broken Sound Parkway NW, Suite 300
Boca Raton, FL 33487-2742

International Standard Book Number-10: 0-8493-3595-7 (Hardcover)
International Standard Book Number-13: 978-0-8493-3595-2 (Hardcover)
Library of Congress Card Number 2005041798

This book contains information obtained from authentic and highly regarded sources. Reprinted material is quoted with permission, and sources are indicated. A wide variety of references are listed. Reasonable efforts have been made to publish reliable data and information, but the author and the publisher cannot assume responsibility for the validity of all materials or for the consequences of their use.

### Library of Congress Cataloging-in-Publication Data

Soy in health and disease prevention / edited by Michihiro Sugano.
     p. cm. -- (Nutrition and disease prevention ; 3)
  Includes bibliographical references and index.
  ISBN 0-8493-3595-7 (alk. paper)
  1. Soyfoods--Health aspects. I. Sugano, Michihiro, 1933- II. Series.

RM666.S59S68 2005
613.2'6--dc22                                        2005041798

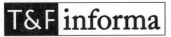

# Preface

This book was written to introduce "the world of the soybean" with respect to its myriad health benefits.

A number of excellent review articles and books are available that cover the nutritional and physiological functions of soybean and its products. The editor is, however, not aware of a book in English devoted to the study of soybean, written fully or mostly by Japanese. As many varieties of soybean products have been consumed for many years in East Asia, much knowledge has accumulated there documenting the health benefits of these products. Japan may be the most experienced country in the use of soybean for fermented foods. Advances in analytical methodologies have disclosed the full details of the chemical composition of soybean, and most soybean ingredients exert diverse physiological functions. Numerous Japanese researchers have been working for many years in every aspect of soybeans, and the Fuji Foundation for Protein Research has been established to support these studies. As a consequence of this research, various soybean books and reviews written in Japanese are available in Japan, and at present soybean is considered to be among the most healthy food items. Five components of soybean are now incorporated in officially approved functional foods called Foods for Specified Health Uses (FOSHU) and they are contributing much to our health. Thus, Japan must be considered a leader in the state-of-the-art of the health aspects of soybean functions.

It seems appropriate to publish a volume in English dealing with soybean as a source of functional and healthy foods. In editing this book, *Soy in Health and Disease Prevention*, it was an easy job to compose its content, as there are many examples available. This book includes several topics that are characteristically studied in our country. Those include FOSHU issues and physiological functions of soybean peptides. The most difficult issue encountered in the preparation of the book was to select contributors, as there are so many top researchers in this field. In other words, I was able to freely select the best contributors. Consequently, I am convinced that the contributors represent the cream of the crop. In addition to the research by Japanese scholars, I asked the most distinguished researchers in their respective fields to contribute. Those are cholesterol-lowering effects of soybean protein and anticancer effects of the trypsin inhibitor. Fortunately, two well-known researchers in these fields, Cesare Sirtori and Ann Kennedy, respectively, accepted my proposal and contributed these chapters. Also important is the chapter by David Kritchevsky that deals with the perspectives of soybean study.

This book encompasses all aspects of soybean from a viewpoint of health benefits. As all the contributors are experts in their respective fields, the latest information is available to understand the diverse health effects of soybean. It also is a good opportunity to learn how Japanese studies are proceeding in this field and how consumers are satisfied with diverse healthy soybean products. The multifunctional properties of soybean will surely bring health to all mankind. Enjoy the world of soybean dispatched from Japan.

This book is recommended for researchers of functional foods and for those who are in functional food industries who have always shown a great deal of interest in new materials for this purpose. The book also is recommended to graduate students to cover fundamental knowledge on functional food study in Japan.

**Michihiro Sugano, Ph.D.**
*Professor Emeritus*
*Kyushu University and*
*Prefectural University of Kumamoto*

# About the Editor

**Michihiro Sugano** received his B.S., M.S., and Ph.D. degrees from the Faculty of Agriculture, Kyushu University (KU), in Fukuoka, Japan. He served as head of the Department of Food Science and Technology, President of Prefectural University of Kumamoto (PUK), and as a member of the Dietary Guideline Examining Committee, Ministry of Health, Labour and Welfare, Japan. He has also served as Vice President of the Japanese Society of Nutrition and Food Science (JSNFS) and has been a director or councillor of a number of food and nutrition-related academic societies in Japan. He is currently professor emeritus of KU and PUK, and director of the Fuji Foundation for Protein Research.

He has published about 440 journal articles, 80 books and book chapters (Japanese and English), and 130 reviews, including several on soybean and lipid metabolism. He has received academic awards from JSNFS, the Agricultural Chemical Society of Japan, the Japanese Oil Chemists' Society, and is a fellow of the American Oil Chemists' Society. His research deals mainly with food functional factors, predominantly regulation of lipid metabolism.

# Contributors

**Yuko Araki**
Department of Clinical Nutrition
Kawasaki University of Medical
  Welfare
Kurashiki, Japan

**Yoshiaki Fujita**
Department of Clinical Nutrition
Kawasaki University of Medical
  Welfare
Kurashiki, Japan

**Tohru Funahashi**
Department of Internal Medicine
  and Molecular Science
Osaka University
Suita, Japan

**Ikuo Ikeda**
Graduate School of Agriculture
Tohoku University
Sendai, Japan

**Katsumi Imaizumi**
Graduate School of Agriculture
Kyushu University
Fukuoka, Japan

**Naoko Ishiwata**
Atomi Junior College
Tokyo, Japan

**Stuart K. Johnson**
Department of Pharmacological
  Science
University of Milan
Milan, Italy

**Ann R. Kennedy**
Division of Oncology Research
University of Pennsylvania School
  of Medicine
Philadelphia, Pennsylvania

**Mituru Kimira**
Tokyo University of Agriculture
Tokyo, Japan

**David Kritchevsky**
Wistar Institute
Philadelphia, Pennsylvania

**Yuji Matsuzawa**
Sumitomo Hospital
Osaka, Japan

**Melissa K. Melby**
Tokyo University of Agriculture
Tokyo, Japan

**Tadashi Ogawa**
Faculty of Health Science
  for Welfare
Kansai University of
  Welfare Science
Kashihara, Japan

**Cesare R. Sirtori**
Department of Pharmacological
  Sciences
University of Milan
Milan, Italy

**Michihiro Sugano**
Professor Emeritus
Kyushu University and
Prefectural University of
  Kumamoto
Fukuoka, Japan

**Hiroyuki Sumi**
Department of Physiological
  Chemistry
Kurashiki University of
  Science and the Arts
Kurashiki, Japan

**Kiyoharu Takamatsu**
Food Science Research Institute
Fuji Oil Co., Ltd.
Izumisano, Japan

**Shoichiro Tsugane**
National Cancer Center
Tokyo, Japan

**Chigen Tsukamoto**
Faculty of Agriculture
Iwate University
Morioka, Japan

**Takahiro Tsuruki**
Kyoto University
Kyoto, Japan

**Shaw Watanabe**
National Institute of Health and
  Nutrition
Tokyo, Japan

**Seiichiro Yamamoto**
National Cancer Center
Tokyo, Japan

**Takashi Yamamoto**
Faculty of Health Management
Nagasaki International
  University
Sasebo, Japan

**Yukio Yamori**
WHO Collaborating Center for
  Research on Primary Prevention
  of Cardiovascular Diseases
Kyoto, Japan

**Chieko Yatagai**
Department of Physiological
  Chemistry
Kurashiki University of
  Science and the Arts
Kurashiki, Japan

**Masaaki Yoshikawa**
Kyoto University
Kyoto, Japan

**Yumiko Yoshiki**
Graduate School of Life Science
Tohoku University
Sendai, Japan

**Xing-Gang Zhuo**
Tokyo University of Agriculture
Tokyo, Japan

# Contents

# 1 Nutritional Implications of Soy*

Michihiro Sugano

## CONTENTS

## 1.1 INTRODUCTION

The soybean plant (*Glycine max*) is the world's most widely cultivated and economically successful legume. Most soybeans cultivated are used as the raw materials for oil milling, and the residues are mainly used as feedstuffs for domestic animals. Although a variety of soy foods have been consumed in East Asia for

---

\* The compositional data of soybean cited in this chapter are from the following source: Resources Council, Science and Technology Agency, Japan, *Standard Tables of Food Composition in Japan*, 5th rev. ed., Printing Bureau of Ministry of Finance, Tokyo, 2000 (in Japanese).

many years, only limited amounts of soybeans are consumed directly in the United States and Europe.

Soybean is a good dietary source of protein and oil. Soybean requires considerably more cooking time than other legumes to have a palatable texture, which may be part of the reason for the use of soybean as processed foods in East Asian countries. Accompanying the scientific understanding that soybean is a healthy food, several approaches have been undertaken to get more soy in the diet.[1] At present, use of soybean protein is probably a suitable approach to increasing soybean consumption.

In addition to protein and oil being major nutrients, soybean contains valuable components, and it is an exceptional foodstuff of which the constituent components are almost totally disclosed chemically. Most of the nutritional and physiological functions of those components have been studied extensively, as summarized in Table 1.1. These functions are discussed in detail in the respective chapters of this book. Several components of soybean are currently approved as Foods for Specified Health Uses (FOSHU) by the Ministry of Health, Labor, and Welfare of Japan. FOSHU are functional foods, and manufacturers are officially allowed to claim their functionality. These include protein, isoflavones, oligosaccharides, germ plant sterols,

## TABLE 1.1
## Major Soybean Components and Their Health Effects

| Components | Functions |
|---|---|
| Protein | Hypocholesterolemic, antiatherogenic, reduces body fat |
| Peptides | Readily absorbed, reduces body fat |
| Lectins | Body defense, anticarcinogenic |
| Trypsin inhibitor | Anticarcinogenic |
| Dietary fiber | Improves digestive tract function, prevents colon cancer, regulates lipid metabolism |
| Oligosaccharides | Bifidus factor, improves digestive tract function |
| Phytin | Regulates cholesterol metabolism, anticarcinogenic, interferes with mineral absorption |
| Saponin | Regulates lipid metabolism, antioxidant |
| Isoflavone | Estrogenic function, prevents osteoporosis, anticarcinogenic |
| Linoleic acid | Essential fatty acid, hypocholesterolemic |
| α-Linolenic acid | Essential fatty acid, hypotriglyceridemic, improves cardiovascular function, antiallergic |
| Lecithin | Improves lipid metabolism, maintains neurofuctions (memory and learning abilities) |
| Tocopherols | Antioxidants, prevents cardiovascular diseases |
| Plant sterols | Hypocholesterolemic, improves prostate cancer |
| Vitamin K | Promotes blood coagulation, prevents osteoporosis |
| Mg | Essential mineral, prevents cardiovascular disorders |

and vitamin K in natto, a fermented soybean. Thus, it is well known that almost all components of soybean have beneficial health effects as characterized by the preventive potential for so-called life-style-related diseases or adult diseases (Table 1.1). Here, it is most probable that the health benefits of soybean reflect a complicated interaction of different components. The anticarcinogenic effect of soybean, for example, may be attributed to this type of interaction rather than to a single component (see Chapter 3). Reflecting on these situations, the phrase "soybean is a meat in the field" that was stressed because of the nutritive value of the rich-in-lysine protein, is now preferably reworded as "soybean is a treasure box of functionality."

In this context, it is important to understand the nutritional superiority of all the components of soybean. In this chapter the chemical components of soybean are discussed to convey fundamental knowledge that will help in understanding the following chapters. A number of good reference books are available.[2–5]

## 1.2  STRUCTURE OF SOYBEAN

Cultivated soybean is composed of approximately 8% hull, 90% cotyledons, and 2% hypocotyl axis. Thus, cotyledon contains the highest percentage of both protein and oil, whereas other components such as isoflavones are concentrated in the hypocotyl axis.

## 1.3  COMPONENTS OF SOYBEAN

As shown in Table 1.2, dry soybean contains 35% protein, 19% oil, 28% carbohydrates (17% dietary fiber), 5% minerals, and several vitamins. There are small but detectable differences in the nutrient composition depending on factors including variety, growing season, geographic location, and environmental stress. For example, soybean harvested in Japan generally contains more protein and less oil than that harvested in the United States. In any case, soybean is a good source of protein and oil.

### 1.3.1  Proteins

Soybean is probably the most efficient protein source in terms of cultivation size and protein content. However, unlike soybean oil, which is used mainly for human consumption, soybean protein has been used exclusively as feedstuffs, although there is a trend toward increasing human consumption of soybean protein.

Dry soybean contains approximately 35% protein, most of which is globulin, a storage protein. The major components of globulin are glycinin and β-conglycinin (or legumins and vicilins, respectively) that collectively correspond to 80% of the storage protein in soybean. These two proteins are called 11S and 7S globulins, respectively, depending on the difference in the sedimentation coefficient. Glycinin, which constitutes most of the total seed protein (over 40%), is a simple protein, while conglycinin is a glycoprotein. Glycinin and conglycinin exhibit

**TABLE 1.2**
**Nutrient Contents of Dried Soybean[a]**

| Component | Content (g/100 g)[a] | Mineral | Content (mg/100 g)[a] | Vitamin | Content (g/100 g)[a] |
|---|---|---|---|---|---|
| Energy (kcal) | 417 (433)[b] | Na | 1 (1) | Retinol (μg) | 0 (0) |
| Moisture | 12.5 (11.7) | K | 1900 (1800) | Carotene (μg) | 6 (7) |
| Protein | 35.3 (33.0) | Ca | 240 (230) | Retinol equivalent (μg) | 1 (1) |
| Fat | | Mg | 220 (230) | Vitamin D (μg) | 0 (0) |
| Carbohydrate | 28.2 (30.8) | P | 580 (480) | Vitamin E (mg) | 3.6 (3.4) |
| Ash | 5.0 (4.8) | Fe | 9.4 (8.6) | Vitamin K (mg) | 18 (34) |
| Dietary fiber | 19.0 (21.7) | Zn | 3.2 (4.5) | Vitamin $B_1$ (mg) | 0.83 (0.88) |
| Total | 17.1 (15.9) | Cu | 0.98 (0.97) | Vitamin $B_2$ (mg) | 0.30 (0.30) |
| Water insoluble | 15.3 (15.0) | Mn | 1.90 (–) | Niacin (mg) | 2.2 (2.1) |
| | | | | Vitamin $B_6$ (mg) | 0.53 (0.46) |
| | | | | Vitamin $B_{12}$ (μg) | 0 (0) |
| | | | | Folic acid (μg) | 230 (220) |
| | | | | Pantothenic acid (mg) | 1.52 (1.49) |
| | | | | Vitamin C (mg) | Tr (Tr) |

[a] Data from Resources Council, Science and Technology Agency, Japan, *Standard Tables of Food Composition in Japan*, 5th rev. ed., Printing Bureau of Ministry of Finance, Tokyo, 2000.
[b] Values in parentheses are for products in the United States.
Tr = trace

differences in nutritional and functional (rheological) properties. In general, glycinin contains three to four times more methionine and cysteine per unit protein than β-conglycinin. Thus, glycinin is more nutritionally valuable.

In addition to these two major proteins, γ-conglycinin and basic 7S globulin are present as minor storage proteins. Currently, β-conglycinin has been isolated at the commercial scale in Japan (Fuji Oil Co., Osaka), and a series of studies are emerging on this preparation. For example, β-conglycinin has been shown to lower serum triglyceride level in humans in 3 months at the dietary level of 5 g/d. Soybean also contains the biologically active protein components hemagglutinin, trypsin inhibitors, α-amylase, and lipoxygenase.

Two types of proteinase inhibitors occur in soybean: the Kaunitz trypsin inhibitor and the Bowman–Birk inhibitor. The former principally inhibits trypsin, while the latter inhibits both trypsin and chymotrypsin. Due to the presence of these protease inhibitors, soybean has to be heated prior to eating to maintain the nutritional quality of the protein. Although both inhibitors are relatively heat labile, the

Bowman–Birk inhibitor is more heat stable than the Kunitz inhibitor. Inhibitor activities are detected in several soybean foods despite heat treatment during preparations (15 to 30% of the activity in raw soybean). Fortunately, no apparent untoward effects have been reported in humans after consuming soybean foods. In contrast, the Bowman–Birk inhibitor appears to be an anticarcinogenic and antiinflammatory agent (see Chapter 12).

## 1.3.2 OIL

Soybean contains approximately 20% oil, of which the triglyceride is the major component. Lecithin, a kind of phospholipid, occurs abundantly in soybean. However, refined edible soybean oil contains more than 99% triglyceride. Soybean oil is a rich source of polyunsaturated fatty acids, not only linoleic acid (approximately 55%), but also α-linolenic acid (approximately 8%) (see Table 1.8). Soybean oil is a good dietary source of these acids for in Japan. However, the occurrence of α-linolenic acid renders the oil unstable, and in the United States, soybean oil is usually lightly hydrogenated to improve the oxidation stability. This is not the case in Japan. The hydrogenated oils contain relatively high amounts of *trans* fatty acids (approximately 5%) as compared to those without hydrogenation (2 to 3%).

Crude soybean oil contains 1 to 3% phospholipids, with 35% phosphatidylcholine, 25% phosphatidylethanolamine, 15% phosphatidyl inositol, and 5 to 10% phosphatidic acid. These phospholipids are removed from the oil mainly during the degumming process and are used as lecithin, a natural food emulsifier. The specific physiological functions of soybean phospholipids are described in Chapter 10.

Soybean contains a relatively high level of plant sterols. Plant sterols are the by-products of the purification of crude soybean oil and are good for various purposes, mainly as a cholesterol-lowering agent. β-Sitosterol, stigmasterol, and campesterol are the major components. Chapter 11 describes the cholesterol-lowering potential of soybean plant sterols.

## 1.3.3 CARBOHYDRATES

Soybean contains approximately 25 to 35% carbohydrates, most of which is nonstarch polysaccharides. It also contains oligosaccharides. Of the oligosaccharides, sucrose (5%), stachyose (4%), and raffinose (1.1%) are major components. Stachyose is a tetraose with a galactose–galactose–glucose–fructose structure, while raffinose is a triose with a structure of galactose–glucose–fructose. Polysaccharides are composed mainly of insoluble dietary fiber (see Table 1.2). Okara (bean curd refuse) contains soluble polysaccharides with galacturonic acid as its underlying structure. In addition to use as a dietary fiber supplement, soluble polysaccharides have been used to modify the physical properties of various foods.[6]

### 1.3.4 MINERALS

As shown in Table 1.2, soy contains approximately 5% minerals. It is relatively rich in K, P, Ca, and Mg. Fe in soybean appears to be well absorbed, similar to Fe in animal products. Thus, even when meat is replaced with soybean protein preparations, the availability of minerals, in particular Fe, is not adversely effected.

### 1.3.5 VITAMINS

Soybean is a better source of B-vitamins compared to cereals, although it lacks $B_{12}$ and vitamin C (Table 1.2). Soybean is also a rich source of tocopherols, an excellent natural antioxidant. Soybean oil contains, in milligrams/kilogram, 116 $\alpha$-tocopherol, 34 $\beta$-tocopherol, 737 $\gamma$-tocopherol, and 275 $\delta$-tocopherol.

## 1.4 COMPOSITION OF SOY PRODUCTS

Table 1.3 to Table 1.5 summarize the nutrient contents of various soybean products. The compositions differ widely within the same product. However, from the standpoint of the serving size of respective foods, all products are at least good sources of either protein or oil, particularly bean curd, fried bean curd, frozen bean curd, natto, and tonyu. Of course, other food items are sources of functional components, such as isoflavones (see Chapters 6 and 7). As shown in Figure 1.1, current nutrition survey shows that the Japanese consume about 60 g/d of soybean, of which about two thirds is consumed as tofu.

## 1.5 NUTRITIONAL ASPECTS OF SOY COMPONENTS

### 1.5.1 PROTEIN

Soybean protein is well digested and absorbed to a similar extent as animal proteins, even in children aged 2 years to 4 years. However, the digestibility differs depending on the source of protein; it is lower with soybean flour and higher with isolated proteins — 84 and 95% in children, respectively, while in adults the absorbability of these protein preparations is comparable, ranging from 91 to 96%. As shown in Table 1.6, the amino acid composition of soybean protein is characterized by the abundance of glutamic acid and aspartic acid, adding up to approximately 45% of total amino acids. Of these amino acids, 50 to 60% occurs as amides, glutamine, and asparagine. Although there are detectable differences in the amino acid composition of glycinin and $\beta$-conglycinin, the composition of soybean protein resembles, with exception of sulfur-containing amino acids (e.g., methionine), that of high-quality animal proteins. The amino acid pattern of soybean protein easily meets with the requirements of individual essential amino acids recommended by the World Health Organization (WHO)/Food and Agriculture Organization (FAO) as shown in Table 1.7. Soybean protein satisfies the requirement for infants aged

**TABLE 1.3**
**Nutrient Contents of Soybean Products (g/100 g)**

| Product[a] | Energy (kcal) | Moisture | Protein | Fat | Carbohydrate | Ash | Dietary Fiber |
|---|---|---|---|---|---|---|---|
| | | | | Nutrient Content (g/100 g) | | | |
| Kinako (parched bean flour[b]) | 437 | 5.0 | 35.5 | 23.4 | 31.0 | 5.1 | 16.9 |
| Tofu (bean curd) | 72 | 86.8 | 6.6 | 4.2 | 1.6 | 0.8 | 0.4 |
| Abra-age (fried bean curd) | 386 | 44.0 | 18.6 | 33.1 | 2.5 | 1.8 | 1.1 |
| Kori-tofu (frozen bean curd) | 529 | 8.1 | 49.4 | 33.3 | 5.7 | 3.6 | 1.8 |
| Natto (fermented soybean) | 200 | 59.5 | 16.5 | 10.0 | 12.1 | 1.9 | 6.7 |
| Okara (tofu refuse) | 111 | 75.5 | 6.1 | 3.6 | 13.8 | 1.0 | 11.5 |
| Tonyu (soymilk) | 46 | 90.8 | 3.6 | 2.0 | 3.1 | 0.5 | 0.2 |
| Yuba (soymilk skin) | 231 | 59.1 | 21.8 | 13.7 | 4.1 | 1.3 | 0.8 |
| Tempe | 202 | 57.8 | 15.8 | 9.0 | 15.4 | 2.0 | 10.2 |
| Miso (bean paste) | 217 | 42.6 | 9.7 | 3.0 | 37.9 | 6.8 | 5.6 |
| Shoyu (soy sauce) | 71 | 67.1 | 7.7 | 0 | 10.1 | 15.1 | 0 |
| Soy protein isolate | 388 | 5.9 | 79.1 | 3.0 | 7.5 | 4.5 | 4.2 |

[a] There are a variety of food items in each product with different nutrient contents.
[b] Full-fat flours.

Data from Resources Council, Science and Technology Agency, Japan, *Standard Tables of Food Composition in Japan*, 5th rev. ed., Printing Bureau of Ministry of Finance, Tokyo, 2000.

**TABLE 1.4**
**Mineral Contents of Soybean Products**

| Product | Mineral Content (mg/100 g)[a] | | | | | | | | |
|---|---|---|---|---|---|---|---|---|---|
|  | Na | K | Ca | Mg | P | Fe | Zn | Cu | Mn |
| Kinako (parched bean flour) | 1 | 1900 | 250 | 240 | 520 | 9.2 | 3.5 | 1.10 | — |
| Tofu (bean curd) | 13 | 140 | 120 | 31 | 110 | 0.9 | 0.6 | 0.15 | 0.38 |
| Abra-age (fried bean curd) | 10 | 55 | 300 | 130 | 230 | 4.2 | 2.4 | 0.21 | 1.41 |
| Kori-tofu (frozen bean curd) | 380 | 30 | 660 | 120 | 880 | 6.8 | 5.2 | 0.55 | 4.50 |
| Natto (fermented soybean) | 2 | 660 | 90 | 100 | 190 | 3.3 | 1.9 | 0.61 | — |
| Okara (tofu refuse) | 5 | 350 | 81 | 40 | 99 | 1.3 | 0.6 | 0.14 | 0.40 |
| Tonyu (soymilk) | 2 | 190 | 15 | 25 | 49 | 1.2 | 0.3 | 0.12 | 0.23 |
| Yuba (soymilk skin) | 4 | 290 | 90 | 80 | 250 | 3.6 | 2.2 | 0.70 | — |
| Tempe | 2 | 730 | 70 | 95 | 250 | 2.4 | 1.7 | 0.52 | 0.80 |
| Miso (bean paste) | 240 | 340 | 80 | 32 | 130 | 3.4 | 0.9 | 0.22 | — |
| Shoyu (soy sauce) | 5700 | 390 | 29 | 65 | 160 | 1.7 | 0.9 | 0.01 | — |
| Soy protein isolate | 1300[b] | 190[b] | 57[b] | 58 | 840 | 9.4 | 2.9 | 1.51 | 0.89 |

[a] Data from Resources Council, Science and Technology Agency, Japan, *Standard Tables of Food Composition in Japan*, 5th rev. ed., Printing Bureau of Ministry of Finance, Tokyo, 2000.
[b] These values differ widely depending on the salt regulation.

2 to 5 years. The nutritional value of soy protein is one of the highest of vegetable proteins (Figure 1.2).

In addition to its nutritive value, soybean protein has a physiological function. Soybean protein, unlike animal proteins, exerts hypocholesterolemic activity. Because of their usability, proteins isolated from soybean have been extensively applied to treat high serum cholesterol. This aspect of soybean protein will be discussed in Chapter 2. In Japan, FOSHU containing soybean protein isolates and related proteins are attracting attention as cholesterol-lowering foods (see Chapters 13, 14, and 16).

Another important point is the regulation of polyunsaturated fatty acid metabolism by dietary protein. Soybean protein, compared to casein, a representative protein source in animal studies, suppresses conversion of linoleic acid to arachidonic acid and hence, the production of eicosanoids,[7] mainly through interference with the $\Delta 6$ desaturation reaction (Figure 1.3), a rate-limiting step in the metabolism of linoleic and $\alpha$-linolenic acids to arachidonic and docosahexaenoic acids. Although this phenomenon has not been confirmed in humans, soybean protein may attenuate the allergic reaction through the reduction of inflammatory eicosanoids.

**TABLE 1.5**
**Vitamin Contents of Soybean Products**

| Product | Retinol (vg) | Carotene (vg) | D (vg) | E (mg) | K (vg) | B$_1$ (mg) | B$_2$ (mg) | Niacin (mg) | B$_6$ (mg) | B$_{12}$ (vg) | Folic (vg) | Pantothenic (mg) | C (mg) |
|---|---|---|---|---|---|---|---|---|---|---|---|---|---|
| | | | | | | | | Vitamin Content (/100 g)[a] | | | | | |
| Kinako (parched bean flour) | 0 | 4 | 0 | 2.4 | 37 | 0.76 | 0.26 | 1.8 | 0.58 | 0 | 250 | 1.33 | Tr |
| Tofu (bean curd) | 0 | 0 | 0 | 0.6 | 13 | 0.07 | 0.03 | 0.1 | 0.05 | 0 | 12 | 0.02 | Tr |
| Abra-age (fried bean curd) | 0 | 0 | 0 | 2.6 | 68 | 0.06 | 0.03 | 0.1 | 0.07 | 0 | 19 | 0.06 | Tr |
| Kori-tofu (frozen bean curd) | 0 | Tr | 0 | 4.4 | 57 | 0.01 | 0.01 | Tr | 0.02 | Tr | 5 | 0.07 | Tr |
| Natto (fermented soybean) | 0 | 0 | 0 | 1.2 | 870[b] | 0.07 | 0.56 | 1.1 | 0.24 | Tr | 12 | 3.60 | Tr |
| Okara (tofu refuse) | 0 | 0 | 0 | 0.7 | 8 | 0.11 | 0.03 | 0.2 | 0.06 | 0 | 14 | 0.31 | Tr |
| Tonyu (soymilk) | 0 | 0 | 0 | 0.3 | 4 | 0.03 | 0.02 | 0.5 | 0.06 | 0 | 28 | 0.28 | Tr |
| Yuba (soymilk skin) | 0 | 10 | 0 | 1.3 | 22 | 0.17 | 0.09 | 0.3 | 0.13 | 0 | 25 | 0.34 | Tr |
| Tempe | 0 | Tr | 0 | 1.8 | 11 | 0.07 | 0.09 | 2.4 | 0.23 | 0 | 49 | 1.08 | Tr |
| Miso (bean paste) | 0 | 0 | 0 | 0.7 | 8 | 0.05 | 0.10 | 1.5 | 0.04 | 0.1 | 21 | Tr | 0 |
| Shoyu (soy sauce) | 0 | 0 | 0 | 0 | 0 | 0.05 | 0.17 | 1.3 | 0.17 | 0.1 | 33 | 0.48 | 0 |
| Soy protein isolate | 0 | 0 | 0 | Tr | Tr | 0.11 | 0.14 | 0.4 | 0.06 | 0 | 270 | 0.37 | Tr |

[a] Data from Resources Council, Science and Technology Agency, Japan, *Standard Tables of Food Composition in Japan*, 5th rev. ed., Printing Bureau of Ministry of Finance, Tokyo, 2000.

[b] Contains menaquinone-7.

Tr = trace.

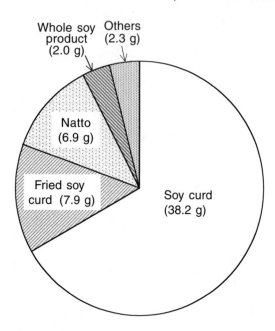

**FIGURE 1.1** Intake of soybean and its products in Japan. Total intake of soybean and soybean products: 57.3 g/d. (Data from The National Nutrition Survey in Japan, 2002.)

In addition, there are a number of studies that indicate the antidiabetic and antiobesity activities of soybean protein. The molecular basis of these functions is described in Chapter 4. Also, several studies show that diets rich in soybean have many known preventive and in some cases therapeutic effects on longevity (see Chapter 6).

Also important is soybean protein's allergic propensity. Soybean allergy is a relatively prevalent hypersensitive disorder, particularly in children under 3 years old. Current technology, however, has made possible the introduction of hypoallergenic soybean products (see Chapter 7).

Lectin is another type of protein. In soybean lectins, hemagglutinin activity is most well known, but in addition to this property, it may have anticarcinogenic activity (see Table 1.1).

### 1.5.2 PEPTIDE

Current studies on food functionality uncovered several methodologies to develop functional foods. Protein is one such component, and it is now well known that peptides exert diverse physiological functions that are unknown in the intact proteins. Because of a good availability of soybean protein preparations, a number of studies have been carried out in Japan. These include, for example, recovery

**TABLE 1.6**
**Amino Acid Compositions of Soybean Protein**

| Product | Protein[b] | Ileu | Leu | Lys | Met | Cys | Phe | Tyr | Thr | Trp | Val | His | Arg | Ala | Asp | Glu | Gly | Pro | Ser |
|---|---|---|---|---|---|---|---|---|---|---|---|---|---|---|---|---|---|---|---|
| Dried soybean | 35.3 | 290 | 470 | 390 | 90 | 99 | 330 | 210 | 230 | 79 | 300 | 170 | 460 | 260 | 710 | 1100 | 260 | 330 | 290 |
| Bean curd | 6.8 | 310 | 510 | 390 | 84 | 100 | 320 | 240 | 230 | 87 | 320 | 170 | 460 | 270 | 710 | 1100 | 260 | 350 | 320 |
| Natto | 16.5 | 260 | 440 | 390 | 90 | 100 | 300 | 240 | 210 | 84 | 290 | 170 | 320 | 240 | 640 | 1100 | 240 | 210 | 250 |
| Bean paste[c] | 9.7 | 280 | 470 | 270 | 66 | 82 | 310 | 210 | 230 | 67 | 310 | 150 | 410 | 270 | 650 | 690 | 250 | 310 | 280 |
| Soymilk | 3.6 | 300 | 490 | 390 | 91 | 100 | 310 | 240 | 240 | 85 | 310 | 170 | 450 | 260 | 410 | 1100 | 260 | 340 | 310 |
| Okara | 4.8 | 280 | 480 | 380 | 95 | 100 | 290 | 190 | 250 | 85 | 320 | 190 | 370 | 280 | 640 | 940 | 290 | 320 | 300 |
| SPI | 78.0 | 300 | 490 | 380 | 78 | 82 | 330 | 230 | 220 | 83 | 300 | 170 | 480 | 250 | 720 | 1200 | 250 | 340 | 310 |

Amino Acid (mg/g Nitrogen)[a]

[a] Data from Resources Council, Science and Technology Agency, Japan, *Standard Tables of Food Composition in Japan*, 5th rev. ed., Printing Bureau of Ministry of Finance, Tokyo, 2000.
[b] g/100 g edible portion.
[c] Bean paste with rice.
SPI = soy protein isolate.

**TABLE 1.7**
**Proposed Patterns for Amino Acid Requirements and Composition of Soybean Proteins**

|  | WHO/FAO[a] | | | Soy Protein | |
| Essential Amino Acid | Age 2–5 years | Age 10–12 years | Adult | Concentrates | Isolates |
|---|---|---|---|---|---|
| Histidine | 19 | 19 | 16 | 25 | 28 |
| Isoleucine | 28 | 28 | 13 | 48 | 49 |
| Leucine | 66 | 44 | 19 | 79 | 82 |
| Lysine | 58 | 44 | 16 | 64 | 64 |
| Methionine + cysteine | 25 | 22 | 17 | 28 | 26 |
| Phenylalanine + tyrosine | 63 | 22 | 19 | 89 | 92 |
| Threonine | 34 | 28 | 9 | 45 | 38 |
| Tryptophan | 11 | 9 | 5 | 45 | 38 |
| Valine | 35 | 25 | 13 | 50 | 50 |

[a] 1985 pattern.

*Source:* Endres, J.G., *Soy Protein Products, Characteristics, Nutritional Aspects, and Utilization*, revised and expanded ed., AOCS Press, Champaign, IL, 2001. With permission.

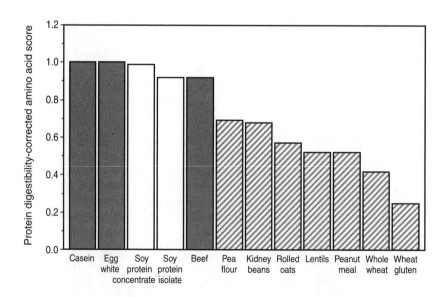

**FIGURE 1.2** Amino acid score of dietary proteins in humans.

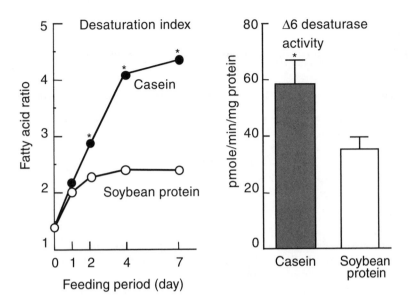

**FIGURE 1.3** Soybean protein lowers liver microsomal $\Delta6$ desaturase activity and liver phospholipid $\Delta6$ desaturation index in rats. Mean ± standard error (SE) (n = 6). *$p < .05$. Desaturation index: (20:3n-6 + 20:4n-6)/18:2n-6. (From Sugano, M. and Koba, K., *Ann. N.Y. Acad. Sci.*, 676, 215–222, 1993. With permission.)

from fatigue, body fat reduction, blood pressure lowering, calming brain function, senility prevention, and so on. Although not all of these effects have been confirmed in human clinical studies, the available information strongly suggests the usefulness of soybean peptide for various health benefits. These points are discussed in Chapters 13 and 14.

### 1.5.3　OIL

Soy oil is characterized by relatively large amounts of the polyunsaturated fatty acids, linoleic acid and $\alpha$-linolenic acid, approximately 55 and 8% of total fatty acids, respectively (Table 1.8). Soy oil, as well as rapeseed oil, is an exceptional source of $\alpha$-linolenic acid. Linoleic acid is an essential fatty acid belonging to the n-6 family of polyunsaturated acids and exerts important nutritional and physiological functions. As an essential fatty acid of the n-3 family, $\alpha$-linolenic acid plays an important role in the regulation of a number of metabolic pathways. However, due to its readily oxidizable nature, $\alpha$-linolenic acid is the cause of the so-called reversed flavor of soybean oil, a kind of rancid flavor. Numerous studies have therefore been carried out to reduce the content of $\alpha$-linolenic acid in soy oil, and current gene technology has made it possible at the expense of the nutritional and physiological benefits of soy oil as shown in Table 1.8.[8]

**TABLE 1.8**
**Fatty Acid Compositions of Soybean Oils (% of Total Fatty Acids)**

| Product | Fatty Acid | | | | |
|---|---|---|---|---|---|
| | 16:0 | 18:0 | 18:1 | 18:2 (n-6) | 18:3 (n-3) |
| Refined edible oil[a] | 10.6 | 3.9 | 23.3 | 53.0 | 7.6 |
| Genetically modified oils[b] | | | | | |
| Low linolenic | 10.1 | 5.3 | 41.1 | 41.2 | 2.2 |
| High oleic | 6.4 | 3.3 | 85.6 | 1.6 | 2.2 |
| Low palmitic | 5.9 | 3.7 | 40.4 | 43.4 | 6.6 |
| Low saturated fatty acid | 3.0 | 1.0 | 31.0 | 57.0 | 9.0 |
| High palmitic | 26.3 | 4.5 | 15.0 | 44.4 | 9.8 |
| High stearic | 12.0 | 21.0 | 63.0 | 1.0 | 3.0 |

[a] Data from Resources Council, Science and Technology Agency, Japan, *Standard Tables of Food Composition in Japan*, 5th rev. ed., Printing Bureau of Ministry of Finance, Tokyo, 2000.
[b] K.S. Liu (1999), collectively modified.

Soybean is also a good source of plant sterols. Sitosterol, campesterol, and stigmasterol are the major constituents of plant sterols in soybean oil. Soy germ oil contains more than three times the plant sterols than soybean oil and contains specific plant sterols including $\Delta7$-stigmastenol, $\Delta7$-avenastanol, and citrostandienol ($\Delta7$) that are rarely present in soybean oil. These sterols appear to exert a strong cholesterol-lowering activity, and vegetable oil fortified with soybean germ oil sterols is now available as FOSHU (see Chapter 16).

### 1.5.4 OLIGOSACCHARIDE

Soybean oligosaccharides serve as a bifidus factor and maintain well-being of the digestive tract. For this purpose, soybean oligosaccharides have been approved as FOSHU (see Chapter 16).

### 1.5.5 VITAMINS

Although soybean is relatively rich in vitamin K, this vitamin further increases during preparation of natto with specific bacteria. Such natto is now approved as FOSHU (see Chapter 15).

### 1.5.6 OTHER COMPONENTS

Soybean contains a relatively large amount of saponins (approximately 2% as glycosides), and these components are currently attracting attention. Soybean saponin is specifically called "soyasapoin" and has unique chemical structures and physiological functions (see Chapter 9).

Isoflavones are the specific components of soybean. Soybean is probably the richest plant source of isoflavones, containing 1 mg/g to 4 mg/g.[9,10] The functions of these components will be discussed in Chapters 7 and 8.

The majority of soybean phosphorus occurs in a phytin form. Phytin, calcium-magnesium salts of inositol-6-phosphate, has attracted attention because of its interference with the absorption of calcium, but it may also exert other functions such as lowering serum cholesterol.

## 1.6  FROM "A MEAT IN THE FIELD" TO "A TREASURE BOX OF FUNCTIONALITY"

Soybean is now regarded as a treasure box of functionality as can be estimated from the functionalities summarized in Table 1.1. For many years, soybean protein has been served as a supplementary source of essential amino acid lysine to improve nutritive values of various vegetable proteins such as rice in East Asia. Improving the dietary protein intake by incorporating more animal foods into diets tended to reduce the role of soybean protein. These dietary changes in turn caused a prevalence of life-style-related diseases.

Under these conditions, the door of functionality has opened as a result of detailed analyses of soybean components. It is said that soybean is full of functionalities with respect to the prevention of life-style-related diseases. These functions are described in detail in the other chapters of this book.

In addition to the nutritional and physiological functions of soybean, soybean protein has physical characteristics, particularly with respect to the ability to process food. Its rheological properties have been well studied, and various soybean protein preparations such as protein isolate, protein concentrate, and textured protein have been commercialized. Thus, the market for soybean protein is extensive in Japan, and the health benefits of these preparations will be immeasurable.

The final chapter (Chapter 17) of this book will give us perspective on issues of soybean protein.

## REFERENCES

1. Watkins, C., Easy ways to get more soy into your diet, *INFORM*, 15, 10–12, 2004.
2. Liu, K., *Soybeans, Chemistry, Technology, and Utilization*, Chapman & Hall, New York, 1997.
3. Endres, J.G., *Soy Protein Products, Characteristics, Nutritional Aspects, and Utilization*, revised and expanded ed., AOCS Press, Champaign, IL, 2001.
4. Descheemaeker, K. and Debruyne, I., Eds., *Soy & Health 2000, Clinical Evidence: Dietetic Application*, Garant, Leuven, Belgium, 2001.
5. Liu, K.S., Ed., *Soybeans as Functional Foods and Ingredients*, AOCS Press, Champaign, IL, 2004.
6. Maeda, H., Soluble soybean polysaccharide, in *Handbook of Hydrocolloids*, Phillips, O.G. and Williams, P.A., Eds., Woodhead Publishing, Cambridge, U.K., 2000, pp. 309–320.

7. Sugano, M. and Koba, K., Effects of dietary protein on lipid metabolism: a multifunctional effect, *Ann. N.Y. Acad. Sci.,* 676, 215–222, 1993.
8. Liu, K.S., Soy oil modification: products, applications, *INFORM,* 10, 868–878, 1999.
9. Wang, H.-J. and Murphy, P.A., Isoflavone content in commercial soybean foods, *J. Agric. Food Chem.,* 42, 1666–1673, 1994.
10. Wang, H.-J. and Murphy, P.A., Isoflavone composition of American and Japanese soybeans in Iowa: effects of variety, crop year, and location, *J. Agric. Food Chem.,* 42, 1674–1677, 1994.

# 2 Soy Proteins, Cholesterolemia, and Atherosclerosis

*Cesare R. Sirtori and Stuart K. Johnson*

## CONTENTS

## 2.1   INTRODUCTION

This review will describe the present state of knowledge of (a) the activity of soy proteins on cholesterolemia, (b) the therapeutic properties of soy proteins for atherosclerosis reduction, (c) the potential cardiovascular health benefits and harmful effects of soy isoflavones (phytoestrogens), and (d) the present knowledge of the beneficial effects of nonsoy legumes on cardiovascular health.

Soy protein consumption successfully reduces cholesterolemia in experimental animals when elevated by dietary means[1,2] as well as in humans with cholesterol elevations of genetic or nongenetic origin.[3-5] This cholesterol reducing effect, potentially leading to a reduced cardiovascular risk, became the basis for the U.S. Food and Drug Administration (FDA) approval of the health claim for the role of soy protein consumption in coronary disease risk reduction.[6]

Evidence is accumulating that the component in soy primarily responsible for reducing cholesterolemia is the protein per se.[3,7] The role in hypocholesterolemia of other minor components of commercial soy protein preparations such as fiber,[8] isoflavones,[9] and saponins[10] have not been supported by convincing experimental and clinical evidence.

Soy proteins appear to elicit their hypocholesterolemic effect mainly by activating liver low-density lipoprotein receptors (LDL-R).[11,12] This mechanism is tentatively attributed to specific protein components such as the 7S globulin and its $\alpha + \alpha'$ subunits.[13]

## 2.2   EPIDEMIOLOGICAL EVIDENCE
## OF CARDIOVASCULAR PROTECTIVE
## EFFECTS OF SOY

An epidemiological association between soy intake and reduced cardiovascular disease risk is well supported by a number of publications. In a recent prospective study of Chinese women, there was a more than 50% reduction of coronary events going from the lowest (<4.50 g/d) to the highest (≥11.19 g/d) quartile of daily soy intake.[14] Soy intake in the general population is clearly linked to reduced cholesterolemia. In particular, Nagata et al.[15] (Table 2.1) reported a progressive reduction of vascular risk in the presence of successive quartiles of soy protein intake in the Japanese population.

Early studies showed that strict vegetarians had a 60% depression of low-density lipoprotein cholesterol (LDL-C) levels and somewhat higher levels of high-density lipoprotein cholesterol (HDL-C) compared to free-living nonvegetarians of a similar age and the same gender.[16] Similar findings were more recently noted in a comparison between vegetarian and nonvegetarian elderly women.[17] A U.K. study

**TABLE 2.1**
**Correlation between Plasma Cholesterol and Soy**
**Protein Intake in a Japanese Population**
**(The Takayama Study)**

| | Quartiles of Soy Protein Intake | | | | |
|---|---|---|---|---|---|
| | 1 | 2 | 3 | 4 | P for Trend |
| Men m mol/L | | | | | |
| Crude | 4.77 | 4.63 | 4.64 | 4.59 | 0.02 |
| Adjusted[a] | 4.83 | 4.66 | 4.63 | 4.52 | 0.0001 |
| Women m mol/L | | | | | |
| Crude | 5.01 | 5.01 | 4.96 | 5.02 | 0.90 |
| Adjusted[b] | 5.01 | 4.89 | 4.79 | 4.78 | 0.0001 |

[a] Adjusted for age, smoking in taking of total energy, total fat, and protein.
[b] Adjusted for age, body mass index (BMI), menopausal status, and intake of vitamin C.

*Source:* Data from Nagata, C., Takatsuka, N., Kurisu, Y., and Shimizu, H. *J. Nutr.,* 128, 209–213, 1998.

of over 10,000 men and women recruited through health food shops, vegetarian societies, and magazines reported an overall mortality rate of about half that of the general population — associated, in particular, with a reduction in ischemic heart and cerebrovascular diseases (risk ratios 0.76 and 0.68, respectively).[18] Recently, a study of a British population (Oxford arm of the European Prospective Investigation into Cancer and Nutrition Study) confirmed the earlier findings by observing that women with a soy protein intake >6 g/d had a 12.4% reduction in LDL-C compared to women who consumed <0.5 g/d.[19]

## 2.3 THE HYPOCHOLESTEROLEMIC EFFECTS OF SOY

### 2.3.1 EARLY OBSERVATIONS

The replacement of animal with vegetable protein for the efficacious dietary treatment of hypercholesterolemia has increased in popularity over the past two decades. The hypothesis that proteins, rather than lipids, are the primary atherogenic dietary components dates back to 1907, when Ignatowski noted a high incidence of vascular diseases in Russian city dwellers on a diet rich in animal foods.[20] This observation was supported by a clear atherogenic response in rabbits fed meat and eggs. However, only a few years later, Anitschkow provided evidence that crystalline cholesterol added to the diets of rabbits could lead to a rapid induction of atheromas.[21] This latter finding overtook the previous observations of Ignatowski, leading to the current predominance of the lipid theory of atherosclerosis.

Only occasional reports on the potential cardiovascular benefit of vegetable proteins in animal or human diets were reported in the first half of past century.[22,23] Then in the 1960s, Howard et al.[24] along with Kritchevsky and Tepper[25] reported an antiatherogenic activity of soy in rabbits.

The increase in research activities on soy and cardiovascular disease prevention was led by the research group of the late K.K. Carroll, who demonstrated differential activities of a variety of vegetable proteins on atherosclerosis in comparison to the prototype animal protein, casein.[26] Huff et al.[27] clearly demonstrated that intact soy protein per se was effective for cholesterol reduction, but a mixture of amino acids corresponding to the composition of the proteins was not.

### 2.3.2 THE EARLY CLINICAL STUDIES

In an attempt to facilitate variation in the composition of diets given to hyper-cholesterolemic patients, Milanese clinicians in the 1970s obtained a new soy protein preparation, "textured vegetable protein" (CROKSOY®) (later found not to contain isoflavones). Surprisingly, the diet supplemented with this soy product was found to be highly effective for cholesterol lowering in the small number of hypercholesterolemic individuals initially treated (Sirtori et al., unpublished observations). The diet was also well tolerated and even appeared to beneficially modify coronary disease symptoms.

The initial findings of the cardiovascular-protective potential of soy protein led to a controlled crossover investigation of 20 hypercholesterolemics who underwent a 6-week inpatient study.[28] This study directly evaluated the effect of a standard low lipid diet containing animal proteins compared to the same diet but with a substitution of the animal protein with CROKSOY®. This study demonstrated that under metabolic ward conditions there was a 20 to 22% reduction in total cholesterol level and a 22 to 25% reduction in LDL-C, without significant changes in triglyceridemia (Figure 2.1). In addition, the reduction in plasma cholesterol was inversely related to the baseline cholesterolemia — a finding later supported by many other studies.[5] Ten more hypercholesterolemic individuals were also given 500 mg of cholesterol without modifying the beneficial effects of the (essentially cholesterol free) soy-supplemented diet.[28] This initial study is probably no longer reproducible due to the prohibitive cost of maintaining patients for 6 weeks in hospital beds. However, it stimulated interest in the potential cardiovascular-protective effects of soy protein and other vegetable protein sources in many other researchers.

A study confirming the hypocholesterolemic effect of soy protein was carried out by Milanese researchers in collaboration with Italian and Swiss clinical centers.[29] This study examined the effect of a low fat dietary regimen with or without soy protein supplementation when given to outpatients under strict dietary control. Hypercholesterolemic outpatients (n = 127) were treated for 8 weeks with the soy protein regimen after a 4-week stabilization period

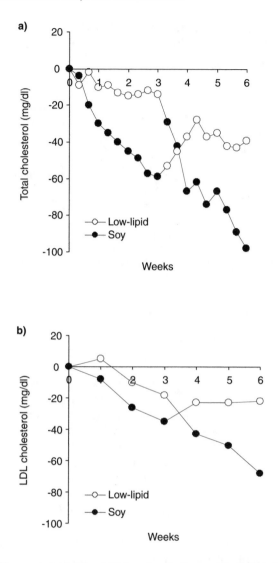

**FIGURE 2.1** Changes in (a) total and (b) low-density lipoprotein (LDL) cholesterol levels (mg/dl) during a randomized crossover investigation of 20 inpatients with severe hyper-cholesterolemia. They were maintained for 3 weeks on a standard low lipid diet with animal proteins preceded or followed by a similar diet with substitution of animal with soy proteins. (Modified from Descovich, G.C. et al., *Lancet*, 2, 709–712, 1980).

on a low lipid diet containing animal protein. A mean reduction in cholester-olemia of 23.1% in the 67 male and 25.3% in the 60 female participants was found, with no significant changes in plasma triglycerides, HDL-C, or body weight. The return of total and LDL-cholesterol levels to their baseline values occurred within 6 to 8 weeks after recommencing the low lipid animal protein diet, but

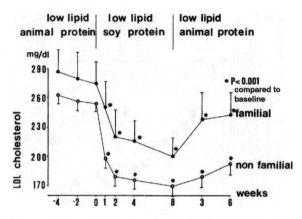

**FIGURE 2.2** Changes in low-density lipoprotein (LDL) cholesterol levels in Type II hypercholesterolemic patients given a soy protein diet for 8 weeks. A more rapid return to baseline is noted in individuals with familial disease. (Modified from Descovich, G.C. et al., *Lancet*, 2, 709–712, 1980).

the reversal was accelerated in participants with familial hypercholesterolemia (FH) (Figure 2.2).

### 2.3.3 CURRENT CONSENSUS

Substitution of animal with soy proteins in the diet of hypercholesterolemic individuals or addition of soy proteins to lipid lowering diets[4] have been repeatedly associated with significant cholesterol reduction.[3] Anderson et al.[5] reported a meta-analysis of 38 studies in both hypercholesterolemics and in normolipidemic volunteers treated for variable lengths of time using diets with partial or total substitution of animal proteins with soy proteins. This meta-analysis confirmed that serum total cholesterol and LDL-C concentrations are modified, dependent on baseline cholesterolemia, from a minimum of −3.3% in subjects with cholesterol in the normal range, up to −19.6% (LDL-C −24%) in clear-cut hypercholesterolemics (Figure 2.3). The finding that the cholesterol-lowering response to the soy protein diet is directly correlated to baseline cholesterolemia is supported by most other clinical reports. An exception may be the case of a soy protein hydrolysate with phospholipids (CSPHP),[30] shown to be an effective hypocholesterolemic agent in mildly hypercholesterolemic individuals. This finding has not, however, been confirmed by further studies.

### 2.3.4 STUDIES IN NORMOLIPIDEMIC AND MILDLY HYPERCHOLESTEROLEMIC SUBJECTS

Normolipidemic or mildly hypercholesterolemic individuals frequently do not have a clear-cut hypocholesterolemic response to a soy protein diet. Bakhit et al.[4] however, performed a well-controlled study in mildly hypercholesterolemic volunteers (mean cholesterol 220 mg/dl) by carefully following guidelines

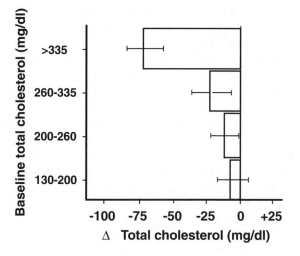

**FIGURE 2.3** Plasma cholesterol changes vs. baseline levels in the meta-analysis from 38 clinical studies of soy proteins in subjects with widely different cholesterolemias. A clearly better response is noted in patients with marked elevations of cholesterolemia. (Modified from Anderson, J.W., Johnstone, B.M., and Cook Newell, M.E., *N. Engl. J. Med.*, 333, 276–282, 1995).

previously optimized in studies with severe hypercholesterolemics. The subjects were given high protein diets of equivalent lipid and fiber contents. In these individuals 25 g/d of soy protein was found to be adequate to exert a significant reduction of LDL-C levels, and this reduction was directly related to the baseline levels (Figure 2.4).

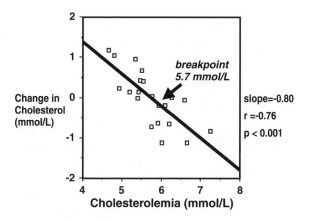

**FIGURE 2.4** First U.S. study of a soy protein diet in subjects with a wide range of cholesterolemia, given an additional 25 g/d of dietary soy protein. Plasma cholesterol reduction occurred only in those with a total cholesterolemia exceeding 5.7 m mol/L (220 mg/dl). (Modified from Bakhit, R.M. et al., *J. Nutr.*, 124, 213–222, 1994).

In normolipidemic but obese individuals, Jenkins et al.[31] showed a significant hypocholesterolemic effect of soy protein when given within an energy restricted diet. When casein was the predominant protein, little change (possibly even a small increase) in total and LDL-C levels occurred, compared to a 20% LDL-C reduction with soy as the predominant protein source.

Meinertz et al.[32] examined whether soy protein intake may improve cholesterol handling in normolipidemics by adding a large amount of cholesterol (500 mg/d) to a diet with a polyunsaturated/saturated fatty acid ratio of 1.43 and containing either casein or soy. The soy protein diet resulted in a 16% lower LDL-C and higher HDL-C levels compared to the casein diet, suggesting that (a) level of cholesterol intake may determine whether plant or animal proteins exert a differential effect on cholesterolemia and (b) responses may be different when (LDL-R) activity is reduced, as in the case of cholesterol addition — a condition not dissimilar from that of some animal models.

### 2.3.5 USE OF SOY PROTEIN-INDUCED HYPOCHOLESTEROLEMIA UNDER SPECIAL CLINICAL CONDITIONS

#### 2.3.5.1 Pediatric Hypercholesterolemia

An important use of the soy protein diet is for the treatment of pediatric hypercholesterolemia. An Italian multicenter study on 18 prepubertal children demonstrated that a reduction in cholesterolemia of around 25% or more is commonly achieved.[33] Indeed, some of these children have remained on the soy protein diet and maintained acceptable levels of cholesterolemia to this day, demonstrating its long-term efficacy. Similar findings have been reported by Widhalm et al.[34] who found beneficial effects of commencing the soy protein regimen at the age of 2 years in 11 infants with FH. Many pediatricians now believe that children with FH should receive the soy protein diet before puberty, a period when drug prescription is not recommended but when the soy protein diet is well accepted by the patients and considered safe.

#### 2.3.5.2 Patients Not Responding to Statins

Researchers at the University of Milan have investigated the possibility that a soy protein diet may favorably affect LDL-C in patients not responding to statins. Statins, the most widely used class of drugs for hypercholesterolemia, reduce cholesterol by inhibiting biosynthesis, but in a significant number of patients, they either do not bring about any significant LDL-C reduction or tolerance to prolonged treatment occurs.[35,36] A soy protein diet could theoretically be helpful for such patients by acting by a different mechanism. In a study by Sirtori et al.[37] a series of patients with unsuccessful statin treatment were given a soy-supplemented diet, resulting in a significant LDL-C reduction (−15%), most marked in patients with the highest baseline levels.

### 2.3.5.3 Kidney Disease

An area for possible clinical application of soy proteins is that of hyperlipidemias secondary to kidney disease, particularly the nephrotic syndrome. In this condition, changing from an animal to a vegetarian soy diet markedly reduces serum cholesterol and also reduces urinary protein excretion.[38]

A recent study by Teixeira et al.[39] concluded that a soy protein isolate-based diet compared to one based on casein can improve both serum lipids and nephropathy biomarkers in Type II diabetic patients with nephropathy. From ongoing long-term studies, it also appears that a change to a soy diet may favorably influence the progression of renal disease.

### 2.3.6 Mechanisms of Action of Soy Protein-Mediated Hypocholesterolemia

#### 2.3.6.1 Soy Protein Components Responsible for Hypocholesterolemic Effects

Considerable debate continues on the relative contribution of soy protein and other components, particularly isoflavones, to the hypocholesterolemic effects of soy protein preparations. Based primarily on studies of monkeys,[40] it was suggested in the 1995 meta-analysis by Anderson et al.[5] that 60% or more of the beneficial effect of soy protein preparations on cholesterolemia could be due to isoflavones (genistein and daidzein and their aglycones and glucosides[41]). Nevertheless, most of the clinical studies of hypercholesterolemics used in the meta-analysis were carried out using soy concentrates or isolates containing negligible isoflavone levels. In addition, soy products demonstrating cholesterol-lowering properties in the clinical studies of Italian and Swiss investigators over the past 20 years[42] have been found to be to be essentially isoflavone-free[43] (Table 2.2).

TABLE 2.2
Normalized Isoflavone Content of Soy Flour and of
Two Batches of the Soy Protein Product Used in the
Italian Clinical Studies

| Product | vg/g Dry Weight | | |
| --- | --- | --- | --- |
| | Daidzein | Genistein | Glycitein |
| Defatted soybean flour | 1142 | 1550 | 168 |
| CROKSOY batch A | 44 | 66 | 34 |
| CROKSOY batch B | 44 | 67 | 34 |

Source: Data from Sirtori, C.R., Gianazza, E., Manzoni, C., Lovati, M.R., and Murphy, P.A., Am. J. Clin. Nutr., 65, 166–167, 1997.

Studies in rats, dating back 20 years, had attempted to establish a link between the hypocholesterolemic effects of soy and activation of liver LDL-R *in vivo*.[44] These early studies clearly demonstrated that animals on a cholesterol and cholic acid dietary regimen with casein (a prototype animal protein) as the major protein source had a dramatic down-regulation of liver LDL-R activity, and this effect was reversed in the presence of soy as the major dietary protein. Based on these findings, researchers at the University of Milan began a detailed investigation of the mechanism of this LDL-R up-regulatory effect of soy protein.

## 2.3.6.2 Evidence from Clinical Studies

A number of hypotheses for the mechanism of the hypocholesterolemic action of soy proteins have been proposed. Among these, effects on cholesterol absorption and elimination by a "fiber-like" mechanism had been suggested by some animal studies but later refuted by a classic cholesterol balance study.[45] This study evaluated both sterol excretion and turnover of labeled cholesterol in hypercholesterolemic patients. In patients consuming soy protein, a significant total and LDL-C reduction (mean −21%) occurred. However, no increase in fecal steroid excretion (either neutral steroids or bile acids) was observed, and there was no change in the plasma-labeled cholesterol decay curve. These findings were in part contradicted by a more recent study of Duane et al.[46] suggesting a modestly higher excretion of neutral sterols and to some extent bile acids during a soy protein regimen. In this study, however, subjects were normocholesterolemic and the plasma cholesterol reductions were negligible.

Anderson et al.[47] carried out a landmark study elucidating the mechanism of plasma cholesterol reduction by both vegetable protein and dietary fiber. A classic oat bran diet (containing the soluble viscous dietary fiber β-glucan) was compared with a bean diet (navy and pinto beans) This study clearly established that both diets can reduce cholesterolemia to a similar extent but that only the oat bran diet leads to a significant increase in fecal sterol elimination (Table 2.3). Cholesterol metabolism therefore appears to be influenced by the bean protein, independent of changes of intestinal steroid absorption and excretion.

Two studies have addressed, directly and indirectly, the potential of soy protein preparations to increase LDL-R expression in humans. In the first study, by Lovati et al.[11] FH patients were treated in a crossover protocol with either animal protein or textured soy protein (with the addition of cholesterol in the latter to balance the two diets). Plasma lipids and LDL degradation by circulating lymphomonocytes (used as mirror images of hepatocytes) were monitored. During the animal protein diet there were minimal changes in LDL-C levels and LDL-R activity, while during the soy protein diet an increase in LDL degradation of about eightfold compared to the animal protein diet was observed (Figure 2.5). This study clearly suggests that some factors in soy protein up-regulate LDL-R–mediated LDL degradation — findings that have been more recently confirmed by a study of Baum et al.[48] in individuals with smaller elevations of cholesterolemia.

## TABLE 2.3
## Effects on Cholesterolemia, Stool Weight, and Fecal Steroid Output of an Oat Bran Diet and of a Similar Diet with Pinto and Navy Beans[a]

|  | Initial | Final |
|---|---|---|
| **Oat Bran** | | |
| Total cholesterol, mg/dl | 289 | 226[b] |
| LDL-cholesterol | 190 | 149[b] |
| Stool weight, g/d | 134 | 191[b] |
| Bile acids mg/d | 109 | 180[b] |
| **Navy and Pinto Beans** | | |
| Total cholesterol, mg/dl | 284 | 244[b] |
| LDL-cholesterol | 221 | 170[b] |
| Stool weight, g/d | 132 | 140 |
| Bile acids, mg/d | 154 | 108 |

[a] Twenty type II hypercholesterolemic patients; 21-d metabolic ward study. The diets only differed in their protein content; soluble fiber contents were similar.

[b] $P < 0.001$ vs. initial.

*Source:* Data from Anderson, J.W. et al., *Am. J. Clin. Nutr.*, 40, 1146–1155, 1984.

Indirect confirmation of the findings of Lovati et al.[11] and Baum et al.[48] has come from a study by Gaddi et al.[49] on cholesterolemic responses after soy protein administration in Type II hypercholesterolemic patients bearing different apo E genotypes. The apo E4 genotype is generally associated with higher cholesterolemia than the apo E2 or E3 genotypes — most likely due to greater suppression of peripheral LDL-R activity by the E4 than the E2 or E3 apoproteins. Apo E2 carriers in this study showed a negligible response to the soy protein diet, whereas there was a clear hypocholesterolemic effect in E3 and E4 carriers. This finding supports the conclusion that patients with already elevated LDL-R activity are less likely to benefit from soy protein dietary regimens.

Finally, a recent clinical study demonstrated that dietary soy protein beneficially effects another well-established protective factor against arterial disease, LDL particle size, independent of the presence of phytoestrogens.[50]

A full understanding of the mechanism of action of soy protein has become vital for selecting the most appropriate forms of soy for treating hypercholesterolemia. There are now a wide variety of soy protein preparations available on the market, including textured soy proteins manufactured from soy flour, more purified soy protein concentrates (approximately 70% protein), and protein isolates (>90% protein).[51] Industrial processing has the potential to modify the

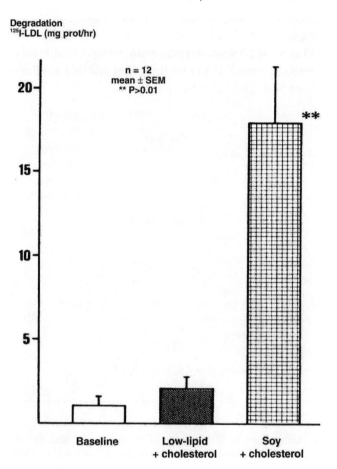

**FIGURE 2.5** Degradation of [125]I-LDL by freshly isolated mononuclear cells from type II hypercholesterolemic patients, before and after dietary treatment with a low lipid diet or with a soy protein diet, with an identical cholesterol content. An almost eightfold increased degradation (reflecting increased LDL-receptor activity) is noted after the soy protein regimen (Modified from Lovati, M.R. et al., *J. Clin. Invest.*, 80, 1498–1502, 1987).

biochemical nature of soy protein, so selection of the most efficacious products for hypercholesterolemia treatment can only be made once the active components and their mechanisms of action have been fully elucidated.

### 2.3.6.3   Role of Soy Polypeptides

The major storage proteins of soybeans are β-conglycinin, otherwise known as 7S globulin, and glycinin, otherwise known as 11S globulin. From early studies, the 7S globulin appeared primarily responsible for the hypocholesterolemic effects of soy protein preparations, while the 11S component appeared essentially inactive.[52,53] To further elucidate the active protein components, a detailed evaluation of the 7S $\alpha + \alpha'$ and $\beta$ subunits, in comparison to the whole 7S complex on the up-regulation of lipoprotein uptake and degradation in Hep G2 cells (a model human hepatoma cell line) was carried out.[54] These studies demonstrated that incubation of cells with the purified $\alpha + \alpha'$ subunits markedly increased uptake and degradation of [125]I-LDL, whereas the $\beta$ subunits were ineffective. In addition, a mutant soy cultivar, Keburi, devoid of the $\alpha'$ subunit, demonstrated no up-regulatory activity on LDL uptake and degradation.[55] It appears, therefore, that the predominant hypocholesterolemic agent is the 7S globulin located within the $\alpha + \alpha'$ subunit.

The peptides responsible for the hypocholesterolemic effect of soy protein were further elucidated by exposing Hep G2 cells to either (a) synthetic peptides with sequences matching the 127–150 position of 7S soy globulin or (b) peptides coming from the in vitro digestion of CROKSOY70®, the commercial isoflavone-poor soy concentrate routinely used for the dietary treatment of hypercholesterolemic patients.[13] Increased [125]I-LDL uptake and degradation occurred after Hep G2 incubation with the addition of the synthetic peptide. Cells exposed to CROKSOY-70 enzyme digestion products showed a marked up-regulation of LDL-R compared to those incubated with undigested CROKSOY70 or to controls with no added soy-derived material. These findings illustrate the potential for 7S-derived peptides to elicit hypocholesterolemic effects should they be absorbed intact in the gut and reach the liver.

Finally, through use of a proteomic approach, clear differences have been found in the protein subcomponents of soy preparations used by European[28,29] compared to U.S. researchers.[56,57] These differences may help explain the variations in the hypocholesterolemic activity attributed to the protein per se by these two groups of researchers. The CROKSOY70 concentrate used by European researchers has undergone some degradation of the 7S globulin during its manufacture but with retention of major 7S fragments and almost intact 11S globulin.[58] In contrast, the SUPRO products, used in the United States, have undergone complete degradation of the 7S globulin with only small peptide fragments remaining — mainly derived from the putatively less hypocholesterolemic 11S globulin.

Very recently a hypocholesterolemic protein subcomponent has been pinpointed more precisely by researchers at the University of Milan, who reported that the isolated 7S globulin $\alpha'$ subunit given to cholesterol-fed rats leads to a strong up-regulation of liver LDL-R activity as well as to dramatic plasma cholesterol and triglyceride reductions[59] (Figure 2.6). These dramatic effects were achieved at only 20 mg/kg/d, a dose that is tenfold lower than that of the standard drug treatment for rats.

The potential of soy 7S globulin as a hypocholesterolemic agent has attracted commercial interest. A recent U.S. patent reports a greater cholesterol-lowering effect in animals fed a 7S-enriched, isoflavone-poor soy product compared to a standard soy isolate.[60] In addition, a similar 7S-enriched product is commercially available in Japan.[61]

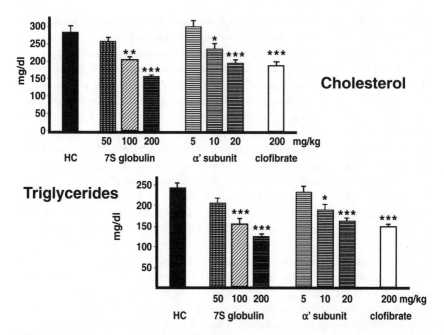

**FIGURE 2.6** Plasma total cholesterol and triglyceride levels in hyperlipidemic rats given a high-cholesterol diet (HC) plus isolated soy 7S globulin, the 7S α′ subunit, or a lipid-lowering drug at a standard rat dose for 28 d. Treatment with the isolated 7S α′ proved about 10 times more effective than clofibrate (* $P < 0.05$; ** $< 0.01$; *** $< 0.001$ compared to HC only). (Modified from Duranti, M. et al., *J. Nutr.*, 134, 1334–1339, 2004.)

### 2.3.7 EVIDENCE OF HYPOCHOLESTEROLEMIC ACTIVITY OF ISOFLAVONES

Isoflavones are compounds with weak estrogenic and antiestrogenic activity,[62] abundant in the Asian diet and present in varying amounts in different soy preparations. Individuals have highly variable gastrointestinal absorption of isoflavones (in some cases close to nil), and absorption is highly dependent on the individual's gut microflora.[63] As inhibitors of tyrosine kinase, isoflavones can negatively regulate cellular LDL-R receptor activity, as clearly demonstrated in experimental systems.[64] Nevertheless, a recent meta-analysis of clinical trials[65] concluded that soy isoflavones have hypocholesterolemic activity — contradicting an earlier meta-analysis that reported no association between changes in cholesterolemia and dietary isoflavones.[66] It should be noted, however, that in most comparative evaluations of soy preparations with and without isoflavones, the isoflavones were eliminated by ethanol extraction, a process that can also denature protein and remove low-molecular-weight peptides that have demonstrated LDL-R–activating properties.[67]

Early primate experiments[57] supported the hypothesis that isoflavones are directly responsible for the hypocholesterolemic properties of soy protein preparations.

This hypothesis has now been refuted by the repetition of the experiments under more appropriately controlled conditions. In one such study, Greaves et al.[7] added a semipurified isoflavone-rich ethanol extract of soy protein to a casein diet, but this diet failed to lower cholesterol levels in ovariectomized cynomolgus monkeys in comparison to a diet with intact soy proteins. The same authors later noted that the addition of the isoflavone-rich extract to casein does not reduce cholesterol absorption.[68]

Further evidence of the lack of a major role of isoflavones in the hypocholesterolemic activity of soy protein preparations comes from a study by Lovati et al.[13] in which the major soy isoflavone, genistein, at concentrations of up to 1 mg/ml, failed to demonstrate any LDL-R stimulatory activity in HepG2 cells. In addition, a soy protein preparation carefully stripped of its isoflavones by column chromatography, without the removal of small peptides or denaturation of the protein, has been shown to maintain all of its hypocholesterolemic properties.[69]

A recent consensus paper[70] indicates that both soy protein and isoflavones may be needed for maximal cholesterol-lowering effect of soy protein preparations and that soy protein should be consumed with a low saturated fat and low cholesterol diet to maximize its effectiveness. It remains, however, difficult to suggest plausible mechanisms whereby soy isoflavones might exert any additional hypocholesterolemic effects to those of the protein. Evidence currently indicates that soy isoflavones at best provide only a minor additional hypocholesterolemic effect above that of the protein, though they may induce additional effects beneficial to cardiovascular disease risk, such as stimulating apo AI production.[71]

## 2.4 ANTIATHEROSCLEROTIC EFFECTS OF SOY PROTEIN PREPARATIONS

The hypothesis that soy protein consumption has antiatherosclerotic effects is supported by the epidemiological association between soy protein intake and reduced cardiovascular disease risk.[15] A number of reports from a variety of animal models indicate that soy protein intake can reduce development and final size of experimentally induced atherosclerosis.[72–74] These studies have attributed the antiatherosclerotic effect to a range of components of the soy protein preparations including the proteins and the isoflavones.

### 2.4.1 ROLE OF PROTEIN IN THE ANTIATHEROGENIC EFFECTS OF SOY PREPARATIONS

A study by Castiglioni et al.[75] provided direct evidence of the antiatherogenic potential of soy proteins by feeding rabbits with focal carotid atheromatous lesions an isoflavone-free soy protein or a casein diet as part of a high lipid regimen. The soy protein group had both a significantly lower cholesterolemia (−47%) and smaller focal lesion size (−39%) than the casein group. Soy protein–fed animals also had a markedly lower rate of copper-mediated LDL oxidation with a far longer lag phase (150 min) than the casein-treated animals (20 min). These findings therefore also suggest that the antioxidant properties of soy protein preparations can, at least in part, be attributed to the protein moiety.

There is evidence that soy 7S globulin, to which most of the cholesterol-lowering activity of soy can be attributed, can also exert an antiatherosclerotic effect. In a recent report[76] male and ovariectomized female apo E knockout and LDL-R knockout mice were treated with either (a) casein and lactalbumin, (b) soy protein isolate with isoflavones, (c) 7S globulin, (d) 11S globulin, (e) soy protein free of 7S, or (f) a hydrolyzed soy product. The 7S-containing diets in all conditions of gender and genetic background were the most antiatheromatous. It should be added, however, that there was no clear evidence of any effect on lipidemia in this study — possibly as a result of the particular animal models used.

### 2.4.2 ROLE OF ISOFLAVONES IN THE ANTIATHEROGENIC EFFECTS OF SOY PROTEIN PREPARATIONS

The evidence that dietary intake of isoflavones can provide hypocholesterolemic effects in humans is essentially negative, but this class of compounds can provide some potentially antiatherogenic physiological effects; for instance, isoflavones do exert some vasodilatory activity in special conditions.[77,78] Walker et al.[79] reported the effects of an acute intravenous administration of genistein (concentrations between 10 and 300 nmol/min, for 6 min) that resulted in a significant increase in forearm arterial flow at the highest doses. This vasodilatory effect was reduced by an NO synthase antagonist. In this study, however, the plasma genistein concentrations were eight- to tenfold higher than those observed after oral intake of high-isoflavone soy proteins.[80] In a randomized double-blind trial, 6 months of treatment with genistein (54 mg/d) significantly increased flow-mediated endothelium-dependent vasodilation in postmenopausal women,[77] along with a significant increase in serum nitrates and a 50% reduction of plasma endothelin-1. This NO-dependent mechanism was supported by the results of a 1-year investigation in postmenopausal women where genistein (54 mg/d) was compared to a standard hormone replacement therapy (1 mg/d 17$\beta$-estradiol and 0.5 mg/d norethisterone acetate).[78] Again, an increase in nitrates and a reduction of endothelin-1 was demonstrated. Flow-mediated vasodilation was, however, not confirmed by another similar study in women given purified isoflavones.[81]

Genistein is known to bind rather weakly to the classical estrogen receptor, estrogen receptor-$\alpha$ (ER-$\alpha$) but binds with much higher affinity to ER-$\beta$[82] and may, therefore, display a more potent effect in the vascular tissues expressing the latter.

There is no experimental evidence currently available on the effects of isoflavones on atherosclerosis, as assessed by the standard clinical procedures of carotid intima-media thickness or coronary angiography, although a study of diabetic and nondiabetic monkeys demonstrated significantly reduced delivery of lipoproteins into arteries after isoflavone-rich soy diets.[83] The relative contributions of the protein and the phytoestrogens to the lipoprotein transport effects were not evaluated.

Another potentially antiatherosclerotic effect attributed to isoflavones is their potential for antioxidant activity. Results of *in vitro* and *in vivo* studies investigating the antioxidant effects of isoflavones have been reviewed by Kurzer et al.[84] who concluded that isoflavones act as antioxidants directly or indirectly by enhancement of the activities of catalase, superoxide dismutase, glutathione peroxidase, and glutathione reductase. In support of the hypothesis that isoflavones have antioxidant potential, a study of 46 surgically postmenopausal nonhuman primates demonstrated that arterial lipid peroxidation levels were ~17% lower in the group fed soy protein isolate containing isoflavones compared with the group fed casein and lactalbumin as the protein sources.[85]

Tikkanen et al.[86] have examined the effects of feeding soy protein containing 60 mg isoflavones per day on copper-induced LDL oxidation in six healthy volunteers. Two weeks of soy protein consumption significantly prolonged the LDL oxidation lag time by ~20 min. These *in vivo* findings confirm *in vitro* data[87,88] demonstrating reduced LDL oxidation in the presence of isoflavones, in particular genistein. Wiseman et al.[89] have evaluated the effect of consuming soy protein containing different levels of isoflavones for 17 d on *in vivo* lipid peroxidation and resistance of LDL to *in vitro* oxidation in 24 men and postmenopausal women. The isoflavone-rich diet induced significantly lower levels (−19.5%) of the F2 isoprostane biomarker of lipid peroxidation, 8-*epi*-prostaglandin $F_{2\alpha}$. In addition, the lag time for copper-mediated LDL oxidation was significantly longer after the high isoflavone diet. However, in a study using purified isoflavones in tablet form (86 mg/d),[90] there was no evidence of reduced LDL oxidation. This lack of effect of purified isoflavones supports the hypothesis that protein[75] or an interaction between protein and isoflavones may be responsible for the antioxidant activity of soy protein preparations.

## 2.5   ALTERNATIVE LEGUMES FOR CARDIOVASCULAR DISEASE RISK REDUCTION

The recent approval of a cardiovascular risk reduction health claim for soy protein by the U.S. FDA[6] and the availability of numerous products derived from soy has no doubt resulted in a wider global consumption of this legume. Nevertheless, in Western Europe, soy protein-based foods are still only used to a modest extent.[91] This appears partly due to these products being foreign to European cuisine and partly due to public concern about the use of genetically modified foods[92] — a classification under which many soy products fall. The potential role of other legumes for coronary disease risk reduction therefore requires investigation.

The potential cardiovascular-protective effect of the consumption of different "pulses" (defined as "the edible seeds of leguminous plants cultivated for food such as peas, beans, lentils, etc.") has been highlighted in a review by Anderson and Major.[93] These authors clearly demonstrated that in clinical trials of nonsoy pulses (using subjects with a wide range of baseline cholesterolemia) there was a mean reduction in total cholesterolemia and LDL-cholesterolemia of 7.2 and 6.2%, respectively, and a rise in HDL-cholesterol of 2.6%.

In response to the potentially harmful effects of soy isoflavones,[94] researchers have recently been focusing on the essentially isoflavone-free seeds of the legume lupin (*Lupinus* spp.) as a novel alternative protein source. By far the most important lupin-producing country is Australia, where Australian sweet lupin (*Lupinus angustifolius*) is a major crop. In Europe lupin is cultivated mostly in France, Poland, Russia, Hungary, and Italy,[95] and here the white lupin (*Lupinus albus*) is an important species. Lupin seeds also have a low content of antinutritional factors, and in modern varieties (sweet lupins), the alkaloids that can impart bitterness have been reduced to very low levels by conventional breeding techniques. Lupins may therefore be more acceptable than soy to the European population.

Preliminary studies with unfractionated lupin kernel and lupin protein and fiber fractions have demonstrated hypocholesterolemic effects in male rats.[96,97] The first report of a hypocholesterolemic effect of lupin fractions in humans was that of Hall et al.[98] who demonstrated beneficial effects on cholesterolemia of the kernel dietary fiber fraction from *L. angustifolius*. The authors of this report, however, suggested that some of the cholesterol-lowering effect could have been due to residual protein in the fiber fraction.

A recent study[99] has demonstrated beneficial effects on cholesterolemia from a daily dose of total protein extract of *L. albus* in rats fed a hypercholesterolemia-inducing diet. Plasma total and very low density lipoprotein (VLDL) + LDL cholesterol concentrations were significantly lower (21% and 30%, respectively) in the lupin-dosed compared to the casein-dosed animals. In an attempt to elucidate the cholesterol-lowering mechanism, the effect of *L. albus* protein fractions on LDL-R activity in HepG2 cells was also evaluated. The total lupin protein extract appeared to be inactive, whereas the conglutin-$\gamma$ subcomponent (a glycoprotein comprising about 5% of the total lupin proteins[100]) had a remarkable up-regulatory effect on LDL-R activity. It therefore appears that lupin protein has potential as a hypercholesterolemic agent.

## 2.6  CONCLUSIONS

Clinical data have confirmed the significant cholesterol-lowering property of soy proteins first reported by University of Milan researchers almost 30 years ago.[28] Experimental and clinical evidence on the cardiovascular benefits of soy consumption has expanded along with technologies for the preparation of more varied and palatable soy preparations for human consumption. These developments have resulted in a dramatic increase in consumption of soy products in the Western world in the past few decades.

A population approach for coronary disease prevention using hypocholesterolemic diets such as ones based on soy protein may be more effective than a patient-based approach with hypocholesterolemic drugs such as statins. The reduction of cardiovascular disease events using dietary intervention may be as high as 30% compared to the 15 to 20% reduction seen using drug therapy.[101]

The effectiveness of the soy protein diet is highly dependent on baseline plasma cholesterol level and the level of intake of other dietary components, in particular, proteins and fats. This variation in response to the soy protein diet offers interesting possibilities for investigations into the mechanism of individual sensitivity to dietary substitution.

Currently the soybean diet appears to be the most potent dietary tool for treating hypercholesterolemia and it provides a unique opportunity for the management of very young hypercholesterolemic patients and opportunities for exploring new mechanisms of plasma cholesterol regulation.

## REFERENCES

1. Kim, D.N., Lee, K.T., Reiner, J.M., and Thomas, W.A., Increased steroid excretion in swine fed high-fat, high-cholesterol diet with soy protein, *Exp. Mol. Pathol.*, 33, 25–35, 1980.
2. Terpstra, A.H.M., Woodward, C.J.H., West, C.E., and Van Boven, J.G., A longitudinal cross-over study of serum cholesterol and lipoproteins in rabbits fed on semipurified diets containing either casein or soya-bean protein, *Br. J. Nutr.*, 47, 213–219, 1982.
3. Sirtori, C.R., Lovati, M.R., Manzoni, C., Gianazza, E., Bondioli, A., Staels, B., and Auwerx, J., Reduction of serum cholesterol by soybean proteins: clinical experience and potential molecular mechanisms. *Nutr. Metab. Cardiovasc. Dis.*, 8, 334–340, 1998.
4. Bakhit, R.M., Klein, B.P., Essex Sorlie, D., Ham, J.O., Erdman, J.W., Jr., and Potter, S.M., Intake of 25 g of soybean protein with or without soybean fiber alters plasma lipids in men with elevated cholesterol concentrations, *J. Nutr.*, 124, 213–222, 1994.
5. Anderson, J.W., Johnstone, B.M., and Cook Newell, M.E., Meta-analysis of the effects of soy protein intake on serum lipids, *N. Engl. J. Med.*, 333, 276–282, 1995.
6. Food and Drug Administration, FDA Food labeling health claims: soybean protein and coronary heart disease. Final rule, *Fed. Regist.*, 64, 57699–57733, 1999.
7. Greaves, K.A., Parks, J.S., Williams, J.K., and Wagner, J.D., Intact dietary soy protein, but not adding an isoflavone-rich soy extract to casein, improves plasma lipids in ovariectomized cynomolgus monkeys, *J. Nutr.*, 129, 1585–1592, 1999.
8. Hunninghake, D.B., Miller, V.T., LaRosa, J.C., Kinosian, B., Jacobson, T., Brown, V., Howard, W.J., Edelman, D.A., and O'Connor, R.R., Long-term treatment of hypercholesterolemia with dietary fiber, *Am. J. Med.*, 97, 504–508, 1994.
9. Clarkson, T.B., Soy, soy phytoestrogens and cardiovascular disease, *J. Nutr.*, 132, 566S–569S, 2002.
10. Oakenfull, D. and Sidhu, G.S., Could saponins be a useful treatment for hypercholesterolaemia?, *Eur. J. Clin. Nutr.*, 44, 79–88, 1990.
11. Lovati, M.R., Manzoni, C., Canavesi, A., Sirtori, M., Vaccarino, V., Marchi, M., Gaddi, G., and Sirtori, C.R., Soybean protein diet increases low density lipoprotein receptor activity in mononuclear cells from hypercholesterolemic patients, *J. Clin. Invest.*, 80, 1498–1502, 1987.

12. Baum, J.A., Teng, H., Erdman, J.W., Jr., Weigel, R.M., Klein, B.P., Persky, V.W., Freels, S., Surya, P., Bakhit, R.M., Ramos, E., Shay, N.F., and Potter, S.M., Long-term intake of soy protein improves blood lipid profiles and increases mononuclear cell low-density-lipoprotein receptor messenger RNA in hypercholesterolemic, postmenopausal women, *Am. J. Clin. Nutr.*, 68, 545–551, 1998.

13. Lovati, M.R., Manzoni, C., Gianazza, E., Arnoldi, A., Kurowska, E., Carroll, K.K., and Sirtori, C.R., Soy protein peptides regulate cholesterol homeostasis in Hep G2 cells, *J. Nutr.*, 130, 2543–2549, 2000.

14. Zhang, X., Shu, X.O., Gao, Y.-T., Yang, G., Li, Q., Li, H., Jin, F., and Zheng, W., Soy food consumption is associated with lower risk of coronary heart disease risk reduction in Chinese women, *J. Nutr.*, 133, 2874–2878, 2003.

15. Nagata, C., Takatsuka, N., Kurisu, Y., and Shimizu, H., Decreased serum total cholesterol concentration is associated with high intake of soy products in Japanese men and women, *J. Nutr.*, 128, 209–213, 1998.

16. Burslem, J., Schonfeld, G., Howald, M.A., Weidman, S., and Miller, J.P., Plasma apoprotein and lipoprotein lipid levels in vegetarians, *Metabolism*, 27, 711–719, 1978.

17. Nieman, D.C., Sherman, K.M., Arabatzis, K., Underwood, B.C., Barbarosa J.C., Johnson, M., Shultz, T.D., and Lee, J., Hematological, anthropometric, and met-abolic comparisons between vegetarian and nonvegetarian women, *Int. J. Sports Med.*, 10, 243–250, 1989.

18. Key, T.J.A., Thorogood, M., Appleby, P.N., and Burr, M.L., Dietary habits and mortality in 11000 vegetarians and health conscious people: results of a 17 year follow up, *BMJ*, 313, 775–779, 1996.

19. Rosell, M.S., Appleby, P.N., Spencer, E.A., and Key, T.J., Soy intake and blood cholesterol concentrations: a cross-sectional study of 1033 pre- and postmeno-pausal women in the Oxford arm of the European Prospective Investigation into Cancer and Nutrition, *Am. J. Clin. Nutr.*, 80, 1391–1396, 2004.

20. Ignatowski, A., Uber die wirkung des tiereschen eiweisses auf die aorta und die parenchymatosen organe der kaninchen, *Virchows Arch. Pathol. Anat. Physiol. Klin. Med.*, 198, 248–270, 1909.

21. Anitschkow, N. and Chalatow, S., Uber experimentelle cholesterinsteatose und ihre bedeutung fur die entstehung einiger pathologisher prozesse, *Zentralbl. Allg. Pathol.*, 24, 1–9, 1913.

22. Clarkson, S. and Newburgh, L.H., The relation between atherosclerosis and ingested cholesterol in the rabbit, *J. Exp. Med.*, 43, 1926.

23. Newburgh, L.H. and Squier, T.L., High protein diet and atherosclerosis in rabbits. A preliminary report, *Arch. Intern. Med.*, 26, 38–40, 1920.

24. Howard, A.N., Gresham, G.A., Jones, D., and Jennings, I. W., The prevention of rabbit atherosclerosis by soya meal, *J. Atheroscler. Res.*, 5, 330–337, 1965.

25. Kritchevsky, D. and Tepper, S.A., Factors affecting atherosclerosis in rabbits fed cholesterol-free diets, *Life Sci.*, 4, 1467–1471, 1965.

26. Carroll, K.K., Hypercholesterolemia and atherosclerosis: effects of dietary protein, *Fed. Proc.*, 41, 2792–2796, 1982.

27. Huff, M.W., Hamilton, R.M., and Carroll, K.K., Plasma cholesterol levels in rabbits fed low fat, cholesterol-free, semipurified diets: effects of dietary proteins, protein hydrolysates and amino acid mixtures, *Atherosclerosis*, 28, 187–195, 1977.

28. Sirtori, C.R., Agradi, E., Conti, F., Mantero, O., and Gatti, E., Soybean-protein diet in the treatment of type-II hyperlipoproteinaemia, *Lancet,* 1, 275–277, 1977.
29. Descovich, G.C., Ceredi, C., Gaddi, A., Benassi, M.S., Mannino, G., Colombo, L., Cattin, L., Fontana, G., Senin, U., Mannarino, E., Caruzzo, C., Bertelli, E., Fragiacomo, C., Noseda, G., Sirtori, M., and Sirtori, C.R., Multicentre study of soybean protein diet for outpatient hyper-cholesterolaemic patients, *Lancet,* 2, 709–712, 1980.
30. Hori, G., Wang, M.-F., Chan, Y.-C., Komtatsu, T., Wong, Y., Chen, T.-H., Yamamoto, K., Nagaoka, S., and Yamamoto, S., Soy protein hydrolyzate with bound phospholipids reduces serum cholesterol levels in hypercholesterolemic adult male volunteers, *Biosci. Biotechnol. Biochem.,* 65, 72–78, 2001.
31. Jenkins, D.J., Wolever, T.M., Spiller, G., Buckley, G., Lam, Y., Jenkins, A.L., and Josse, R.G., Hypocholesterolemic effect of vegetable protein in a hypocaloric diet, *Atherosclerosis,* 78, 99–107, 1989.
32. Meinertz, H., Nilausen, K., and Faergeman, O., Soy protein and casein in cholesterol-enriched diets: effects on plasma lipoproteins in normolipidemic subjects, *Am. J. Clin. Nutr.,* 50, 786–793, 1989.
33. Gaddi, A., Descovich, G.C., Noseda, G., Fragiacomo, C., Nicolini, A., Montanari, G., Vanetti, G., Sirtori, M., Gatti, E., and Sirtori, C.R., Hypercholesterolaemia treated by soybean protein diet, *Arch. Dis. Childhood,* 62, 274–278, 1987.
34. Widhalm, K., Brazda, G., Schneider, B., and Kohl, S., Effect of soy protein diet versus standard low fat, low cholesterol diet on lipid and lipoprotein levels in children with familial or polygenic hypercholesterolemia, *J. Pediatr.,* 123, 30–34, 1993.
35. Pazzucconi, F., Dorigotti, F., Gianfranceschi, G., Campagnoli, G., Sirtori, M., Franceschini, G., and Sirtori, C.R., Therapy with HMG CoA reductase inhibitors: characteristics of the long-term permanence of hypocholesterolemic activity, *Atherosclerosis,* 117, 189–198, 1995.
36. Rubinstein, A. and Weintraub, M., Escape phenomenon of low-density lipoprotein cholesterol during lovastatin treatment, *Am. J. Cardiol.,* 76, 184–186, 1995.
37. Sirtori, C.R., Pazzucconi, F., Colombo, L., Battistin, P., Bondioli, A., and Descheemaker, K., Double-blind study of the addition of high-protein soya milk v. cows' milk to the diet of patients with severe hypercholesterolaemia and resistance to or intolerance of statins, *Br. J. Nutr.,* 82, 91–96, 1999.
38. D'Amico, G., Gentile, M.G., Manna, G., Fellin, G., Ciceri, R., Cofano, F., Petrini, C., Lavarda, F., Perolini, S., and Porrini, M., Effect of vegetarian soy diet on hyperlipidaemia in nephrotic syndrome, *Lancet,* 339, 1131–1134, 1992.
39. Teixeira, S.R., Tappenden, K.A., Carson, L., Jones, R., Prabhudesai, M., Marshall, W.P., and Erdman, J.W., Jr., Isolated soy protein consumption reduces urinary albumin excretion and improves the serum lipid profile in men with type 2 diabetes mellitus and nephropathy, *J. Nutr.,* 134, 1874–1880, 2004.
40. Anthony, M.S., Clarkson, T.B., Hughes C.L., Jr., Morgan, T.M., and Burke, G.L., Soybean isoflavones improve cardiovascular risk factors without affecting the reproductive system of peripubertal rhesus monkeys, *J. Nutr.,* 126, 43–50, 1996.
41. Wang, H.J. and Murphy, P.A., Isoflavone content in commercial soybean foods, *J. Agric. Food Chem.,* 42, 1666–1673, 1994.
42. Sirtori, C.R., Lovati, M.R., Manzoni, C., Monetti, M., Pazzucconi, F., and Gatti, E., Soy and cholesterol reduction: clinical experience, *J. Nutr.,* 125, 598S–605S, 1995.

43. Sirtori, C.R., Gianazza, E., Manzoni, C., Lovati, M.R., and Murphy, P.A., Role of isoflavones in the cholesterol reduction by soy proteins in the clinic, *Am. J. Clin. Nutr.,* 65, 166–167, 1997.

44. Sirtori, C.R., Galli, G., Lovati, M.R., Carrara, P., Bosisio, E., and Kienle, M.G., Effects of dietary proteins on the regulation of liver lipoprotein receptors in rats, *J. Nutr.,* 114, 1493–1500, 1984.

45. Fumagalli, R., Soleri, L., Farina, R., Musanti, R., Mantero, O., Noseda, G., Gatti, E., and Sirtori, C.R., Fecal cholesterol excretion studies in type II hypercholesterolemic patients treated with the soybean protein diet, *Atherosclerosis,* 43, 341–353, 1982.

46. Duane, W.C., Effects of soybean protein and very low dietary cholesterol on serum lipids, biliary lipids, and fecal sterols in humans, *Metabolism,* 48, 489–494, 1999.

47. Anderson, J.W., Story, L., Sieling, B., Chen, W.J., Petro, M.S., and Story, J., Hypocholesterolemic effects of oat-bran or bean intake for hypercholesterolemic men, *Am. J. Clin. Nutr.,* 40, 1146–1155, 1984.

48. Baum, J.A., Teng, H., Erdman J.W., Jr., Weigel, R.M., Klein, B.P., Persky, V.W., Freels, S., Surya, P., Bakhit, R.M., Ramos, E., Shay, N.F., and Potter, S.M., Long-term intake of soy protein improves blood lipid profiles and increases mononuclear cell low-density-lipoprotein receptor messenger RNA in hypercholesterolemic, postmenopausal women, *Am. J. Clin. Nutr.,* 68, 545–551, 1998.

49. Gaddi, A., Ciarrocchi, A., Matteucci, A., Rimondi, S., Ravaglia, G., Descovich, G.C., and Sirtori, C.R., Dietary treatment for familial hypercholesterolemia: differential effects of dietary soy protein according to the apolipoprotein E phenotypes, *Am. J. Clin. Nutr.,* 53, 1191–1196, 1991.

50. Desroches, S., Mauger, J.-F., Ausman, L.M., Lichtenstein, A.H., and Lamarche, B., Soy protein favorably affects LDL size independently of isoflavones in hypercholesterolemic men and women, *J. Nutr.,* 134, 574–579, 2004.

51. Lucas, E.W. and Riaz, M.N., Soy protein products: processing and use, *J. Nutr.,* 125, 573S–580S, 1995.

52. Lovati, M.R., Manzoni, C., Corsini, A., Granata, A., Frattini, R., Fumagalli, R., and Sirtori, C.R., Low density lipoprotein receptor activity is modulated by soybean globulins in cell culture, *J. Nutr.,* 122, 1971–1978, 1992.

53. Lovati, M.R., Manzoni, C., Corsini, A., Granata, A., Fumagalli, R., and Sirtori, C.R., 7S globulin from soybean is metabolized in human cell cultures by a specific uptake and degradation system, *J. Nutr.,* 126, 2831–2842, 1996.

54. Lovati, M.R., Manzoni, C., Gianazza, E., and Sirtori, C.R., Soybean protein products as regulators of liver low-density lipoprotein receptors. I. Identification of active β-conglycinin subunits, *J. Agric. Food Chem.,* 46, 2474–2480, 1998.

55. Manzoni, C., Lovati, M.R., Gianazza, E., and Sirtori, C.R., Soybean protein products as regulators of liver low-density lipoprotein receptors. II. $\alpha - \alpha'$ rich commercial soy concentrate and $\alpha'$ deficient mutant differently affect low-density lipoprotein receptor activation, *J. Agric. Food Chem.,* 46, 2481–2484, 1998.

56. Crouse J.R., 3rd, Morgan, T., Terry, J.G., Ellis, J., Vitolins, M., and Burke, G.L., A randomized trial comparing the effect of casein with that of soy protein containing varying amounts of isoflavones on plasma concentrations of lipids and lipoproteins, *Arch. Intern. Med.,* 159, 2070–2076, 1999.

57. Anthony, M.S., Clarkson, T.B., Bullock, B.C., and Wagner, J.D., Soy protein versus soy phytoestrogens in the prevention of diet-induced coronary artery atherosclerosis of male cynomolgus monkeys, *Arterioscler. Thromb. Vasc. Biol.,* 17, 2524–2531, 1997.

58. Gianazza, E., Eberini, I., Arnoldi, A., Wait, R., and Sirtori, C.R., A proteomic investigation of isolated soy proteins with variable effects in experimental and clinical studies, *J. Nutr.*, 133, 9–14, 2003.
59. Duranti, M., Lovati, M.R., Dani, V., Barbiroli, A., Scarafoni, A., Castiglioni, S., Ponzone, C., and Morazzoni, P., The α′ subunit from soybean 7S globulin lowers plasma lipids and upregulates liver β-VLDL receptors in rats fed a hyper-cholesterolemic diet, *J. Nutr.*, 134, 1334–1339, 2004.
60. Bringe, N.A., High β-conglycinin products and their use, U.S. Patent 6,171,640, 2001.
61. Hirokumi, K., Motohiko, H., Kiyohara, T., and Makoto, K., Triglyceride-lowering effect of soybean β-conglycinin in humans, *Therap. Res.*, 23, 85–89, 2002.
62. Adlercreutz, H., Hockerstedt, K., Bannwart, C., Bloigu, S., Hamalainen, E., Fotsis, T., and Ollus, A., Effect of dietary components, including lignans and phytoestrogens, on enterohepatic circulation and liver metabolism of estrogens and on sex hormone binding globulin (SHBG), *J. Steroid Biochem.*, 27, 1135–1144, 1987.
63. Xu, X., Harris, K.S., Wang, H.J., Murphy, P.A., and Hendrich, S., Bioavailability of soybean isoflavones depends upon gut microflora in women, *J. Nutr.*, 125, 2307–2315, 1995.
64. Grove, R.I., Mazzucco, C.E., Radka, S.F., Shoyab, M., and Kiener, P.A., Oncos-tatin M up-regulates low density lipoprotein receptors in HepG2 cells by a novel mechanism, *J. Biol. Chem.*, 266, 18194–18199, 1991.
65. Zhuo, X.G., Melby, M.K., and Watanabe, S., Soy isoflavone intake lowers serum LDL cholesterol: a meta-analysis of 8 randomised control trials in humans, *J. Nutr.*, 134, 2395–2400, 2004.
66. Weggemans, R.M. and Trautwein, E.A., Relation between soy-associated isofla-vones and LDL and HDL cholesterol concentrations in humans: a meta-analysis, *Eur. J. Clin. Nutr.*, 57, 940–946, 2003.
67. Lovati, M.R., Manzoni, C., Agostinelli, P., Ciappellano, S., Mannucci, L., and Sirtori, C.R., Studies on the mechanism of the cholesterol lowering activity of soy proteins. Soy protein extract reduces plasma cholesterol and increases liver β-VLDL receptors in mice, *Nutr. Metab. Cardiovasc. Dis.*, 1, 18–24, 1991.
68. Greaves, K.A., Wilson, M.D., Rudel, L.L., Williams, J.K., and Wagner, J.D., Consumption of soy protein reduces cholesterol absorption compared to casein alone or supplemented with an isoflavone extract or conjugated equine estrogen in ovariectomized cynomolgous monkeys, *J. Nutr.*, 130, 820–826, 2000.
69. Fukui, K., Tachibana, N., Wanezaki, S., Tsuzaki, S., Takamatsu, K., Yamamoto, T., Hashimoto, Y., and Shimoda, T., Isoflavone-free soy protein prepared by col-umn chromatography reduces plasma cholesterol in rats, *J. Agr. Food Chem.*, 50, 5717–5721, 2002.
70. Erdman, J.W., Soy protein and cardiovascular disease: a statement for healthcare professionals from the Nutrition Committee of the AHA, *Circulation*, 102, 2555–2559.
71. Lamon-Fava, S., Genistein activates apolipoproteins A-I gene expression in the human hepatoma cell line HepG2, *J. Nutr.*, 130, 2489–2492, 2000.
72. Carroll, K.K., Hypercholesterolemia and atherosclerosis: effects of dietary protein, *Fed. Proc.*, 41, 2792–2796, 1982.
73. Ni, W., Tsuda, Y., Sakono, M., and Imaizumi, K., Dietary soy protein isolate, compared with casein, reduces atherosclerotic lesion area in apolipoprotein E-deficient mice, *J. Nutr.*, 128, 1884–1889, 1998.

74. Cos, E., Ramjiganesh, T., Roy, S., Yoganathan, S., Nicolosi, R.J., and Fernandez, M.L., Soluble fiber and soybean protein reduce atherosclerotic lesions in guinea pigs. Sex and hormonal status determine lesion extension, *Lipids,* 36, 1209–1216, 2001.

75. Castiglioni, S., Manzoni, C., D'Uva, A., Spiezie, R., Monteggia, E., Chiesa, G., Sirtori, C.R., and Lovati, M.R., Soy proteins reduce regression of a focal lesion and lipoprotein oxidiability in rabbits fed a cholesterol-rich diet, *Atherosclerosis,* 171, 163–170, 2003.

76. Adams, M.R., Golden, D.L., Franke, A.A., Potter, S.M., Smith, H.S., and Anthony, M.S., Dietary soy β-conglycinin (7S globulin) inhibits atherosclerosis in mice, *J. Nutr.,* 134, 511–516, 2004.

77. Squadrito, F., Altavilla, D., Morabito, N., Crisafulli, A., D'Anna, R., Corrado, F., Ruggeri, P., Campo, G.M., Calapai, G., Caputi, A.P., and Squadrito, G., The effect of the phytoestrogen genistein on plasma nitric oxide concentrations, endothelin-1 levels and endothelium dependent vasodilation in postmenopausal women, *Atherosclerosis,* 163, 339–347, 2002.

78. Squadrito, F., Altavilla, D., Crisafulli, A., Saitta, A., Cucinotta, D., Morabito, N., D'Anna, R., Corrado, F., Ruggeri, P., Frisina, N., and Squadrito, G., Effect of genistein on endothelial function in postmenopausal women: a randomized, double-blind, controlled study, *Am. J. Med.,* 114, 470–476, 2003.

79. Walker, H.A., Dean, T.S., Sanders, T.A.B., Jackson, G., Ritter, J.M., and Cho-wienczyk, P.J., The phytoestrogen genistein produces acute nitric oxide-dependent dilation of human forearm vasculature with similar potency to 17[β]-estradiol, *Circulation,* 103, 258–262, 2001.

80. Adlercreutz, H., Markkanen, H., and Watanabe, S., Plasma concentrations of phyto-oestrogens in Japanese men, *Lancet,* 342, 1209–1210, 1993.

81. Simons, L.A., von Konigsmark, M., Simons, J., and Celermajer, D.S., Phytoestrogens do not influence lipoprotein levels or endothelial function in healthy, post-menopausal women, *Am. J. Cardiol.,* 85, 1297–1301, 2000.

82. Mäkelä, S., Savolainen, H., Aavik, E., Myllarniemi, M., Strauss, L., Taskinen, E., Gustafsson, J.A., and Hayry, P., Differentiation between vasculoprotective and uterotrophic effects of ligands with different binding affinities to estrogen receptors α and β, *Proc. Natl. Acad. Sci. USA,* 96, 7077–7082, 1999.

83. Wagner, J.D., Zhang, L., Greaves, K.A., Shadoan, M.K., and Schwenke, D.C., Soy protein reduces the arterial low-density lipoprotein (LDL) concentration and delivery of LDL cholesterol to the arteries of diabetic and nondiabetic male cynomolgus monkeys, *Metabolism,* 49, 1188–1196, 2000.

84. Kurzer, M.S. and Xu, X., Dietary phytoestrogens, *Annu. Rev. Nutr.,* 17, 353–381, 1997.

85. Wagner, J.D., Cefalu, W.T., Anthony, M.S., Litwak, K.N., Zhang, L., and Clarkson, T.B., Dietary soy protein and estrogen replacement therapy improve cardiovascular risk factors and decrease aortic cholesteryl ester content in ovariectomized cyno-molgus monkeys, *Metabolism,* 46, 698–705, 1997.

86. Tikkanen, M.J., Wahala, K., Ojala, S., Vihma, V., and Adlercreutz, H., Effect of soybean phytoestrogen intake on low density lipoprotein oxidation resistance, *Proc. Natl. Acad. Sci. USA,* 95, 3106–3110, 1998.

87. Kapiotis, S., Hermann, M., Held, I., Seelos, C., Ehringer, H., and Gmeiner, B.M., Genistein, the dietary-derived angiogenesis inhibitor, prevents LDL oxidation and protects endothelial cells from damage by atherogenic LDL, *Arterioscler. Thromb. Vasc. Biol.,* 17, 2868–2874, 1997.

88. Kerry, N. and Abbey, M., The isoflavone genistein inhibits copper and peroxyl radical mediated low density lipoprotein oxidation *in vitro, Atherosclerosis,* 140, 341–347, 1998.

89. Wiseman, H., O'Reilly, J.D., Adlercreutz, H., Mallet, A.I., Bowey, E.A., Rowland, I.R., and Sanders, T.A.B., Isoflavone phytoestrogens consumed in soy decrease F2-isoprostane concentrations and increase resistance of low-density lipoprotein to oxidation in humans, *Am. J. Clin. Nutr.,* 72, 395–400, 2000.

90. Samman, S., Lyons Wall, P.M., Chan, G.S., Smith, S.J., and Petocz, P., The effect of supplementation with isoflavones on plasma lipids and oxidisability of low density lipoprotein in premenopausal women, *Atherosclerosis,* 147, 277–283, 1999.

91. Keinan Boker, L., Peeters, P.H.M., Mulligan, A.A., Navarro, C., and Slimani, N., Consumption of soybean products in 10 European countries, in *4th International Symposium on Role of Soybean in Preventing and Treated Chronic Disease, San Diego, CA, Nov.* 4–7, 2001 (Abstract).

92. Baker, G.A. and Burnham, T.A., Consumer response to genetically modified foods: market segment analysis and implications for producers and policy makers, *J. Agric. Resour. Econ.,* 26, 387–403, 2001.

93. Anderson, J.W. and Major, A.W., Pulses and lipaemia, short- and long-term effect: potential in the prevention of cardiovascular disease, *Br. J. Nutr.,* 88(Suppl 3), S263–271, 2002.

94. Sirtori, C.R., Risks and benefits of soy phytoestrogens in cardiovascular diseases, cancer, climacteric symptoms and osteoporosis, *Drug Saf.,* 24, 665–682, 2001.

95. www.fao.org/waicent/portal/statistics_en.asp. Accessed June 2003.

96. Rahman, M.H., Hossain, A., Siddiqua, A., and Hossain, I., Hemato-biochemical parameters in rats fed *Lupinus angustifolius* L. (sweet lupin) seed protein and fiber fractions, *J. Clin. Biochem. Nutr.,* 20, 99–111, 1996.

97. Chango, A., Villaume, C., Bau, H.M., Schwertz, A., Nicolas, J., and Mejean, L., Effects of casein, sweet white lupin and sweet yellow lupin on cholesterol metabolism in rats, *J. Sci. Food Agric.,* 76, 303–309, 1998.

98. Hall, R.S., Johnson, S.K., Baxter, A.L., and Ball, M.J., Lupin kernel fibre enriched foods beneficially modify serum lipids in men, *Eur. J. Clin. Nutr.,* 59, 325–333, 2005.

99. Sirtori, C.R., Lovati, M.R., Manzoni, C., Castiglioni, S., Duranti, M., Magri, C., Morandi, S., D'Agostina, A., and Arnoldi, A., Proteins of white lupin seed, a naturally isoflavone-poor legume, reduce cholesterolemia in rats and increase LDL receptor activity in HepG2 cells, *J. Nutr.,* 134, 18–23, 2004.

100. Duranti, M., Restani, P., Poniatowska, M., and Cerletti, P., The seed globulins of Lupinus albus, *Phytochemistry,* 20, 2071–2075, 1981.

101. Yusuf, S. and Anand, S., Cost of prevention. The case of lipid lowering, *Circulation,* 93, 1774–1776, 1996.

# 3 Soy and Breast Cancer Prevention

*Seiichiro Yamamoto and Shoichiro Tsugane*

## CONTENTS

## 3.1 INTRODUCTION

Breast cancer incidence is higher in Western countries than in Asian countries. In addition, migrant populations from Asia to the United States have increased incidence of breast cancer[1] (Figure 3.1). As for Japan, breast cancer mortality is higher in metropolitan areas but shows steadily increasing trends for all prefectures[2] (Figure 3.2). This evidence suggests that the difference in life-style

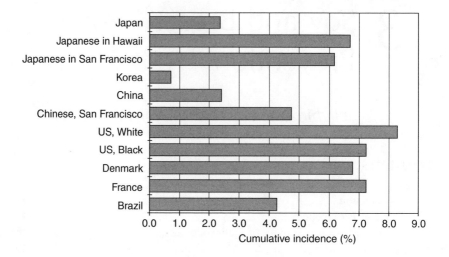

**FIGURE 3.1** Cumulative incidence of breast cancer in the world.

between the Western countries and Asia, in particular, the difference in eating habits, may be associated with the difference in incidence of breast cancer. Attention has been paid to soybean products since they are widely consumed in Asia but rarely consumed in Western countries (at least until quite recently). There is a 10- to 100-fold difference in consumption between Japan and the Western countries (Table 3.1).[3-13]

Known risk factors of breast cancer are reproductive factors (early age at menarche, nulliparous, little parity, late age at first pregnancy, late natural menopause), dietary factors (high total fat, saturated and animal fat, meat, alcohol, and less carotenoid consumption), family history of breast cancer, benign breast disease history, and body size (rapid growth, greater adult height, high body mass, and adult weight gain), and low physical activity.[14] Most of these risk factors seem to be related to steroid hormone concentration in the body. Soy has attracted attention due to its ingredient, isoflavone, which is a class of phytoestrogen (plant estrogen) and has a potential effect on estrogen circulation in the human body.

## 3.2 SOY AND ISOFLAVONE

Since most research concerning the effect of soy intake on breast cancer has been dedicated to soy itself or to isoflavone, we will mainly focus on the effect of soy and isoflavone on breast cancer unless stated otherwise.

Soy primarily contains three isoflavones, daidzein (4′7-dihydroxyisoflavone), genistein (4′,5,7-trihydroxyisoflavone), and glycitein (7,4′-dihydroxy-6-methoxyisoflavone), and their respective β-glycosides, daidzin, genistin, and glycitin

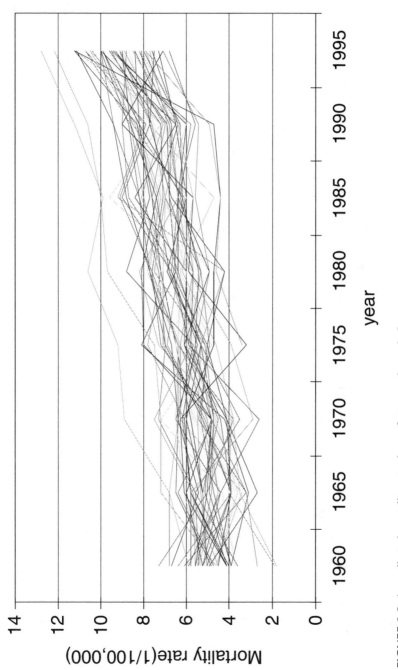

**FIGURE 3.2** Age-adjusted mortality rates by prefecture and year in Japan.

**TABLE 3.1**
**Comparison of Isoflavone Intake, Concentration in Blood, and Urine Excretion of Isoflavone in Various Populations**

| Intake (mg/d) | Author | Publication Year | Method of Assessment | Statistics | No. of Subjects | Daidzein | Genistein |
|---|---|---|---|---|---|---|---|
| Japanese men | Yamamoto et al. | 2001 | 28-d DR | A-mean | 102 | 15.8 | 25.4 |
| Japanese women | Yamamoto et al. | 2001 | 28-d DR | A-mean | 113 | 13.4 | 21.6 |
| Japanese | Wakai et al. | 2000 | 1-d DR | Median | 1230 | 12.1 | 19.6 |
| Japanese | Wakai et al. | 2000 | 16-d weighed DR | Median | 88 | 9.5 | 14.9 |
| Japanese | Arai et al. | 2000 | 3-d DR | A-mean | 115 | 16.6 | 30.5 |
| Japanese women in United States | Huang et al. | 2000 | 48-h dietary recall | A-mean | 51 | 7.3 | 11.1 |
| Chinese in Singapore | Seow et al. | 1998 | In-person interview FFQ | A-mean | 147 | 2.4 | 2.4 |
| U.S. Caucasian women | Huang et al. | 2000 | 48-h dietary recall | A-mean | 18 | 1.0 | 2.0 |
| U.S. Caucasian men | Strom et al. | 1999 | Self-administered FFQ | A-mean | 107 | $22.8 \times 10^{-3}$ | $29.7 \times 10^{-3}$ |
| **Blood Concentration (nmol/l)** | | | | | | | |
| Japanese men | Yamamoto et al. | 2001 | TR-FIA | G-mean | 93 | 68.3 | 352.8 |
| Japanese women | Yamamoto et al. | 2001 | TR-FIA | G-mean | 109 | 62.5 | 247.0 |
| Japanese women | Arai et al. | 2000 | TR-FIA | A-mean | 115 | 111.7 | 307.5 |
| Japanese men | Adlercreutz et al. | 1993 | GC-MS | G-mean | 14 | 107.0 | 276.0 |
| Finnish men | Adlercreutz et al. | 1993 | GC-MS | G-mean | 14 | 6.2 | 6.3 |
| Finnish women | Wang | 2000 | TR-FIA | A-mean | 80 | 3.8 | 3.2 |
| Finnish omnivorous women | Adlercreutz et al. | 1994 | GC-MS | G-mean | 14 | 4.2 | 4.9 |
| Finnish vegetarian women | Adlercreutz et al. | 1994 | GC-MS | G-mean | 14 | 18.5 | 17.1 |

*(continued)*

**Urine Excretion (µmol/day)**

| Group | Author | Year | Method | Mean | | | |
|---|---|---|---|---|---|---|---|
| Japanese men | Yamamoto et al. | 2001 | HPLC | G-mean | 33 | 10.4 | 8.5 |
| Japanese women | Yamamoto et al. | 2001 | HPLC | G-mean | 60 | 11.1 | 8.5 |
| Japanese women | Arai et al. | 2000 | HPLC | A-mean | 115 | 23.3 | 13.2 |
| Japanese men | Adlercreutz et al. | 1991 | GC-MS | G-mean | 9 | 2.2 | NA |
| Japanese women | Adlercreutz et al. | 1991 | GC-MS | G-mean | 10 | 2.6 | NA |
| Japanese women in United States | Huang et al. | 2000 | HPLC | A-mean | 51 | 6.9 | 3.8 |
| U.S. Caucasian women | Huang et al. | 2000 | HPLC | A-mean | 18 | $860 \times 10^{-3}$ | $400 \times 10^{-3}$ |
| U.S. omnivorous women | Adlercreutz et al. | 1986 | GC-MS | G-mean | | $320 \times 10^{-3}$ | NA |
| U.S. lacto-vegetarian women | Adlercreutz et al. | 1986 | GC-MS | G-mean | | $1260 \times 10^{-3}$ | NA |
| U.S. macrobiotics women | Adlercreutz et al. | 1986 | GC-MS | G-mean | | $3460 \times 10^{-3}$ | NA |
| Finnish omnivorous men | Adlercreutz et al. | 1991 | GC-MS | A-mean | 10 | $134 \times 10^{-3}$ | $184 \times 10^{-3}$ |
| Finnish omnivorous women | Adlercreutz et al. | 1986 | GC-MS | G-mean | | $219 \times 10^{-3}$ | NA |
| Finnish lacto-vegetarian women | Adlercreutz et al. | 1986 | GC-MS | G-mean | | $275 \times 10^{-3}$ | NA |

FFQ, food frequency questionnaire; DR, dietary record; A-mean, arithmetic mean; G-mean, geometric mean; TR-FIA, time-resolved fluoroimmunoassay; GC-MS, gas chromatography-mass spectrometry; NA, not available.

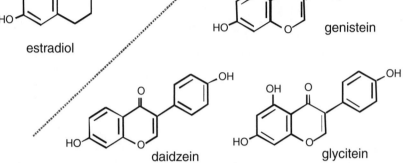

**FIGURE 3.3** Estrogens and isoflavones.

(Figure 3.3). Glycitein content in soy is relatively small. Unfermented soy includes mainly β-glycoside, but fermented soybean products (e.g., miso) include more aglycon. This review mainly focuses on genistein because it has the strongest affinity to estrogen receptors and the actions of other isoflavones are not very different from those of genistein.

### 3.2.1 ESTROGENIC ACTIVITY OF ISOFLAVONE

The estrogenic effect of isoflavone (binding affinity to estrogen receptors) has been investigated under various conditions and shown to be relatively weak: 1/100 to 1/10,000 of 17β-estradiol.[15–18] Genistein has severalfold higher activities than daidzein. The estrogenic activity of isoflavone depends on the tissue, partly because of the different distribution of estrogen receptor type (ER-α and ER-β) expression among tissues. Expression of ER-α is reported to be rich in adrenal, kidney, and testes. ER-β is rich in thymus, bladder, lungs, bone, prostate, and vasculature, and both are expressed in the breast and uterus.[19] Isoflavone may act differently in different tissues as selective estrogen receptor modulater (SERM) like raloxifene.[20]

In discussing the effect of isoflavone, we have to consider the physiological level of isoflavone and estrogen. The serum genistein level is below 10 n$M$ (2.7 ng/ml) for Western people who rarely eat soybean products and 300 n$M$ (810 ng/ml) for Japanese who eat soybean products every day (Table 3.1). Our unpublished results show that more than 10% of the subjects exceed serum genistein levels of 1000 n$M$ (order of micrograms per milliliter)

(Yamamoto et al. 2001, unpublished results). Serum E2 levels rapidly increase at menarche, and peak in the twenties, and decrease with age. For simplicity, we can consider that serum E2 level is ~100 pg/ml, ~300 pg/ml, and ~200 pg/ml for at follicular phase, ovular phase, and luteal phase, respectively, and below 50 pg/ml for postmenopausal women (100 pg/ml = 0.37 n$M$). E2 level varies across ethnic groups: it is lower in Asians than in Caucasians and African-Americans.[21] Serum E2 levels vary, but their variation is not as large as that of serum isoflavone. Even if its binding affinity is low, serum isoflavone may compete with endogenous estrogen in Japanese people because their isoflavone concentration is very high.

Experimental results show that intake of isoflavone lowers serum estrogen levels and prolongs menstrual cycle lengths, especially follicular phase lengths[22-26] for premenopausal women. This may be mediated by decreasing serum follicle-stimulating hormone and luteinizing hormone levels caused by isoflavones. Lower estrogen levels and longer menstrual cycles length reduce lifetime exposure to estrogens. This is consistent with the observation that breast cancer patients have shorter menstrual cycles.[27,28] Furthermore, longer menstrual cycles without lengthening luteal phases might be also favorable since the mitotic activity of the breast tissue is fourfold higher in the luteal phase compared with the follicular phase.[29,30] Estrogen levels are lower in Asian women than in Western women,[21] and isoflavone intake also lowers serum estrogen levels for postmenopausal women.[31] However, other studies do not show the prolongation of menstrual cycles or lowering of estrogen levels.[32,33] Isoflavone also lowers serum estrogen levels by simulating sex hormone–binding globulin production[34,35] and inhibiting aromatase.[36-38]

## 3.3 *IN VITRO* STUDIES

Thousands of *in vitro* studies have been dedicated to examining the effects of soy and isoflavones on cancer. Initially, isoflavone was hypothesized to have effects on cancer cell growth via its estrogenic or antiestrogenic properties because of its similarity to the structure to estrogen. Many studies have been conducted using human and rodent breast cancer cell lines. Isoflavone has a cell growth inhibition effect in high (5 µ$M$ to 100 µ$M$) concentrations for both estrogen-dependent (MCF-7) and estrogen-independent (MDA-468) breast cancer cell lines but has a cell growth stimulation effect in relatively low (<1 µ$M$) concentrations.[39-43]

### 3.3.1 Physiological Environment

The prevailing hypothesis has been that isoflavone exerts antiestrogenic effects when placed in a high estrogen environment, such as exists in premenopausal women, and estrogenic effects in a low estrogen environment, as in postmenopausal women.[44] This hypothesis should be cautiously interpreted if estrogen and isoflavone concentrations in the human body are considered.

The physiological concentration of isoflavone is below 10 n$M$ for Western people and 300 n$M$ (or at most a micromolar level) for Japanese people. This concentration corresponds to the level that shows cell growth stimulation and the level which is much lower than that showing cell inhibition *in vitro*. However, the results above are in an estrogen-free environment. Variation of estrogen concentration is not so large, and an estrogen-free environment is not realistic, even for postmenopausal women. Therefore, taking different environments into account, the cell-stimulating effect of an *in vitro* study may not be applicable. While several reports show genistein's stimulating effect on cancer cell growth in an estrogen environment,[45] others show no additional stimulating effect or even inhibition of an estrogen-stimulating effect on cancer cells in the environment with physiological isoflavone concentrations.[41,43,46,47]

### 3.3.2 Cell Growth Inhibition by Genistein

Genistein, a tyrosine kinase inhibitor (TKI),[48] and many studies show that its cell growth inhibition is mediated by this TKI activity. Although genistein is a potent protein tyrosine kinase (PTK) inhibitor, its mechanism of action is not known. Since genistein inhibits epidermal growth factor (EGF)–stimulated cell growth without any inhibition of EGF autophosphorylation, genistein's PTK inhibition does not have a direct effect on tyrosine kinase but rather indirect effects mediated by other mechanisms.[49,50] Growth inhibition was also associated with the inhibition of DNA topoisomerases, ribosomal S6 kinase activity, and phospatidylinisitol breakdown.[51–54]

In addition to cell growth inhibition, genistein inhibits proliferation, induces differentiation and apoptosis, and arrests cell cycle progression at G2-M in ER positive and negative human breast cancer cell lines.[46,49,55–65] Due to the similarity of these effects, genistein activity might be mediated by the TGF-$\beta$1 signaling pathway.[50]

Isoflavone also inhibits angiogenesis[66] and antioxidant effects.[67] However, these *in vitro* effects occur in concentrations that exceed the physiological levels in humans and the effects in humans are not clear.

### 3.3.3 Summary

In addition to its antiestrogenic effects such as suppressing estrogen levels and prolonging menstrual cycles, isoflavone may contribute to breast cancer risk reduction by its effect on cancer cell growth inhibition. These are either antiestrogenic or nonhormal effects since isoflavone inhibits ER-positive and ER-negative breast cancer cell growth. Since most of the effects are observed in the supraphysiological concentrations, further studies are needed to elucidate the effect in more physiological environments in *in vitro, in vivo,* and human studies. Coexistence of estrogen and other substances and high concentrations achieved by heavy isoflavone intake may interact to reduce cancer risk.

## 3.4  ANIMAL STUDIES

Animal experiments examining the effect of soy or its ingredients on breast cancer development are not as numerous as *in vitro* studies. Animal studies are listed in Table 3.2.[68–82] This list is not exhaustive but is collected from previous reviews[83,84] and a PubMed literature search. The rodent studies on the effect of a soy diet on mammary tumor development started in the 1970s. The list summarizes not only isoflavone effects but also other soy effects on mammary cancer development.

### 3.4.1  Overall Results

Overall results show moderate effects. Various tumor induction methods were used including x-irradiation, dimethylbenz[a] anthracene (DMBA), *N*-methyl-*N*-nitrosourea (MNU), and 2-amino-1-methyl-6-phenylimidazo[4,5-b] pyridine (PhIP). Examined substances were raw soybean, soybean protein, soy powder, SPI, genistein, daidzein, isoflavone mixture, SPI-depleted isoflavone, miso, and fermented soymilk via diet or injection. Administration of these substances achieved serum isoflavone concentrations similar to or higher than those in the Japanese population. Most of the studies show reduced tumor multiplicity and prolongation of latency, but a few studies show statistically significant decreases of tumor incidence.

### 3.4.2  Early Exposure

Compared with the modest effect on adult animals, results of early exposure are much more impressive. Lamartiniere's group intensively examined the effect of early genistein exposure. They first investigated the effect of supraphysiological levels of genistein exposure[85–88] and later, physiological levels of genistein exposure[89] during neonatal (2 to 9 d postpartum) and prepubertal (until 3 weeks postpartum) periods on the subsequent DMBA-induced mammary tumors and showed statistically significant reduction and latency delay in tumor development. They investigated the effect of prepubertal genistein exposure on EGF signaling pathways and found that in 50-d-old rats it reduces EGF receptor expression specifically in the epithelial cells of the terminal end buds.[90] Reduction of EGF receptor mass in the target tissue of adult animals may alter signal transduction, mammary gland differentiation, and cell proliferation.[91] The studies showed no effect on the rate of fertility in dams or offspring number of males or females, anogenital distances, time of vaginal opening or testes descent, body weights at all ages, proportion of time spent in the phases of the estrous cycle or of follicular development, or reproductive tract alterations (ovaries, uteri, and vagina).[89] On the contrary, another group found that in utero exposure to genistein induces mammary tumors in the offspring,[92] but this may not be applicable to humans, because Japanese people eat soybean products during pregnancy. Lamartiniere et al.[93] concluded that "differentiation effects are believed to occur via an imprinting mechanism that determines the 'blueprint' from which the mammary cells respond to

**TABLE 3.2**
**Experimental Studies of Isoflaovone in Rodents**

| Author, Year | Animal | Induction Method | Treatment Groups | Results and Comments |
|---|---|---|---|---|
| Carroll, 1975 | SD rats | DMBA | Control (casein), soy protein diet | No difference in number of tumors |
| Troll et al., 1980 | SD rats | x-irradiation | control (casein), raw soybean (500 g/kg diet) diet | Reduction of tumor incidence ($P < .01$) |
| Gridley et al., 1983 | C3H/HeJ mice | Spontaneous | Protein diet (milk, beef, fish, soybean, either 11 or 33% by weight) | Age at first tumor appearance varied (48–84 d); tumors in the soy group appeared late but increased rapidly |
| Barnes et al., 1990 | SD rats | MNU | Control (AIN-76A), soy powder/SPI +AIN-76A diet | Tumor appearance was inhibited by soy powder and SPI; soy powder delayed latency but had no effect on reproductive apparatus |
| Baggott, 1990 | SD rats | DMBA | Control (AIN-76A), miso+AIN-76A diet | Tumor incidence was decreased and delayed significantly in miso group |
| Hawrylewicz et al., 1991 | SD rats | MNU | Control (casein), SPI diet | Tumor incidence was decreased and delayed significantly in SPI group but increased with methionine supplementation |
| Constantinou et al., 1996 | SD rats | MNU | Control, daidzein, genistein injection | Genistein, not daidzein, reduced multiplicity Neither affected incidence significantly TopoII and PTK activity are similar among the groups |
| Gotoh et al., 1998 | CD/Crj rats | MNU | Control diet MF, soybean, miso-supplemented diet | Soybean and miso significantly reduced multiplicity but not incidence |
| Appelt and Reicks, 1999 | SD rats | DMBA | Control (casein), soy diet | Tumor incidence and antioxidant/phase II enzyme activities are significantly inversely associated with isoflavone concentration |

| Reference | Animal | Carcinogen | Diet/Treatment | Results |
|---|---|---|---|---|
| Ohta et al., 2000 | SD rats | PhIP | Control (high fat basal diet), fermented soymilk, isoflavone mixture | Significant decrease in multiplicity, but not in incidence, observed in fermented soy-milk and 0.04% isoflavone mixture group |
| Cohen et al., 2000 | F-344 rats | MNU | Control (AIN-93G), soy protein, isoflavone-depleted soy protein AIN-93G diet | No significant differences were observed in tumor incidence, latency, multiplicity, or volume |
| Constantinou et al., 2001 | SD rats | DMBA | Control (AIN-76A), daidzein, genistein, daidzein + genistein, SPI, SPI-depleted isoflavone supplemented diet | No difference in tumor incidence; significant decreases in multiplicity were observed in daidzein, SPI, and SPI-depleted isoflavone group |
| Day et al., 2001 | ER-alpha WT/KO mice | DMBA | Casein with 0/1 g genistein/kg diet | Malignant adenocarcinoma observed only in the group with ER-$\alpha$ WT and genistein diet; dietary intake was reduced in genistein group and led to subsequent significant weight loss |
| Jin and MacDonald, 2002 | MMTV-neu mice | Spontaneous | AIN-93G diet with no isoflavone, daidzein, genistein, isoflavone mixture | MMTV-neu mouse spontaneously develops mammary tumors due to overexpression of ErbB-2/neu/Her2 oncogene; tumor latency was delayed in isoflavone-fed group, but number and size of the tumors were not different |
| Yang, 2003 | MMTV-neu mice | Spontaneous | Control (casein) vs. soy diet, E2, tamoxifen, placebo pellet implantation | Soy-fed group developed tumors at later age than casein-fed group in E2 and placebo pellet group; no difference in incidence or latency was observed in the tamoxifen-treated mice by dietary group |

future hormonal and/or xenobiotic exposure." Prepubertal periods in rats correspond to adolescence in humans, and this is consistent with findings that the breast cancer risk of Japanese Americans is similar to that of U.S.-born Americans when they migrated at younger ages.[94]

### 3.4.3 IN VIVO STUDIES IN HUMANS

Many intervention studies have been conducted to determine the effect of soy or isoflavone intake on biomarkers in humans such as serum sex hormone or sex hormone–binding globulin levels and menstrual length,[22–25,32,95–105] urinary production of potentially carcinogenic estrogen metabolites,[96,98,103] and nipple aspirate and tissue.[32,98] Since the results are not consistent and the association of these biomarkers and breast cancer is not evident, these data are difficult to interpret.

## 3.5 EPIDEMIOLOGICAL STUDIES

### 3.5.1 LEVEL OF EVIDENCE IN EPIDEMIOLOGICAL STUDIES

Before reviewing the epidemiological studies, it is necessary to know there is an evidence level in epidemiological studies (Table 3.3). Consider the study to see the association between soy-rich food and breast cancer. The highest evidence comes from the randomized controlled trial with sufficient statistical power to show the difference in breast cancer incidence between the soy-rich food group and no soy-rich food group to which subjects are randomized. The second highest evidence comes from the prospective cohort study where subjects are asked or measured about their soy food intake at the study baseline and followed up for years to see if they develop breast cancer. The third highest evidence comes from retrospective case-control studies where breast cancer patients and controls are asked or measured about their soy food intake. Other possible evidence can come from an ecological study where nation- or region-specific average intakes are compared with their breast cancer incidences. Time-series analysis is used to compare trends of soy food intake and those of breast cancer incidence in a nation or region. The unit of the data is individual for the first three study designs (randomized controlled trial, cohort study, case-control study) and population for the latter two study designs. The higher the evidence level, the more funds, time, and subjects are needed.

### 3.5.2 POPULATION-LEVEL STUDIES OF SOYBEAN INTAKE AND BREAST CANCER

An example of a time-series analysis is shown in Figure 3.4, which plots soy food consumption per capita and breast cancer mortality by year in Japan. The intake data come from the National Nutrition Survey in Japan, and mortality data come from the vital statistics of Japan.[2] Breast cancer showed an increased tendency, with no difference in soybean intake levels over 20 years. No association between these items is observed. The second set of results came from the ecological study by

**TABLE 3.3**
**Evidence Level and Epidemiological Study Design**

| Evidence Level | | Study Design | Data Collection | Unit | No. of Subjects | Period | Cost |
|---|---|---|---|---|---|---|---|
| High | Randomized controlled trial | Randomize subjects into two groups (isoflavone and placebo) and compare subsequent cancer incidence | Prospective | Individual | 1,000–100,000 | 10 years | >$10 million |
| ∅ | Cohort study | Investigate food intake of large healthy population and follow up several to >10 years and examine association between intake and incidence | Prospective | Individual | 10,000–1,000,000 | 10 years | $10 million |
| | Case-control study | Select case subjects and corresponding healthy controls and compare their past diet | Retrospective | Individual | 100–1000 | 2–3 years | $1 million |
| → | Ecological study | Compare country-specific intake and incidence among countries | Cross sectional | Population | <100 Populations | 0 | 0 |
| Low | Time series | Investigate the change of dietary habits and incidence in one population | Cross sectional | Population | 1 population | 0 | 0 |

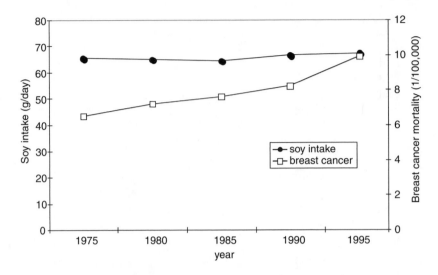

**FIGURE 3.4** Time series analysis of soy intake and breast cancer in Japan.

prefectures in Japan (Figure 3.5). Soybean intake and mortality data are both averaged for the period 1975 to 1995 by prefectures (http://nihn-jst.nih.go.jp:8888/nns/owa/nns_main.hm01). The scatterplot shows a slight inverse association but it is not impressive. This slight association is possibly due to a small difference in

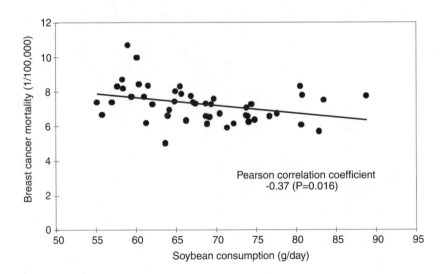

**FIGURE 3.5** Soy bean consumption and breast cancer mortality by prefectures in Japan. Updated from Nagata 2000.[106]

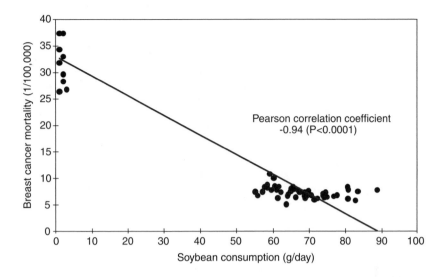

**FIGURE 3.6** Soy bean consumption and breast cancer mortality by prefectures in Japan and selected Western countries. (Soy intake for Westerns is assumed to be close to 0.).

soy food intake and breast cancer incidence among prefectures in Japan. Figure 3.6 is based on hypothetical data with actual breast cancer mortality rates[107] and hypothetical soybean intake data in Western countries. Since the intake of soybean in Western countries is known to be very low, arbitrary values close to 0 are assigned to the intake data. This is a hypothetical figure that many soy and breast cancer researchers bear in mind. Although it is hypothetical, Figure 3.6 shows the importance of international collaborative studies.

### 3.5.3 INDIVIDUAL-LEVEL STUDIES OF SOYBEAN INTAKE AND BREAST CANCER

To date, 15 individual-level epidemiological studies have evaluated associations between soy or isoflavone consumption and breast cancer risk (Table 3.4)[108–122] Among the studies that reported results for premenopausal women, four case-control studies conducted on Singapore Chinese,[115] Japanese,[116] Asian American,[118] and Chinese[120] populations found statistically significant inverse associations between soy consumption and breast cancer risk. Two prospective studies conducted on American[111] and Japanese[112] and four case-control studies conducted on Chinese,[117] American and Canadian,[119] non-Asian American,[121] and Asian American[122] populations found no such association. Of the studies that reported results for post-menopausal women, two case-control studies conducted on Chinese[120] and Asian American[122] populations and one prospective Japanese study[112] found statistically significant inverse associations. Two prospective American studies[109,111] and five case-control studies conducted on Singapore Chinese,[115] Japanese,[116] Chinese,[117]

## TABLE 3.4
## Summary of Epidemiological Studies Investigating Dietary Soybean Products and Breast Cancer

| Author, Publication Year | Population | Number of Subjects | Exposure Comparison Category | Menopausal Status | Relative Risk (95% Confidence Intervals) |
|---|---|---|---|---|---|
| **Cohort Study** | | | | | |
| Hirayama, 1990 | Japanese | 241 cases 2,140,369 person-years | Miso soup Daily vs. nondaily | Combined | 0.85 (0.68–1.06) |
| Greenstein et al., 1996 | American | 1,018 cases 34,388 women | Soy or tofu: consumers vs. nonconsumers | Post | 0.76 (0.50–1.18) |
| Key et al., 1999 | Japanese | 427 cases 488,989 person-years | Miso soup $\Pi$5 vs. $\Sigma$1 time/week | Combined | 0.87 (0.68–1.12) |
| Horn-Ross et al., 2002 | American | 711 cases 222,249 person-years | Genistein Fifth vs. first quintile | Combined | 1.0 (0.7–1.3) |
| Yamamoto et al., 2003 | Japanese | 179 cases 209,354 person-years | Genistein Fourth vs. first quartile | Pre Post | 0.66 (0.25–1.7) 0.32 (0.14–0.71) |
| Keinan-Boker et al., 2004 | Dutch | 280 cases 80,215 person-years | Isoflavone Fourth vs. first quartile | Combined[a] | 0.98 (0.65–1.48) |
| **Case-Control Study** | | | | | |
| Hirohata et al., 1985 | Japanese | 212 cases 212 controls | Fat from soybean products Mean intake | Combined | Not significant |
| Lee et al., 1992 | Singapore Chinese | 200 cases 420 controls | Total soya products $\Pi$55.0 vs. <20.3 g/d | Pre Post | 0.4 (0.2–0.9) 1.1 (0.5–2.3) |

*(continued)*

| Study | Population | Cases/controls | Exposure | Menopausal status | OR (95% CI) |
|---|---|---|---|---|---|
| Hirose et al., 1995 | Japanese | 1,186 cases / 23,163 controls | Tofu, >3 vs. $\Sigma$3 times/week | Pre / Post | 0.81 (0.65–0.99) / 1.17 (0.92–1.49) |
| Yuan et al., 1995 | Chinese | 834 cases / 834 controls | Soy protein 18 g/d | Combined[a] | 1.0 (0.7–1.4) |
| Wu et al., 1996 | Asian American | 597 cases / 966 controls | Tofu, 1 time/week | Pre / Post | 0.84 (0.70–0.99) / 0.86 (0.66–1.13) |
| Witte et al., 1997 | American and Canadian | 140 cases / 222 controls | Tofu or soybean, 1 serving/week vs. none | Pre | 0.5 (0.2–1.1) |
| Dai et al., 2001 | Chinese | 1,459 cases / 1,556 controls | Soy protein >139.1 vs. $\Sigma$18.6 g/week | Combined[a] | 0.66 (0.46–0.95) |
| Horn-Ross et al., 2001 | Non-Asian American | 1,326 cases / 1,657 controls | Isoflavones, Per 1000 µg/d | Pre / Post | 1.00 (0.98–1.02) / 0.99 (0.97–1.01) |
| Wu et al., 2002 | Asian-American | 501 cases / 594 controls | Isoflavones, >12.68 vs. $\Sigma$1.79 mg/1000 kcal | Pre / Post | 0.60, $P > .05$ / 0.39, $P < .05$ |

[a] Results were not substantially different when analyzed separately by menopausal status.

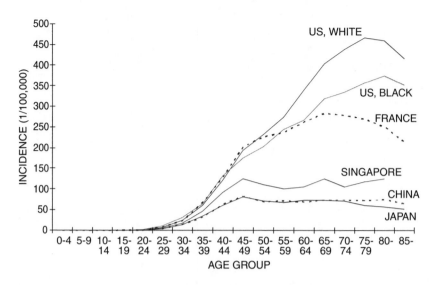

**FIGURE 3.7** Age-specific breast cancer incidence throughout the world.

Asian American,[118] and non-Asian American[121] populations found no such associations. Two other prospective studies and one case-control study conducted of Japanese populations[109,110,114] and a Dutch cohort study[113] reported combined results for pre- and postmenopausal women and found no statistically significant association between soy consumption and breast cancer risk. Yamamoto et al.[112] showed an inverse association in postmenopausal women, and this observation is consistent with the disparity of age-specific incidence between Asian and Western countries (Figure 3.7). Only one study investigated early exposure to soybean (age 13 to 15 years) and breast cancer and found a significant inverse association.[123] Early exposure should be investigated in future epidemiological research.

The results of individual-level studies seem inconsistent even in the same study design (Figure 3.8). However, relative risks by study design and menopausal status and ethnic group give us some idea. Recent case-control studies tend to show inverse associations in Asian ethnic groups both for pre- and postmenopausal women (Figure 3.9). Studies of Western subjects do not show any trend. In cohort studies, although sufficient data are not provided by menopausal status, similar trends as in case-control studies are shown for Asian and Western ethnic groups (Figure 3.10).

If we assume that the association between soy intake and breast cancer risk exists, possible reasons of the lack of associations observed in the previous studies could be the result of recall bias in case-control studies, errors in exposure measurements, or small exposure variation in Western subjects. In particular, association between disease and exposure can be detected more easily when exposure has wide variability. For example, while the most recent study of Japanese[112] estimated relative risk to be 0.46 by comparing the highest (>25.3 mg/d

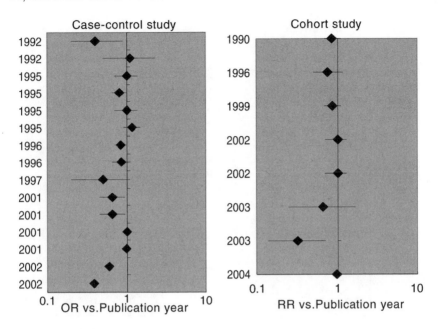

**FIGURE 3.8** Relative risk of soy product in breast cancer in epidemiological studies by design and publication year.

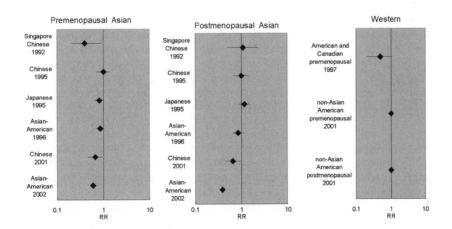

**FIGURE 3.9** Relative risk of soy product in breast cancer in case-control studies by ethnicity, menopausal status, and publication year.

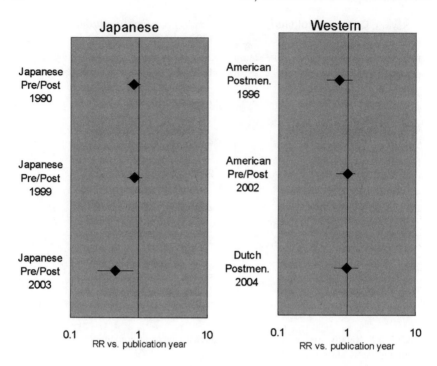

**FIGURE 3.10** Relative risk of soy product in breast cancer in cohort studies by ethnicity and publication year.

for genistein) and the lowest quartiles (<6.9 mg/d for genistein), the most recent study of Western subjects[113] estimated relative risk to be 0.98 by comparing the highest (>0.54 mg/d for isoflavone) and the lowest quartiles (<0.28 mg/d for isoflavone). The latter comparison is only within the lowest quartile in the former. Indeed, median isoflavone intake among the Japanese study participants[3] was seven times higher than that among Chinese in Singapore, 15 times higher than that among U.S. non-Asian (African-American, Latina, and White) women, and 700 times higher than that among U.S. Caucasians[7,8,124] (Table 3.1). Two other Japanese prospective studies, which did not show the association, may also have a high level but small variation in soy intake because soy intake was uniformly high when the cohorts were established in the 1960s and 1970s.[108,110]

If we assume the association does not exist, several possibilities may explain the observed associations. One is, of course, chance. Another possibility is the failure to control potential confounding factors. Low breast cancer incidence may be associated with other Asian dietary habits such as eating more rice, pickles, vegetables, and fish and less bread and butter; other Asian life-style factors; and genetic predispositions. There remains the possibility of residual confounding even if they are controlled for in the multivariate models. The fact that the recent results tend to be significant might only reflect of the publication bias.

Several studies showed an inverse association between serum isoflavone level and urinary excretion and breast cancer even in the Western population.[125–128] These results should be interpreted with caution when the samples were collected after the diagnosis, since they may reflect possible changes after breast cancer development.

In order to obtain more confirmative evidence from epidemiological studies, it is necessary to conduct studies with more cases, those clarifying the difference in effects among various soybean products, and those investigating breast cancer and biomarkers of soybean intake such as serum isoflavones and urine isoflavones that were collected before the onset of disease.[129]

### 3.5.4 RANDOMIZED CONTROLLED TRIALS

There have not been randomized controlled trials (RCTs) that investigate the effect of soy and isoflavone on breast cancer incidence, although RCTs with other end points have been conducted.[104,105] Such studies would require huge resources including money, time, subjects, and staffs. To conduct RCTs, more probable evidence of isoflavone's effects on humans is necessary. Since genistein is not a patented chemical structure and is not considered a viable pharmaceutical product, the Chemopreventive Agent Development Research Group (CADRG), Division of Cancer Prevention, National Cancer Institute in the United States assessed the preclinical toxicity of purified soy isoflavone products (trade name PTI G-2535: unconjugated isoflavone and PTI G-4660: conjugated isoflavone, Protein Techonologies International) and conducted phase 1 clinical trials under an Investigational New Drug Application to the Food and Drug Administration (FDA) to evaluate their safety and pharmacokinetics in rats, dogs, and humans. No clinical or histological signs of toxicity or teratology were observed.[131,132] Also, genotoxicity and carcinogenicity were investigated *in vitro, in vivo,* and in human studies. Some mutagenicity was found *in vitro* and *in vivo,* but significant genotoxicity was not found in humans.[132,133] CADRG is sponsoring other early phase clinical trials, and the results are forthcoming (http://www3.cancer.gov/prevention/ agents/Soy_Isoflavones.html). Isoflavone intervention may be effective for populations at high risk for breast cancer, with low habitual soybean intake.

### 3.6 SUMMARY

*In vitro* experiments show that isoflavone inhibits cell growth in supraphysiological concentrations but stimulates cell growth in physiological concentrations in an estrogen-free environment. On the contrary, animal experiments show modest effects on reduction of tumor multiplicity and prolongation of latency. Results of epidemiological studies are not consistent, but recent studies of Asian ethnic groups tend to show inverse trends between soybean and isoflavone intake and breast cancer incidence for both pre- and postmenopausal women. Neonatal and prepubertal exposure to soy and isoflavone in animals and exposure in adolescent humans shows consistent inverse effects.

Although most of the effects are not clarified, soy and its ingredients, mainly isoflavone, have some effect on breast cancer development via various pathways with highest probability. Further studies are warranted, especially *in vitro* studies to elucidate isoflavone's mechanism of action in physiological environments with respect to estrogen and isoflavone circulation, *in vivo* and human studies focusing on early exposure, studies to investigate the interaction with other substances, epidemiological studies using biomarkers, epidemiological studies to determine the effect of soy and isoflavone intake on breast cancer patients, and intervention studies to determine the effect on biomarkers in humans. If these results are promising, randomized controlled studies to determine the effect of soy on breast cancer incidence should be conducted in the future, especially in low–soy intake and high–breast cancer risk populations.

## ACKNOWLEDGMENTS

The authors thank Dr. Mark Messina, Dr. Jing-Rong Zhou, Dr. Ken Kobayashi, and Dr. Tomoyuki Hanaoka for their valuable comments on the earlier version of the manuscript.

## REFERENCES

1. Parkin, D.M., Whelan, S.L., Ferlay, J., Raymond, L., and Young, J., Eds., *Cancer Incidence in Five Continents*, Vol. 7, IARC, Lyon, 1997.
2. Statistics and Information Department, Minister's Secretariat, Ministry of Health and Welfare, Japan, Age-Adjusted Death Rates by Prefecture, Special Report on Vital Statistics, 1990.
3. Yamamoto, S., Sobue, T., Sasaki, S., Kobayashi, M., Arai, Y., Uehara, M., Adlercreutz, H., Watanabe, S., Takahashi, T., Iitoi, Y., Iwase, Y., Akabane, M., and Tsugane, S., Validity and reproducibility of a self-administered food-frequency questionnaire to assess isoflavone intake in a Japanese population in comparison with dietary records and blood and urine isoflavones, *J. Nutr.*, 131, 2741–2747, 2001.
4. Wakai, K., Egami, I., Kato, K., Kawamura, T., Tamakoshi, A., Lin, Y., Nakayama, T., Wada, M., and Ohno, Y., Dietary intake and sources of isoflavones among Japanese, *Nutr. Cancer*, 33, 139–145, 2000.
5. Arai, Y., Watanabe, S., Kimira, M., Shimoi, K., Mochizuki, R., and Kinae, N., Dietary intakes of flavonols, flavones and isoflavones by Japanese women and the inverse correlation between quercetin intake and plasma LDL cholesterol concentration, *J. Nutr.*, 130(9), 2243–2250, 2000.
6. Huang, M.H., Harrison, G.G., Mohamed, M.M., Gornbein, J.A., Henning, S.M., Go V.L., and Greendale, G.A., Assessing the accuracy of a food frequency questionnaire for estimating usual intake of phytoestrogens, *Nutr. Cancer*, 37(2), 145–154, 2000.
7. Seow, A., Shi, C.-Y., Franke, A.A., Hankin, J.H., Lee, H.-P., and Yu, M.C., Isoflavonoid levels in spot urine are associated with frequency of dietary soy intake in a population-based sample of middle-aged and older Chinese in Singapore, *Cancer Epidemiol. Biomarkers Prev.*, 7, 135–140, 1998.

8.  Strom, S.S., Yamamura, Y., Duphorne, C.M., Spitz, M.R., Babaian, R.J., and Pillow, P.C. et al., Phytoestrogen intake and prostate cancer: a case-control study using a new database, *Nutr. Cancer,* 33, 20–25, 1999.

9.  Adlercreutz, H., Markkanen, H., and Watanabe, S., Plasma concentration of phyto-oestorogen in Japanese men, *Lancet,* 342, 1209–1210, 1993.

10. Adlercreutz, H., Fotsis, T., Watanabe, S., Lampe, J., Wahala, K., Makela, T., and Hase, T., Determination of lignans and isoflavonoids in plasma by isotope dilution gas chromatography-mass spectrometry, *Cancer Detect. Prev.,* 18, 259–271, 1994.

11. Adlercreutz, H., Honjo, H., Higashi, A., Fotsis, T., Hamalainen, E., Hasegawa, T., and Okada, H., Urinary excretion of lignans and isoflavonoid phytoestrogens in Japanese men and women consuming a traditional Japanese diet, *Am. J. Clin. Nutr.,* 54, 1093–1100, 1991.

12. Adlercreutz, H., Fotsis, T., Bannwart, C., Wahala, K., Makela, T., Brunow, G., and Hase, T., Determination of urinary lignans and phytoestrogen metabolites, potential antiestrogens and anticarcinogens, in urine of women on various habitual diets, *J. Steroid Biochem.,* 25, 791–797, 1986.

13. Adlercreutz, H., Fotsis, T., Bannwart, C., Wahala, K., Brunow, G., and Hase, T., Isotope dilution gas chromatographic-mass spectrometric method for the determination of lignans and isoflavonoids in human urine, including identification of genistein, *Clin. Chim. Acta,* 199, 263–278, 1991.

14. World Cancer Research Fund/American Institute for Cancer Research, Food, nutrition and the prevention of cancer: a global perspective, 1997.

15. Breinholt, V. and Larsen, C., Detection of weak estrogenic flavonoids using a recombinant yeast strain and modified MCF 7 cell proliferation assay, *Chem. Res. Toxicol.,* 11, 622–629, 1998.

16. Miksicek, R.J., Commonly occurring plant flavonoids have estrogenic activity, *Mol. Pharmacol.,* 44(1), 37–43, 1993.

17. Markiewicz, L., Garey, J., Adlercreutz, H., and Gurpide, E., *In vitro* bioassays of non-steroidal phytoestrogens, *J. Steroid Biochem. Mol. Biol.,* 45(5), 399–405, 1993.

18. Folman, Y. and Pope, G.S., The interaction in the immature mouse of potent oestrogens with coumestrol, genistein and other utero-vaginotrophic compounds of low potency, *J. Endocrinol.,* 34(2), 215–25, 1966.

19. Kuiper, G.G.J.M., Carlsson, B., Grandien, K., Enmark, E., Haggblad, J., Nilson, S., and Gustafsson, J.A., Comparison of the ligand binding specificity and transcript tissue distribution of estrogen receptors $\alpha$ and $\beta$, *Endocrinology,* 138, 863–870, 1997.

20. Ettinger, B., Black, D.M., Mitlak, B.H., Knickerbocker, R.K., Nickelsen, T., Genant, H.K., Christiansen, C., Delmas, P.D., Zanchetta, J.R., Stakkestad, J., Gluer, C.C., Krueger, K., Cohen, F.J., Eckert, S., Ensrud, K.E., Avioli, L.V., Lips, P., and Cummings, S.R., Reduction of vertebral fracture risk in postmenopausal women with osteoporosis treated with raloxifene: results from a 3-year randomized clinical trial. Multiple Outcomes of Raloxifene Evaluation (MORE) Investigators, *JAMA,* 282(7), 637–645, 1999; Erratum: *JAMA,* 282(22), 2124, 1999.

21. Randolph, J.F, Jr., Sowers, M., Bondarenko, I.V., Harlow, S.D., Luborsky, J.L., and Little, R.J., Change in estradiol and follicle-stimulating hormone across the early menopausal transition: effects of ethnicity and age, *J. Clin. Endocrinol. Metab.,* 89(4), 1555–1561, 2004.

22. Cassidy, A., Bingham, S., and Setchell, K.D.R., Biological effects of a diet of soy protein rich in isoflavones on the menstrual cycle of premenopausal women, *Am. J. Clin. Nutr.*, 60, 333–340, 1994.

23. Cassidy, A., Bingham, S., and Setchell, K., Biological effects of isoflavones in young women: importance of the chemical composition of soybean products, *Br. J. Nutr.*, 74, 587–601, 1995.

24. Lu, L.J.W., Anderson, K.E., Grady, J.J., and Nagamani, M., Effects of soya consumption for one month on steroid hormones in premenopausal women: implications for breast cancer risk reduction, *Cancer Epidemiol. Biomarkers Prev.*, 5, 63–70, 1996.

25. Nagata, C., Takatsuka, N., Inaba, S., Kawakami, N., and Shimizu, H., Effect of soymilk consumption on serum estrogen concentrations in premenopausal Japanese women, *J. Natl. Cancer Inst.*, 90, 1830–1835, 1998.

26. Watanabe, S., Terashima, K., Sato, Y., Arai, S., and Eboshida, A., Effects of isoflavone supplement on healthy women, *Biofactors*, 12(1–4), 233–241, 2000.

27. Olsson, H., Landin-Olsson, M., and Gullberg, B., Retrospective assessment of menstrual cycle length in patients with breast cancer, in patients with benign breast disease, and in women without breast disease, *J. Natl. Cancer Inst.*, 70(1), 17–20, 1983.

28. Yuan, J.M., Yu, M.C., Ross, R.K., Gao, Y.T., and Henderson, B.E., Risk factors for breast cancer in Chinese women in Shanghai, *Cancer Res.*, 48(7), 1949–1953, 1988.

29. Treolar, A.E., Boynton, R.E., Behn, B.G., and Brown, B.W., Variation of the human menstrual cycle throughout reproductive life, *Int. J. Fertil.*, 12, 77–126, 1970.

30. Ferguson, D.J.P. and Anderson, T.J., Morphological evaluation of cell turnover in relation to the menstrual cycle in the "resting" human breast, *Br. J. Cancer*, 44, 177–181, 1981.

31. Duncan, A.M., Underhill, K.E.W., Xu, X., Lavalleur, J., Phipps, W.R., and Kurzer, M.S., Modest hormonal effects of soy isoflavones in postmenopausal women, *J. Clin. Endocrinol. Metab.*, 84, 3479–3484, 1999.

32. Petrakis, N.L., Barnes, S., King, E.B., Lowenstein, J., Wiencke, J., Lee, M.M., Miike, R., Kirk, M., and Coward, L., Stimulatory influence of soy protein isolate on breast secretion in pre- and postmenopausal women, *Cancer Epidemiol. Biomarkers Prev.*, 5(10), 785–794, 1996.

33. Pino, A.M, Valladares, L.E., Palma, M.A., Mancilla, A.M., Yanez, M., and Albala, C., Dietary isoflavones affect sex hormone-binding globulin levels in postmenopausal women, *Clin. Endocrinol. Metab.*, 85, 2797–2800, 2000.

34. Adlercreutz, H., Western diet and western diseases: some hormonal and biochemical mechanisms and associations, *Scand. J. Clin. Lab. Invest.*, 50(Suppl.) 201, 3–23, 1990.

35. Mousavi, Y. and Adlercreutz, H., Genistein is an effective stimulator of sex hormone-binding globulin production in hepatocarcinoma human liver cancer cells and suppresses proliferation of these cells in culture, *Steroids*, 58(7), 301–304, 1993.

36. Adlercreutz, H., Bannwart, C., Wahala, K., Makela, T., Brunow, G., Hase, T., Arosemena, P.J., Kellis, J.T., Jr., and Vickery, L.E., Inhibition of human aromatase by mammalian lignans and isoflavonoid phytoestrogens, *J. Steroid Biochem. Mol. Biol.*, 44, 147–153, 1993.

37. Campbell, D.R. and Kurzer, M.S., Flavonoid inhibition of aromatase enzyme activity in human preadipocytes, *J. Steroid Biochem. Mol. Biol.*, 46, 381–388, 1993.

38. Kao, Y.C., Zhou, C., Sherman, M., Laughton, C.A., and Chen, S., Molecular basis of the inhibition of human aromatase (estrogen synthetase) by flavone and

isoflavone phytoestrogens: a site-directed mutagenesis study, *Environ. Health Perspect.*, 106, 85–92, 1998.

39. Peterson, G. and Barnes, S., Genistein inhibits of the growth of human breast cancer cells: independence from estrogen receptors and the multi-drug resistance gene, *Biochem. Biophys. Res. Commun.*, 179, 661–667, 1991.

40. Peterson, G. and Barnes, S., Genistein inhibits both estrogen and growth factor-stimulated proliferation of human breast cancer cells, *Cell Growth Differ.*, 7, 1345–1351, 1996.

41. Zava, D.T. and Duwe, G., Estrogenic and antiproliferative properties of genistein and other flavonoids in human breast cancer cells *in vitro*, *Nutr. Cancer*, 27(1), 31–40, 1997.

42. Makela, S., Davis, V.L., Tally, W.C., Korkman, J., Salo, L., Vihko, R., Santti, R., and Korach, K.S., Dietary estrogens act through estrogen receptor-mediated processes and show no antiestrogenicity in cultured breast cancer cells, *Environ. Health Perspect.*, 102(6–7), 572–578, 1997.

43. Miodini, P., Fioravanti, L., Di, Fronzo, G., and Cappelletti, V., The two phyto-oestrogens genistein and quercetin exert different effects on oestrogen receptor function, *Br. J. Cancer*, 80(8), 1150–1155, 1999.

44. Anderson, J.J.B., Anthony, M., Messina, M., and Garner, S.C., Effects of phyto-oestrogens on tissues, *Nutr. Res. Rev.*, 12, 75–116, 1999.

45. Wang, C. and Kurzer, M.S., Effects of phytoestrogens on DNA synthesis in MCF-7 cells in the presence of estradiol or growth factors, *Nutr. Cancer*, 31(2), 90–100, 1998.

46. Wang, T.T., Sathyamoorthy, N., and Phang, J.M., Molecular effect of genistein on estrogen receptor mediated pathways, *Carcinogenesis*, 17, 271–275, 1996.

47. Sathyamoorthy, N. and Wang, T.T., Differential effects of dietary phyto-oestrogens daidzein and equol on human breast cancer MCF-7 cells, *Eur. J. Cancer*, 33(14), 2384–2389, 1997.

48. Akiyama, T., Ishida, J., Nakagawa, S., Ogawara, H., Watanabe, S., Itoh, N., Shibuya, M., and Fukami, Y., Genistein, a specific inhibitor of tyrosine-specific protein kinases, *J. Biol. Chem.*, 262(12), 5592–5595, 1987.

49. Peterson, G., Evaluation of the biochemical targets of genistein in tumor cells, *J. Nutr.*, 125(3 Suppl.), 784S–789S, 1995.

50. Kim, H., Peterson, T.G., and Barnes, S., Mechanisms of action of the soy isofla-vone genistein: emerging role for its effects via transforming growth factor beta signaling pathways, *Am. Clin. Nutr.*, 68(6 Suppl.), 1418S–1425S, 1998.

51. Okura, A., Arakawa, H., Oka, H., Yoshinari, T., and Monden, Y., Effect of genistein on topoisomerase activity and on the growth of [Val 12]Ha-ras-transformed NIH 3T3 cells, *Biochem. Biophys. Res. Commun.*, 157(1), 183–189, 1988.

52. Imoto, M., Yamashita, T., Sawa, T., Kurasawa, S., Naganawa, H., Takeuchi, T., Bao-quan, Z., and Umezawa, K., Inhibition of cellular phosphatidylinositol turn-over by psi-tectorigenin, *FEBS Lett.*, 230(1–2), 43–46, 1988.

53. Markovits, J., Linassier, C., Fosse, P., Couprie, J., Pierre, J., Jacquemin-Sablon, A., Saucier, J.M., Le, Pecq, J.B., and Larsen, A.K., Inhibitory effects of the tyrosine kinase inhibitor genistein on mammalian DNA topoisomerase II, *Cancer Res.*, 49(18), 5111–5117, 1989.

54. Linassier, C., Pierre, M., LePecq, J.B., and Pierre, J., Mechanisms of action in NIH-3T3 cells of genistein, an inhibitor of EGF receptor tyrosine kinase activity, *Biochem. Pharmacol.*, 39(1), 187–193, 1990.

55. Watanabe, T., Shiraishi, T., Sasaki, H., and Oishi, M., Inhibitors for protein-tyrosine kinases, ST638 and genistein: induce differentiation of mouse erythro-leukemia cells in a synergistic manner, *Exp. Cell Res.,* 183(2), 335–342, 1989.

56. Constantinou, A., Kiguchi, K., and Huberman, E., Induction of differentiation and DNA strand breakage in Human HL-60 and K562 leukemia cells by genistein, *Cancer Res.,* 50, 2618–2624, 1990.

57. Watanabe, T., Kondo, K., and Oishi, M., Induction of *in vitro* differentiation of mouse erythroleukemia cells by genistein, an inhibitor of tyrosine protein kinases, *Cancer Res.,* 51(3), 764–768, 1991.

58. Barnes, S., Effect of genistein on *in vitro* and *in vivo* models of cancer. *J. Nutr.,* 125(3 Suppl), 777S–783S, 1995.

59. Constantinou, A. and Huberman, E., Genistein, an inducer of tumor cell differentiation: possible mechanism of action, *Proc. Soc. Exp. Biol. Med.,* 208, 109–115, 1995.

60. Jing, Y. and Waxman, S., Structural requirements for differentiation-induction and growth-inhibition of mouse erythroleukemia cells by isoflavones, *Anticancer Res.,* 15, 1147–1152, 1995.

61. Shimokado, K., Umezawa, K., and Ogata, J., Tyrosine kinase inhibitors inhibit multiple steps of the cell cycle of vascular smooth muscle cells, *Exp. Cell Res.,* 220, 266–273, 1995.

62. Kuo, S.M., Antiproliferative potency of structurally distinct dietary flavonoids on human colon cancer cells, *Cancer Lett.,* 110, 41–48, 1996.

63. Kuzumaki, T., Matsuda, A., Ito, K., and Ishikawa, K., Cell adhesion to substratum and activation of tyrosine kinases are essentially required for G1/S phase transition in BALB/c 3T3 fibroblasts, *Biochem. Biophys. Acta.,* 1310, 185–192, 1996.

64. Constantinou, A.I., Krygier, A.E., and Mehta, R.R., Genistein induces maturation of cultured human breast cancer cells and prevents tumor growth in nude mice, *Am. J. Clin. Nutr.,* 68(Suppl.), 1426S–1430S, 1998.

65. Shao, Z.M., Alpaugh, M.L., Fontana, J.A., and Barsky, S.H., Genistein inhibits proliferation similarly in estrogen receptor-positive and negative human breast carcinoma cell lines characterized by P21WAF1/CIPI induction, G2/M arrest, and apoptosis, *J. Cell. Biochem.,* 69, 44–54, 1998.

66. Fotsis, T., Peppe, R.M., Adlercreutz, H., Fleischmann, G., Hase, T., Montesano, R., and Schweigerer, L., Genistein, a dietary-derived inhibitor of *in vitro* angio-genesis, *Proc. Natl. Acad. Sci. USA,* 90(7), 2690–2694, 1993.

67. Wei, H., Bowen, R., Cai, Q., Barnes, S., and Wang, Y., Antioxidant and antipro-motional effects of the soybean isoflavone genistein, *Proc. Soc. Exp. Biol. Med.,* 208(1), 124–130, 1995.

68. Carroll, K.K., Experimental evidence of dietary factors and hormone-dependent cancers, *Cancer Res.,* 35(11 Pt. 2), 3374–3383, 1975.

69. Troll, W., Wiesner, R., Shellabarger, C.J., Holtzman, S., and Stone, J.P., Soybean diet lowers breast tumor incidence in irradiated rats, *Carcinogenesis,* 1(6), 469–472, 1980.

70. Gridley, D.S., Kettering, J.D., Slater, J.M., and Nutter, R.L., Modification of spontaneous mammary tumors in mice fed different sources of protein, fat and carbohydrate, *Cancer Lett.,* 19(2), 133–146, 1983.

71. Barnes, S., Grubbs, C., Setchell, K.D., and Carlson, J., Soybeans inhibit mammary tumors in models of breas, *Prog. Clin. Biol. Res.,* 347, 239–253, 1990.

72. Baggot, J.E., Ha, T., Vaughn, W.H., Juliana, M.M., Hardin, J.M., and Grubbs, C.J., Effect of miso (Japanese soybean paste) and NaCl on DMBA-induced rat mammary tumors, *Nutr. Cancer,* 14(2), 103–109, 1990.

73. Hawrylewicz, E.J., Huang, H.H., and Blair, W.H., Dietary soybean isolate and methionine supplementation affect mammary tumor progression in rats, *J. Nutr.,* 121(10), 1693–1698, 1991.

74. Constantinou, A.I., Mehta, R.G., and Vaughan, A., Inhibition of N-methyl-N-nitrosourea-induced mammary tumors in rats by the soybean isoflavones, *Anticancer Res.,* 16(6A), 3293–3298, 1996.

75. Gotoh, T., Yamada, K., Yin, H., Ito, A., Kataoka, T., and Dohi, K., Chemoprevention of N-nitroso-N-methylurea-induced rat mammary carcinogenesis by soy foods or biochanin A, *Jpn. J. Cancer Res.,* 89(2), 137–142, 1998.

76. Appelt, L.C. and Reicks, M.M., Soy induces phase II enzymes but does not inhibit dimethylbenz[a]anthracene-induced carcinogenesis in female rats, *J. Nutr.,* 129(10), 1820–1826, 1999.

77. Ohta, T., Nakatsugi, S., Watanabe, K., Kawamori, T., Ishikawa, F., Morotomi, M., Sugie, S., Toda, T., Sugimura, T., and Wakabayashi, K., Inhibitory effects of Bifidobacterium-fermented soy milk on 2-amino-1-methyl-6-phenylimidazo[4,5-b]pyridine-induced rat mammary carcinogenesis, with a partial contribution of its component isoflavones, *Carcinogenesis,* 21(5), 937–941, 2000.

78. Cohen, L.A., Zhao, Z., Pittman, B., and Scimeca, J.A., Effect of intact and isoflavone-depleted soy protein on NMU-induced rat mammary tumorigenesis, *Carcinogenesis,* 21(5), 929–935, 2000.

79. Constantinou, A.I., Lantvit, D., Hawthorne, M., Xu, X, van Breemen, R.B., and Pezzuto, J.M., Chemopreventive effects of soy protein and purified soy isoflavones on DMBA-induced mammary tumors in female Sprague-Dawley rats, *Nutr. Cancer,* 41(1–2), 75–81, 2001.

80. Day, J.K., Besch-Williford, C., McMann, T.R., Hufford, M.G., Lubahn, D.B., and MacDonald, R.S., Dietary genistein increased DMBA-induced mammary adenocarcinoma in wild-type, but not ER alpha KO, mice, *Nutr. Cancer,* 39(2), 226–232, 2001.

81. Jin, Z. and MacDonald, R.S., Soy isoflavones increase latency of spontaneous mammary tumors in mice, *J. Nutr.,* 132(10), 3186–3190, 2002.

82. Yang, J., Nakagawa, H., Tsuta, K., and Tsubura, A., Influence of perinatal genistein exposure on the development of MNU-induced mammary carcinoma in female Sprague-Dawley rats, *Cancer Lett.,* 149(1–2), 171–179, 2000.

83. Messina, M.J., Persky, V., Setchell, K.D.R., and Barnes, S., Soy intake and cancer risk: a review of the *in vitro* and *in vivo* data, *Nutr. Cancer,* 21, 113–131, 1994.

84. Adlercreutz, H., Phytoestrogens and breast cancer, *J. Steroid Biochem. Mol. Biol.,* 83, 113–118, 2003.

85. Lamartiniere, C.A., Moore, J.B., Brown, N.M., Thompson, R., Hardin, M.J., and Barnes, S., Genistein suppresses mammary cancer in rats, *Carcinogenesis,* 16(11), 2833–2840, 1995.

86. Lamartiniere, C.A., Moore, J., Holland, M., and Barnes, S., Neonatal genistein chemoprevents mammary cancer, *Proc. Soc. Exp. Biol. Med.* 208(1), 120–123, 1995.

87. Murrill, W.B., Brown, N.M., Zhang, J.X., Manzolillo, P.A., Barnes, S., and Lamartiniere, C.A., Prepubertal genistein exposure suppresses mammary cancer and enhances gland differentiation in rats, *Carcinogenesis,* 17(7), 1451–1457, 1996.

88. Lamartiniere, C.A., Murrill, W.B., Manzolillo, P.A., Zhang, J.X., Barnes, S., Zhang, X., Wei, H., and Brown, N.M., Genistein alters the ontogeny of mammary gland development and protects against chemically-induced mammary cancer in rats, *Proc. Soc. Exp. Biol. Med.*, 217(3), 358–364, 1998.

89. Fritz, W.A., Coward, L., Wang, J., and Lamartiniere, C.A., Dietary genistein: perinatal mammary cancer prevention, bioavailability and toxicity testing in the rat, *Carcinogenesis*, 19(12), 2151–2158, 1998.

90. Brown, N.M., Wang, J., Cotroneo, M.S., Zhao, Y.X., and Lamartiniere, C.A., Prepubertal genistein treatment modulates TGF-alpha, EGF and EGF-receptor mRNAs and proteins in the rat mammary gland, *Mol. Cell Endocrinol.* 144(1–2), 149–165, 1998.

91. Lamartiniere, C.A., Protection against breast cancer with genistein: a component of soy, *Am. J. Clin. Nutr.*, 71(6 Suppl.), 1705S–1707S; discussion 1708S–1709S, 2000.

92. Hilakivi-Clarke, L., Cho, E., Onojafe, I., Raygada, M., and Clarke, R., Maternal exposure to genistein during pregnancy increases carcinogen-induced mammary tumorigenesis in female rat offspring, *Oncol. Rep.*, 6(5), 1089–1095, 1999.

93. Lamartiniere, C.A., Cotroneo, M.S., Fritz, W.A., Wang, J., Mentor-Marcel, R., and Elgavish, A., Genistein chemoprevention: timing and mechanisms of action in murine mammary and prostate, *J. Nutr.*, 132(3), 552S–558S, 2002.

94. Shimizu, H., Ross, R.K., Bernstein, L., Yatani, R., Henderson, B.E., and Mack, T.M., Cancers of the prostate and breast among Japanese and white immigrants in Los Angeles County, *Br. J. Cancer*, 63(6), 963–966, 1991.

95. Baird, D.D., Umbach, D.M., Lansdell, L., Hughes, C.L., Setchell, K.D., Weinberg, C.R., Haney, A.F., Wilcox, A.J., and Mclachlan, J.A., Dietary intervention study to assess estrogenicity of dietary soy among postmenopausal women, *J. Clin. Endocrinol. Metab.*, 80(5), 1685–1690, 1995.

96. Xu, X., Duncan, A.M., Merz, B.E., and Kurzer, M.S., Effects of soy isoflavones on estrogen and phytoestrogen metabolism in premenopausal women, *Cancer Epidemiol. Biomarkers Prev.*, 7(12), 1101–1108, 1998.

97. Martini, M.C., Dancisak, B.B., Haggans, C.J., Thomas, W., and Slavin, J.L., Effects of soy intake on sex hormone metabolism in premenopausal women, *Nutr. Cancer*, 34(2), 133–139, 1999.

98. Hargreaves, D.F., Potten, C.S., Harding, C., Shaw, L.E., Morton, M.S., Roberts, S.A., Howell, A., and Bundred, N.J., Two-week dietary soy supplementation has an estrogenic effect on normal premenopausal breast, *J. Clin. Endocrinol. Metab.*, 84(11), 4017–4024, 1999.

99. Duncan, A.M., Merz, B.E., Xu, X., Nagal, T.C., Phipps, W.R., and Kurzer, M.S., Soy isoflavones exert modest hormonal effects in premenopausal women, *J. Clin. Endocrinol. Metab.*, 84, 192–197, 1999.

100. Lu, L.J.W., Anderson, K.E., Grady, J.J., Kohen, F., and Nagamani, M., Decreased ovarian hormones during a soya diet: implications for breast cancer prevention, *Cancer Res.*, 6, 4112–4121, 2000.

101. Lu, L.J., Cree, M., Josyula, S., Nagamani, M., Grady, J.J., and Anderson, K.E., Increased urinary excretion of 2-hydroxyestrone but not 16-alpha-hydroxyestrone in premenopausal women during a soya diet containing isoflavones, *Cancer Res.*, 60(5), 1299–1305, 2000.

102. Wu, A.H., Stanczyk, F.Z., Hendrich, S., Murphy, P.A., Zhang, C., Wan, P., and Pike, M.C., Effects of soy foods on ovarian function in premenopausal women, *Br. J. Cancer*, 82(11), 1879–1886, 2000.

103. Xu, X., Duncan, A.M., Wangen, K.E., and Kurzer, M., Soy consumption alters endogenous estrogen metabolism in postmenopausal women, *Cancer Epidemiol. Biomarkers Prev.,* 9, 781–786, 2000.
104. Mackey, R., Ekangaki, A., and Eden, J.A., The effects of soy protein in women and men with elevated plasma lipids, *Biofactors,* 12(1–4), 251–257, 2000.
105. Habito, R.C., Montalto, J., Leslie, E., and Ball, M.J., Effects of replacing meat with soyabean in the diet on sex hormone concentrations in healthy adult males, *Br. J. Nutr.,* 84(4), 557–563.
106. Nagata, C., Ecological study of the association between soy product intake and mortality from cancer and heart disease in Japan, *Int. J. Epidemiol.,* 29(5), 832–836, 2000.
107. World Health Organization Statistics, Mortality Database.
108. Hirayama, T., Life-style and mortality: a large-scale census-based cohort study in Japan, in *Contributions to Epidemiology and Biostatistics,* Vol. 6, Wahrendorf, J, Ed., Karger, Basel, 1990.
109. Greenstein, J., Kushi, L., Zheng, W., Fee, R., Campbell, D., Sellers, T. et al., Risk of breast cancer associated with intake of specific foods and food groups, *Am. J. Epidemiol.,* 143, S36, 1996
110. Key, T.J., Sharp, G.B., Appleby, P.N., Beral, V., Goodman, M.T., and Mabuchi, K., Soya foods and breast cancer risk: a prospective study in Hiroshima and Nagasaki, Japan, *Br. J Cancer,* 81, 1248–1256, 1999.
111. Horn-Ross, P.L., Hoggatt, K.J., West, D.W., Krone, M.R., Stewart, S.L., Anton-Culver, H., et al., Recent diet and breast cancer risk: the California Teachers Study (USA), *Cancer Causes Control,* 13, 407–415, 2002.
112. Yamamoto, S., Sobue, T., Kobayashi, M., Sasaki, S., and Tsugane, S., Japan Public Health Center-Based Prospective Study on Cancer Cardiovascular Diseases Group. Soy, isoflavones, and breast cancer risk in Japan, *J. Natl. Cancer Inst.,* 95, 906–913, 2003.
113. Keinan-Boker, L., van Der Schouw, Y.T., Grobbee, D.E., and Peeters, P.H., Dietary phytoestrogens and breast cancer risk, *Am. J. Clin. Nutr.,* 79(2), 282–288, 2004.
114. Hirohata, T., Shigematsu, T., Nomura, A.M.Y., Nomura, Y., Horie, A., and Hirohata, I., Occurrence of breast cancer in relation to diet and reproductive history: a case-control study in Fukuoka, Japan, *J. Natl. Cancer Inst. Monogr.,* 69, 187–190, 1985.
115. Lee, H.P., Gourley, L., Duffy, S.W., Esteve, J., Lee, J., and Day, N.E., Risk factors for breast cancer by age and menopausal status: a case-control study in Singapore, *Cancer Causes Control.,* 3, 313–322, 1992.
116. Hirose, K., Tajima, K., Hamajima, N., Inoue, M., Takezaki, T., Kuroishi, T., et al., A large-scale, hospital-based case-control study of risk factors of breast cancer according to menopausal status, *Jpn. J. Cancer Res.,* 86, 146–154, 1995.
117. Yuan, J.-M., Wang, Q.-S., Ross, R.K., Henderson, B.E., and Yu, M.C., Diet and breast cancer in Shanghai and Tianjin, China, *Br. J. Cancer,* 71, 1353–1358, 1995.
118. Wu, A.H., Ziegler, R.G., Horn-Ross, P.L., Nomura, A.M.Y., West, D.W., Kolonel, L.N. et al., Tofu and risk of breast cancer in Asian-Americans, *Cancer Epidemiol. Biomarkers Prev.,* 5, 901–906, 1996.
119. Witte, J.S., Ursin, G., Siemiatycki, J., Thompson, W.D., Paganini-Hill, A., and Haile, R.W., Diet and premenopausal bilateral breast cancer: a case-control study, *Breast Cancer Res. Treat.,* 42, 243–251, 1997.

120. Dai, Q., Shu, X.-O., Jin, F., Potter, J.D., Kushi, L.H., Teas, J. et al., Population-based case-control study of soyfood intake and breast cancer risk in Shanghai, *Br. J. Cancer*, 85, 372–378, 2001.

121. Horn-Ross, P.L., John, E.M., Lee, M., Stewart, S.L., Koo, J., Sakoda, L.C. et al., Phytoestrogen consumption and breast cancer risk in multiethnic population. The Bay Area Cancer Study, *Am. J. Epidemiol.*, 154, 434–441, 2001.

122. Wu, A.H., Wan, P., Hankin, J., Tseng, C.-C., Yu, M.C., and Pike, M.C., Adolescent and adult soy intake and risk of breast cancer in Asian-Americans, *Carcinogenesis*, 23, 1491–1496, 2002.

123. Shu, X.O., Jin, F., Dai, Q., Wen, W., Potter, J.D., Kushi, L.H., Ruan, Z., Gao, Y.T., and Zheng, W., Soyfood intake during adolescence and subsequent risk of breast cancer among Chinese women, *Cancer Epidemiol. Biomarkers Prev.*, 10(5), 483–488, 2001.

124. Horn-Ross, P.L., Lee, M., John, E.M., and Koo, J., Sources of phytoestrogen exposure among non-Asian women in California, USA, *Cancer Causes Control.*, 11, 299–302, 2000.

125. Ingram, D., Sanders, K., Kolybaba, M., and Lopez, D., Case-control study of phyto-oestrogens and breast cancer, *Lancet*, 350(9083), 990–994, 1997.

126. Zheng, W., Dai, Q., Custer, L.J., Shu, X.O., Wen, W.Q., Jin, F., and Franke, A.A., Urinary excretion of isoflavonoids and the risk of breast cancer, *Cancer Epidemiol. Biomarkers Prev.*, 8(1), 35–40.

127. Murkies, A., Dalais, F.S., Briganti, E.M., Burger, H.G., Healy, D.L., Wahlqvist, M.L., and Davis, S.R., Phytoestrogens and breast cancer in postmenopausal women: a case control study, *Menopause*, 7(5), 289–296, 2000.

128. Dai, Q., Franke, A.A., Yu, H., Shu, X.O., Jin, F., Hebert, J.R., Custer, L.J., Gao, Y.T., and Zheng, W., Urinary phytoestrogen excretion and breast cancer risk: evaluating potential effect modifiers endogenous estrogens and anthropometrics, *Cancer Epidemiol. Biomarkers Prev.*, 12(6), 497–502, 2003.

129. den Tonkelaar, I., Keinan-Boke, R.L., Veer, P.V., Arts, C.J., Adlercreutz, H., Thijssen, J.H., and Peeters, P.H., Urinary phytoestrogens and postmenopausal breast cancer risk, *Cancer Epidemiol. Biomarkers Prev.*, 10(3), 223–228, 2001.

130. Busby, M.G., Jeffcoat, A.R., Bloedon, L.T., Koch, M.A., Black, T., Dix, K.J., Heizer, W.D., Thomas, B.F., Hill, J.M., Crowell, J.A., and Zeisel, S.H., Clinical characteristics and pharmacokinetics of purified soy isoflavones: single-dose administration to healthy men, *Am. J. Clin. Nutr.*, 75(1), 126–136, 2002.

131. Misra, R.R., Hursting, S.D., Perkins, S.N., Sathyamoorthy, N., Mirsalis, J.C., Riccio, E.S., and Crowell, J.A., Genotoxicity and carcinogenicity studies of soy isoflavones, *Int. J. Toxicol.*, 21(4), 277–285, 2002.

132. Miltyk, W., Craciunescu, C.N., Fischer, L., Jeffcoat, R.A., Koch, M.A., Lopaczynski, W., Mahoney, C., Jeffcoat, R.A., Crowell, J., Paglieri, J., and Zeisel, S.H., Lack of significant genotoxicity of purified soy isoflavones (genistein, daidzein, and glycitein) in 20 patients with prostate cancer, *Am. J. Clin. Nutr.*, 77(4), 875–882, 2003.

# 4 Adipocytokines

## Tohru Funahashi and Yuji Matsuzawa

## CONTENTS

## 4.1  INTRODUCTION

Obesity and diabetes mellitus are major health problems worldwide. These patho-genetic conditions greatly increase the chance an individual will suffer cardio-vascular disease (CVD). Ingestion of vegetable protein instead of animal protein is thought to be associated with decreased risk of CVD. However, the effects of soy protein on obesity and diabetes in humans have not been consistent. Recent advances in adipocyte biology have revealed that adipose tissue functions as a huge endocrine organ. Obesity, diabetes, and the effects of a vegetable protein diet on these disorders must be reconsidered from the new point of view.

## 4.2  VISCERAL OBESITY AND METABOLIC SYNDROME

CVD is now the leading cause of mortality worldwide.[1] Many epidemiological and experimental studies have revealed that hypercholesterolemia and elevated low-density lipoprotein (LDL) level are the strongest risk factor for CVD and the pathogenetic role of oxidized LDL in the development of atherosclerotic vascular change. Many clinical trials of LDL-lowering therapies have demonstrated how much reduction of LDL-cholesterol can lead to how much reduction of CVD prevalence. However, hypercholesterolemia can only partly explain the prevalence of CVD. Multiple risk factor syndrome, which is a cluster of hyperglycemia, hypertriglyceridemia, low high-density lipoprotein (HDL) cholesterol level, and high blood pressure, is a common cause of CVD. These risks sometimes cluster by chance because they are very common abnormal measures. However, some unidentified upstream factor may trigger these risks and subsequent atherosclerotic vascular change. This cascading condition has been referred to as syndrome X, deadly quartet, or visceral fat syndrome.[2,3,4] The name "syndrome X" changed to metabolic syndrome X to distinguish it from cardiac syndrome X with positive exercise testing and normal coronary angiogram, and now it is called the metabolic syndrome. Insulin resistance has been considered an upstream factor for clustering of multiple risks. However, the molecular mechanism clustering metabolic and circulatory disorders in an individual and high atherogeneity of the metabolic syndrome have not been fully clarified.

Many clinical studies have suggested that absolute quantity of total body fat alone cannot explain the development of obesity-related diseases, but body fat distribution is a more important determinant for the morbidity of obesity. Introduction of the computerized tomography (CT) scan method for the assessment of body fat distribution enabled us to evaluate the adipose tissue in the intra-abdominal cavity. Accumulation of visceral adipose tissue is associated with the occurrence of diabetes mellitus, hyperlipidemia, hypertension, and CVD.[5–9] Thus, visceral obesity may be located upstream of the cascade of the metabolic syndrome.

## 4.3   MOLECULAR ASPECTS OF ADIPOSE TISSUE AND ADIPOCYTOKINES

To elucidate the biological functions of subcutaneous and visceral fat tissue and to clarify the molecular links between visceral obesity and the metabolic syndrome, we analyzed depot-specific expression profiles of the genes in adipose tissue. When the analysis was completed, only 60% of the genes were "known" human genes found in the nonexpressed sequence tags (EST) division of the GenBank.[10] The remaining 40% were unidentified and novel. Unexpectedly, we found that the genes encoded secretory proteins in adipose tissue with high frequency. Most of them were for biologically active substances.[11] In subcutaneous adipose tissue, approximately 20% of the known genes encoded secretory protein (Figure 4.1). Its frequency came up to 30% in visceral adipose tissue. Leptin and tumor necrosis factor (TNF)-$\alpha$ are well recognized as bioactive substances produced by adipose tissues to control or to modify the functions of other organs. We conceptualized these adipose-derived bioactive substances as "adipocytokines," although some of them are not cytokines according to the classic description.

The visceral fat cDNA library contains cDNAs for plasminogen-activator-inhibitor-type (PAI)-1 and heparin binding EGF (epidermal growth factor)-like growth factor (HB-EGF).[12,13] PAI-1 mRNA was overexpressed in visceral fat during the development of obesity in ventromedial hypothalamic (VMH)-lesioned rats but remained unchanged in the subcutaneous fat. Plasma PAI-1 concentration was correlated positively with the amount of visceral fat determined by CT scan in humans. Elevated PAI-1 in circulation is a risk factor for thrombotic disorders.[14] PAI-1 produced and secreted by accumulated visceral fat may contribute to the

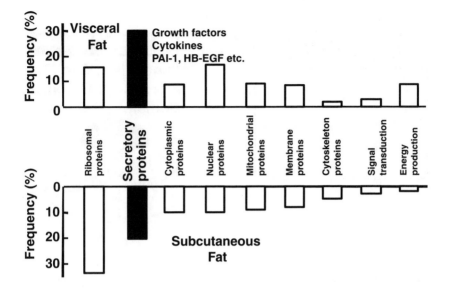

**FIGURE 4.1** High frequency of genes for secretory proteins in adipose tissue.

development of thrombotic disorders. Thus, there is a direct connection between visceral fat and vascular injury independent of multiple risk factors (adipo-vascular axis). This may partly explain high atherogeneity in visceral obesity. Forty percent of the genes expressed in adipose tissue were unknown. This encouraged us to pull out an unidentified adipocytokine.

## 4.4 DISCOVERY OF ADIPONECTIN

Among the genes analyzed in the human adipose cDNA library, the gene expressed most abundantly and specifically in adipose tissue was unidentified in GeneBank database.[15] The gene, adipose most abundant gene transcript-1(apM-1), encoded a single 244-amino acid peptide with a signal-sequence presumably secretory protein. The protein consisted of an N-terminal collagen-like motif and a C-terminal globular domain with significant homology with collagen X, VIII, and complement factor C1q (Figure 4.2).[15] In a solid phase binding assay, the protein bound to collagen I, III, and V. These are the groups of collagens present in the subendothelial intima. We raised an antibody against the protein and stained a balloon-injured rat carotid artery with this antibody. The injured vascular wall was stained positively by this antibody, while no staining was found in the noninjured vascular wall.[16] We named the protein with adhesive property "adiponectin." ACRP30 and AdipoQ, independently identified as the genes up-regulated during the differentiation of the murine adipocyte-cell line, were the mouse homologues of adiponectin.[17,18]

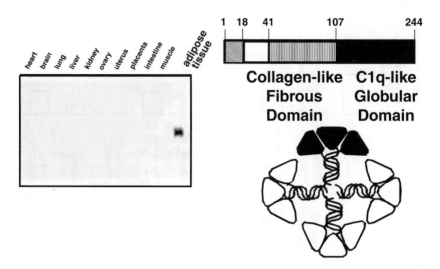

**FIGURE 4.2** Structure and adipose tissue-specific expression of adiponectin gene. (From Matsuzawa, Y. et al., *Arterioscler. Thromb. Vasc. Biol.*, 24: 29–33, 2004. With permission.)

We established the enzyme-linked immunosorbent assay for adiponectin and determined plasma adiponectin levels in humans.[19] Plasma levels of adiponectin were extremely high, with the range between 5 and 30 µg/ml on average. Interestingly, plasma levels were low in obese subjects in spite of adiponectin's limited expression in adipose tissue. In particular, plasma adiponectin concentration was correlated negatively with the amount of visceral fat, in clear contrast to PAI-1.[19]

## 4.5 EFFECTS OF ADIPONECTIN ON ATHEROSCLEROSIS AND DIABETES

Adiponectin binds to injured vascular walls, and its concentration is decreased in visceral obesity. To elucidate the functions of this molecule, we investigated the effects of adiponectin on the cellular components of the vascular wall. During the early process of atherosclerotic vascular change, vascular endothelial cells express adhesion molecules such as endothelial leukocyte adhesion molecule-1 (E-selectin), vascular cell adhesion molecule-1 (VCAM-1), and intracellular adhesion molecule-1 (ICAM-1) on their cell surface and attach circulating monocytes. Monocytes invade beneath the endothelial cells and transform into macrophages. Macrophages take up oxidized LDL through scavenger receptors and become foam cells. Macrophages also secrete various cytokines such as interleukin-6 (IL-6), TNF-α, platelet-derived growth factor (PDGF), and HB-EGF. PDGF and HB-EGF stimulate vascular smooth muscle cells in media to migrate into intima and to accelerate proliferation.

The physiological concentration of adiponectin suppressed TNF-α-induced activation of NFκB through the inhibition of IκB phosphorylation, resulting in the suppression of adhesion molecule expression including ICAM-1, VCAM-1, and E-selectin.[20,21] In macrophages, adiponectin inhibited the expression of the class 1A scavenger receptor, resulting in the decreased uptake of oxidized LDL and the inhibition of foam cell formation.[22] Adiponectin also dramatically inhibited the expression and secretion of TNF-α selectively among cytokines produced by macrophages. In vascular smooth muscle cells, adiponectin suppressed PDGF and HB-EGF-induced proliferation and migration of the cells. This was achieved partly by direct binding of adiponectin with PDGF-BB and generally by the inhibition of growth factor-stimulated signal transduction through p42/44 extracellular signal-related kinase (ERK).[23] These observations suggest that adiponectin has potential antiatherogenic activities.

Our hypothesis is shown in Figure 4.3. Adiponectin is produced by adipocytes and is present abundantly in circulating plasma. When the inflammatory stimuli and chemical substances damage the endothelial barrier, adiponectin accumulates in the injured vascular wall and protects against the development of atherogenic vascular changes. Adiponectin may work as "firefighters" in the vascular wall. Reduction of plasma adiponectin caused by visceral fat accumulation will cause a small fire to become bigger and bigger because of the lack of firefighters. Clinical observation showed that the plasma adiponectin level was low in the subjects with

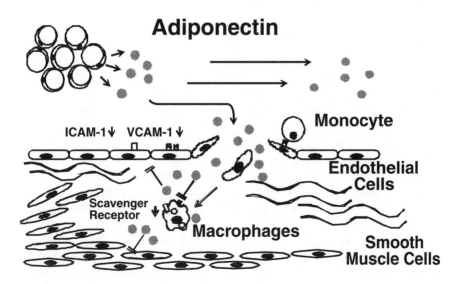

**FIGURE 4.3** Molecular mechanism of antiatherogenic functions of adiponectin. (From Matsuzawa, Y. et al., *Arterioscler. Thromb. Vasc. Biol.*, 24: 29–33, 2004. With permission.)

CVD, even though body mass indexes were adjusted.[20] Those with plasma adiposectin levels below 4 µg/ml had twice the risk for CVD.[24] Among the subjects with renal insufficiency, those with hypoadiponectinemia had a higher incidence of later CVD death during the 4-year observation period.[25] A recent nested case-control study of 18,225 males aged 40 to 75 years who were free of CVD at entry demonstrated that the subjects in the highest compared with the lowest quintile of adiponectin levels had a significantly decreased risk of myocardial infarction (MI), even after adjustment for family history of MI, body mass index, alcohol consumption, physical activity, and history of diabetes and hypertension.[26] These data suggest that hypoadiponectinemia is a novel risk factor for CVD.

The incidence of CVD is three- to fivefold higher in subjects with Type II diabetes compared to the general population. The diabetic subjects with macroangiopathy had low plasma levels of adiponectin. The diabetic women showed lower plasma adiponectin concentrations compared nondiabetic subjects, even though they did not have CVD.[27] The National Institution of Health (NIH) in Phoenix also demonstrated that plasma levels of adiponectin are lower in diabetic Pima Indians, a unique cohort with a high prevalence of obesity and Type II diabetes.[28] Approximately 80% of Pima Indians suffer from Type II diabetes during their lives. These researchers also showed that plasma adiponectin concentration is correlated positively with insulin sensitivity evaluated by glucose clamp test.[28] A case-control study revealed that the subjects with high concentrations of plasma adiponectin at baseline showed a low risk of later onset of Type II diabetes, even in Pima Indians.[29] A series of studies demonstrated that hypoadiponectinemia is a novel risk factor both for CVD and diabetes.

## 4.6 GENETIC HYPOADIPONECTINEMIA

In order to clarify whether primary hypoadiponectinemia causes metabolic disturbances including insulin resistance and atherosclerotic vascular changes, we investigated the clinical profiles of subjects with mutations in their adiponectin gene. We found four types of mutations or polymorphisms, in which the substitution of amino acids was predicted.[30,31,32] Among these genetic polymorphisms, plasma adiponectin concentration in the subjects carrying the mutation with a substitution of isoleucine at amino acid 164 to threonine was remarkably low. Interestingly, these subjects frequently also had hypertension, hyperlipidemia-impaired glucose tolerance, or diabetes. Furthermore, two thirds of the subjects already suffered from CVD. Thus, genetic hypoadiponectinemia is part of the genetic background of the metabolic syndrome.

To confirm this concept, we generated mice disrupting adiponectin gene. The knockout (KO) mice were apparently normal and showed normal glucose tolerance when fed laboratory chow. However, they developed insulin resistance and elevated plasma glucose levels when they were fed a high fat, high sucrose diet. The adenovirus-mediated supplementation of adiponectin improved this insulin resistance.[33]

When the vascular walls of KO mice were injured by catheter wire, they exhibited severe neointimal thickening, even under the normal diet. These data suggest that adiponectin plays an important role in the protection against vascular remodeling, and this effect occurs independently of insulin resistance.[34]

We overexpressed adiponectin using an adenovirus vector in apolipoprotein E-deficient mice, which spontaneously developed fatty streak lesions similar to human atherosclerotic plaque. Exogenous adiponectin accumulated in the fatty streak lesions.[35] Expression of VCAM-1, class A scavenger receptor, and TNF-α mRNA in the aorta was reduced without affecting the class B scavenger receptor (CD36) mRNA level. The size of lipid droplets in the fatty-streak lesion became smaller, and plaque area was narrower compared with the control mice. These observations confirm that adiponectin suppresses the development of atherosclerotic vascular changes.

The above observations from cell experiments and clinical evidence, together with the data from the genetic hypoadiponectinemia in humans and mice, strongly suggest that decreases in adiponectin with antiatherogenic and antidiabetic functions play an important role in the development of the metabolic syndrome. Although the observations from the subjects with genetic hypoadiponectinemia contribute to our understanding of the function of this molecule, this disorder is rare in the general population. Commonly, accumulation of visceral fat leads to a decrease of plasma adiponectin concentration (Figure 4.4). Furthermore, dysregulation of various adipocytokines occurs in visceral obesity as described above. PAI-1 and HB-EGF are overexpressed in visceral obesity. Thus, accumulation of visceral fat is a pathogenic condition leading to atherosclerotic vascular diseases not only by accompanying multiple coronary risk factors but also by accompanying the dysregulation of multiple adipocytokines.

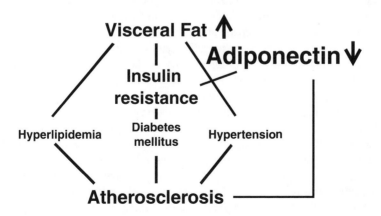

**FIGURE 4.4** Concept of metabolic syndrome. Importance of visceral fat accumulation and hypoadiponectinemia.

## 4.7 SOY PROTEIN AND ADIPOCYTOKINES

Ingestion of vegetable protein instead of animal protein is thought to be associated with lower risk of CVD. Several studies have reported the cholesterol-lowering, antilipogenic, and antihypertensive effects of soy protein. Antiobesity and antidiabetic effects of soy protein diets are still controversial. There are few reports on the antidiabetic effect of soy protein diets in addition to the effect of body weight reduction. Soy proteins used in the studies are purified, semipurified ethanol extracted soy protein isolates (SPI), or SPI hydrolysate (SPI-H). The active component of soy protein diets on reducing the risks of CVD remain unclear. It may be the protein itself. Soy protein contains low methionine and has an amino acid pattern containing a high level of sulfur. Alternatively, other components may be active. Several studies have reported that small peptides resulting from limited digestion are effective. Further, soy protein contains isoflavones, which exhibit estrogenic and distinct physiological activities.

The effects of soy protein on the functions of adipose tissue have not been studied. Not only the total calorie value of a diet, but also its composition may affect the expression of adipocytokines in adipose tissue. We investigated the effects of a soy protein diet on the expression of adipose genes and plasma concentrations in rodents. First, we examined the effect of a calorie-restricted diet containing SPI on the expression and plasma levels of adiponectin in KKAy obese mice and compared them with those of mice on an isocaloric casein-protein diet.[36] The total body weight, fat content, and weight of liver and fat of the mice in the SPI and casein groups were significantly lower than those in the initial group. Adipose adiponectin mRNA levels were higher in the calorie-restricted group than the initial group. Plasma adiponectin concentrations were significantly higher in each calorie-restricted group than those of the initial group. However, we did not observe any differences between soy protein and casein protein groups under acute calorie restriction.

In the second set of experiments, we sought to clarify the effect of the soy protein diet itself, compared to a casein diet under non-calorie-restricted conditions, on the expression of hepatic and adipose genes related to lipid metabolism and the expression of the genes for adipocytokines in male Wistar rats.[37] Body weights were not significantly different between the SPI and casein groups at the end of the experimental period. Hepatic fatty acid synthase and acyl-CoA carboxylase mRNA expression was suppressed in the SPI group. The mRNA level of acyl-CoA oxidase, which catalyzes β oxidation of fatty acids, was not different in the two groups. The mRNA expression of sterol regulatory element binding protein (SREBP)-1, which regulates many of the genes for fatty acid synthesis and activates the entire program of fatty acid synthesis, was suppressed in the livers of the SPI group compared to that of casein group. Triglyceride content of the livers in the SPI group was less than in the casein group. The mRNA levels of SREBP-2, an isoform of SREBP-1, preferentially controls the genes for cellular cholesterol homeostasis such as HMG-CoA reductase and LDL receptor, HMG-CoA reductase, and LDL receptor, were not different between the two groups, and the cholesterol content of the livers in the SPI group was similar to that in the casein group.

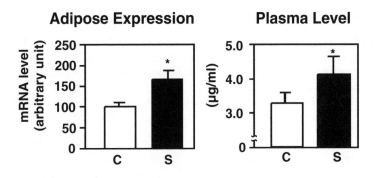

**FIGURE 4.5** Effect of soy protein diet on the expression and plasma concentration of adiponectin. (From Nagasawa, A. et al., *Biochem. Biophys. Res. Commun.*, 311, 909–914, 2003. With permission.)

We determined the mRNA expression levels of various adipocytokines in adipose tissue. The mRNA expression levels in adipose tissue and plasma concentrations of adiponectin were higher in rats of the SPI group than those in the casein group (Figure 4.5). However, PAI-1 and leptin mRNA levels were lower in the SPI group than those in the casein group. No significant difference was found in angiotensinogen and TNF-$\alpha$ mRNA levels between the two groups. These results suggest divergent regulation of adipocytokine expression by the SPI diet. The molecular mechanisms of the soy protein diet–enhanced expression of adiponectin remain unclear. One possible mechanism is that the soy protein diet promotes the conversion of large adipocytes to smaller ones exhibiting appropriate adipocytokine-producing activities. We analyzed the mRNA levels of the genes related to lipid metabolism in adipose tissue. The mRNA levels of fatty acid synthase were significantly lower in the liver of the SPI group compared to those in the casein group. However, SREBP-1 mRNA levels in adipose tissue were similar to those in the SPI and casein groups. The mRNA levels of malic enzyme, acyl-CoA carboxylase, acyl-CoA synthase, LPL, and GLUT-4 were not different in the two groups. Although the body weights were not significantly different between the SPI and casein groups, the triglyceride content of the adipose tissue in the SPI group was significantly lower than that in the casein group. SPI may also affect the differentiation of adipocytes. PPAR-$\gamma$ is a nuclear receptor that controls the differentiation of adipocytes. Administration of PPAR-$\gamma$ ligands changes the plasma concentration of adipocytokines.[38] The soy protein diet did not influence the expression of PPAR-$\gamma$ in adipose tissue. However, it is possible that SPI contains substances with PPAR-$\gamma$ ligand activity.

A soy protein diet increases the expression and plasma concentration of adiponectin and decreases the expression of PAI-1 in adipose tissue without any changes in body weight in rodents. These changes may yield beneficial effects for the prevention of CVD in humans. Further studies to clarify the effect of soy protein diets on the production of adipocytokines in humans are necessary.

# REFERENCES

1. World Health Organization, *World Health Report 2002: Reducing Risks Promoting Healthy Life,* World Health Organization, 2002.
2. Reaven, G.M., Role of insulin resistance in human disease, *Diabetes,* 37, 1595–1607, 1988.
3. Kaplan, N.M., The deadly quartet: upperbody obesity, glucose intolerance, hypertriglyceridemia and hypertention, *Arch. Intern. Med.,* 149, 1514–1520, 1989.
4. Matsuzawa, Y.M., Pathophysiology and molecular mechanism of visceral fat syndrome: the Japanese case, *Diabet./Metab. Rev.,* 13, 3–13, 1997.
5. Fujioka, S., Matsuzawa, Y., Tokunaga, K., and Tarui, S., Contribution of intra-abdominal fat accumulation to the impairment of glucose and lipid metabolism, *Metabolism,* 36, 54–59, 1987.
6. Kanai, H., Matsuzawa, Y., Kotani, K., Keno, Y., Kobatake, T., Nagai, Y., Fujioka, S., Tokunaga, K., and Tarui, S., Close correlation of intraabdominal fat accumulation to hypertension in obese women, *Hypertension,* 16, 484–490, 1990.
7. Despres, J.P., Moorjani, M., Ferland, M., Tremblay, A., Lupien, P.J., Nadeau, A., Pinault, S., Theriault, G., and Bouchard, C., Adipose tissue distribution and plasma lipoprotein levels in obese women. Importance of intraabdominal fat, *Arteriosclerosis,* 9, 203–210, 1989.
8. Despres, J.P., Nadeau, A., Tremblay, A., Ferland, M., Moorjani, S., Lupien, P.J., Theriault, G., Pinault, S., and Bouchard, C., Role of deep abdominal fat in the association between regional adipose tissue distribution and glucose tolerance in obese women, *Diabetes,* 38, 304–309, 1989.
9. Nakamura, T., Tokunaga, K., Shimomura, I., Nishida, M., Yoshida, S., Kotani, K., Islam, A.H.M.W., Keno, Y., Kobatake, T., Nagai, Y., Fujioka, S., Tarui, S., and Matsuzawa, Y., Contribution of visceral fat accumulation to the development of coronary artery disease in non-obese subjects, *Atherosclerosis,* 107, 239–246, 1994.
10. Maeda, K., Okubo, K., Shimomura, I., Mizuno, K., Matsuzawa, Y., and Matsubara, K., Analysis of expression profile of genes in the human adipose tissue, *Gene,* 190, 227–235, 1997.
11. Funahashi, T., Nakamura, T., Shimomura, I., Maeda, K., Kuriyama, H., Takahashi, M., Arita, Y., Kihara, S., and Matsuzawa, Y., Role of adipocytokines on the pathogenesis of atherosclerosis in visceral obesity, *Int. Med.,* 38, 202–206, 1999.
12. Shimomura, I., Funahashi, T., Takahashi, M., Maeda, K., Kotani, K., Nakamura, T., Yamashita, S., Miura, M., Fukuda, Y., Takemura, K., Tokunaga, K., Matsuzawa, Y., Enhanced expression of PAI-1 in visceral fat: possible contribution to vascular disease in obesity, *Nat. Med.,* 2, 1–5, 1996.
13. Matsumoto, S., Kishida, K., Maeda, N., Nagaredani, H., Matsuda, M., Nishizawa, H., Kihara, S., Funahashi, T., Matsuzawa, Y., Yamada, A., Yamashita, S., Tamura, S., and Kawata, S., Increased plasma HB-EGF associated with obesity and coronary artery disease, *Biochem. Biophys. Res. Commun.,* 292, 781–786, 2002.
14. Paganelli, F., Alessi, M.C., Morange, P., Maixent, J.M., Levy, S., and Vague, I.J., Relationship of plasmanogen activator inhibitor-1 levels following thrombolytic therapy with rt-PA as compared to streptokinase and patency of infarct related coronary artery, *Thromb. Haemast.,* 82, 104–108, 1999.

15. Maeda, K., Okubo, K., Shimomura, I., Funahashi, T., Matsuzawa, Y., and Matsubara, K., cDNA cloning and expression of a novel adipose specific collagen-like factor, apM 1 (adipose most abundant gene transcript-1), *Biochem. Biophys. Res. Commun.*, 221, 286–289, 1996.

16. Okamoto, Y., Arita, Y., Nishida, M., Muraguchi, M., Ouchi, N., Takahashi, M., Igura, T., Inui, Y., Kihara, S., Nakamura, T., Yamashita, S., Miyagawa, J., Funahashi, T., and Matsuzawa, Y., An adipocyte-derived plasma protein, adiponectin, adheres to injured vascular walls, *Horm. Metab. Res.*, 32, 47–50, 2000.

17. Scherer, E.P., Williams, S., Fogliano, M., Baldin, G., and Lodish, H.F., A novel serum protein similar to C1q produced exclusively in adipocytes, *J. Biol. Chem.*, 270, 26740–26744, 1995.

18. Hu, E., Liang, P., and Spiegelman, B.M., AdipoQ is a novel adipose-specific gene dysregulated in obesity, *J. Biol. Chem.*, 271, 10697–10703, 1996.

19. Arita, Y., Kihara, S., Ouchi, N., Takahashi, M., Maeda, K., Miyagawa, J., Hotta, K., Shimomura, I., Nakamura, T., Miyaoka, K., Kuriyama, H., Nishida, M., Muraguchi, H., Ohmoto, Y., Funahashi, T., and Matsuzawa, Y., Paradoxical decrease of an adipose-specific protein, adiponectin, in obesity, *Biochem. Biophys. Res. Commun.*, 257, 79–83, 1999.

20. Ouchi, N., Kihara, S., Arita, Y., Maeda, K., Kuriyama, H., Okamoto, Y., Hotta, K., Nishida, M., Takahashi, M., Nakamura, T., Yamashita, S., Funahashi, T., and Matsuzawa, Y., Novel modulator for endothelial adhesion molecules: adipocyte-derived plasma protein, *Circulation,* 100, 2473–2476, 1999.

21. Ouchi, Y., Kihara, S., Arita, Y., Okamoto, Y., Maeda, K., Kuriyama, H., Hotta, K., Nishida, M., Takahashi, M., Muraguchi, M., Ohmoto, Y., Nakamura, T., Yamashita, S., Funahashi, T., and Matsuzawa, Y., Adiponectin, adipocyte-derived plasma protein, inhibits endothelial NFκB signaling through cAMP-dependent pathway, *Circulation,* 102, 1296–1301, 2000.

22. Ouchi, Y., Kihara, S., Arita, Y., Nishida, M., Matsushima, A., Okamoto, Y., Ishigami, M., Kuriyama, H., Kishda, K., Nishizawa, H., Hotta, K., Muraguchi, M., Ohmoto, Y., Yamashita, S., Funahashi, T., and Matsuzawa, Y., Adipocyte-derived plasma protein, adiponectin, suppress lipid accumulation and class A scavenger receptor expression in human monocyte-derived macrophages, *Circulation,* 103, 1057–1063, 2001.

23. Arita, Y., Kihara, S., Ouchi, Y., Kuriyama, H., Okamoto, Y., Kumada, M., Hotta, K., Nishida, M., Takahashi, M., Nakamura, T., Shimomura, I., Muraguchi, M., Ohmoto, Y., Funahashi, T., and Matsuzawa, Y., Adipocyte-derived plasma protein, adiponectin, acts as a platelet-derived growth factor-BB-binding protein and regulates growth factor-induced common postreceptor signal in vascular smooth muscle cell, *Circulation,* 105, 2893–2898, 2002.

24. Kumada, M., Kihara, S., Sumitsuji, S., Kawamoto, T., Matsumoto, S., Ouchi, N., Arita, Y., Okamoto, Y., Shimomura, I., Hiraoka, H., Nakamura, T., and Matsuzawa, Y., Association of hypoadiponectinemia with coronary artery disease in men, *Arterioscler. Thromb. Vasc. Biol.*, 23, 85–89, 2003.

25. Zoccali, C., Mallamaci, F., Tripepi, G., Benedetto, F.A.Q., Cutrupi, S., Parlongo, S., Malatino, L.S., Monanno, G., Seminara, G., Rapisarda, F., Fatuzzo, P., Buemi, M., Nicocia, G., Tanaka, S., Kihara, S., Funahashi, T., and Matsuzawa, Y., Adiponectin, metabolic risk factors, and cardiovascular events among patients with end-stage renal disease, *J. Am. Soc. Nephrol.*, 13, 134–141.

26. Pischon, T., Girman, C.J., Hotamisligil, G.S., Rifai, N., Hu, F.B., and Rimm, E.B., Plasma adiponectin levels and risk of myocardial infarction in men, *JAMA,* 291, 1730–1737, 2004.

27. Hotta, K., Funahashi, T., Arita, Y., Takahashi, M., Matsuda, M., Okamoto, Y., Iwahashi, H., Kuriyama, H., Maeda, K., Nishida, M., Kihara, S., Sakai, N., Nakajima, T., Muraguchi, M., Ohmoto, Y., Nakamura, T., Yamashita, S., and Matsuzawa, Y., Plasma concentrations of a novel adipose-specific protein, adiponectin, in type 2 diabetic patients, *Arterioscler. Thromb. Vasc. Med.,* 20, 1595–1599, 2000.

28. Weyer, C., Funahashi, T., Tanaka, S., Hotta, K., Matsuzawa, Y., Pratley, R.E., and Tataranni, P.A., Hypoadiponectinemia in obesity and type 2 diabetes: close association with insulin resistance and hyperinsulinemia, *J. Clin. Endocrinol. Metab.,* 86, 1930–1935, 2001.

29. Lindsay, R.S., Funahashi, T., Hanson, R.L., Matsuzawa, Y., Tanaka, S., Tataranni, P.A., Knowler, W.C., and Krakoff, J., Adiponectin and development of type 2 diabetes in the Pima Indian population, *Lancet,* 360, 57–58, 2002.

30. Takahashi, M., Arita, Y., Yamagata, Y., Okutomi, K., Horie, M., Shimomura, I., Hotta, K., Kuriyama, H., Ouchi, Y., Maeda, K., Nishida, M., Kihara, H., Nakamura, S., Yamashita, S., Funahashi, T., and Matsuzawa, Y., Genomic structure and mutation in adipose-specific gene, adiponectin, *Int. J. Obes. Relat. Disord.,* 24, 861–868, 2000.

31. Kondo, H., Shimomura, I., Matsukawa, Y., Kumada, M., Takahashi, M., Matsuda, M., Ouchi, Y., Kihara, S., Kawamoto, T., Sumotuji, S., Funahashi, T., and Matsuzawa, Y., Association of adiponectin mutation, with type 2 diabetes: a candidate gene for the insulin resistance syndrome, *Diabetes,* 51, 2325–2328, 2002.

32. Ohashi, K., Ouchi, N., Kihara, S., Funahashi, T., Nakamura, T., Sumitsuji, S., Kawamoto, T., Matsumoto, S., Nagaretani, H., Kumada, M., Okamoto, Y., Nishizawa, H., Kishida, K., Maeda, N., Hiraoka, H., Iwashima, Y., Ishikawa, K., Ohishi, M., Katsuya, T., Rakugi, H., Ogihara, T., and Matsuzawa, Y., Adiponectin I164T mutation is associated with the metabolic syndrome and coronary artery disease, *J. Am. Coll. Cardiol.,* 43, 1195–1200, 2004.

33. Maeda, N., Shimomura, I., Kishida, K., Nishizawa, H., Matsuda, M., Nagaretani, H., Furuyama, N., Kondo, H., Takahashi, M., Arita, Y., Komuro, R., Ouchi, N., Kihara, S., Tochino, Y., Okutomi, K., Horie, M., Takeda, S., Aoyama, T., Funahashi, T., and Matsuzawa, Y., Diet-induced insulin resistance in mice lacking adiponectin/ACRP30, *Nat. Med.,* 8, 731–737, 2002.

34. Matsuda, M., Shimomura, I., Sata, M., Arita, Y., Nishida, M., Marda, N., Kumada, M., Okamoto, Y., Nagaretani, H., Nishizawa, H., Kishida, K., Komuro, R., Ouchi, N., Kihara, S., Nagai, R., Funahashi, T., and Matsuzawa, Y., Role of adiponectin in preventing vascular stenosis. The missing link of adipo-vascular axis, *J. Biol. Chem.,* 277, 37487–37491, 2002.

35. Okamoto, Y., Kihara, S., Ouchi, N., Nishida, M., Arita, Y., Kumada, M., Ohashi, K., Sakai, N., Shimomura, I., Kobayashi, H., Terasaka, N., Fuahashi, T., and Matsuzawa, Y., Adiponectin reduces atherosclerosis in apolipoprotein E-deficient mice, *Circulation,* 26, 2767–2770, 2002.

36. Nagasawa, A., Fukui, K., Funahashi, T., Maeda, N., Shimomura, I., Kihara, S., Waki, M., Takamatsu, K., and Matsuzawa, Y., Effects of soy protein diet on the expression of adipose genes and plasma adiponectin, *Horm. Metab. Res.,* 34, 635–639, 2002.

37. Nagasawa, A., Fukui, K., Kojima, M., Kishida, K., Maeda, N., Nagaretani, H., Hibuse, T., Nishizawa, H., Kihara, S., Waki, M., Takamatsu, K., Funahashi, T., and Matsuzawa, Y., Divergent effects of soy protein diet on the expression of adipocytokines, *Biochem. Biophys. Res. Commun.,* 311, 909–914, 2003.

38. Maeda, N., Takahashi, M., Funahashi, T., Kihara, S., Nishizawa, H., Kishida, K., Nagaretani, H., Matsuda, M., Komuro, R., Ouchi, N., Kuriyama, H., Hotta, K., Nakamura, T., Shimomura, I., and Matsuzawa, Y., PPARγ ligands increase expression and plasma concentration of adiponectin, an adipose-derived protein, *Diabetes,* 50, 2094–2099, 2001.

# 5 Systematic Review of Intervention Studies Using Isoflavone Supplements and Proposal for Future Studies

*Shaw Watanabe, Xing-Gang Zhuo, Melissa K. Melby, Naoko Ishiwata, and Mituru Kimira*

## CONTENTS

## ABSTRACT

Many studies have reported beneficial health effects of isoflavones (IFs) on estrogen-related cancer, cardiovascular disease, lipid profiles, climacteric symptoms, and osteoporosis in humans. However, results have been mixed and are difficult to compare due to differences in study populations (e.g., men vs. women, pre- vs. postmenopausal women, equol producers and nonproducers), IF origin (soy vs. clover), IF form (extracted IF in aglycone form vs. with protein and various precursors), IF dose, and lack of other important data such as dietary intake.

To more precisely characterize the various health effects and limitations of clinical intervention studies carried out to date, we performed a systematic review of studies using extracted IF supplements in humans. Of the 22 articles identified, 6 studies were further selected for lipid analysis. Several studies of IF supplementation reported significant effects on prostate cancer, cardiovascular disease, osteoporosis, antioxidant status, hot flashes, menstrual cycle and associated hormones, and selected cognitive functions. Other studies reported no significant effects on prostate cancer, cardiovascular disease, menstrual cycle and associated hormones, reproductive health, and insulin resistance.

These conflicting and nonsignificant findings most likely result from data and study design limitations, and thus we propose a set of minimum requirements and guidelines for future research to enable comparison between studies and meta-analysis of future results. These issues include subject selection and characteristics, equol producer status, IF source, IF dose, IF components, intervention duration, blood or urinary levels of IFs, and dietary sources of IFs. Selection of a proper end point and its biological plausibility are also important.

**Keywords:** isoflavones, supplement, intervention, epidemiology.

## 5.1   INTRODUCTION

Early evidence suggesting that IFs play a role in the prevention of estrogen-related cancer[1,2] and cardiovascular disease led to a rapid increase in studies of IFs and health. Recently, following concerns about the use of hormone replacement therapy (HRT) at menopause, IFs are increasingly being investigated as an alternative to HRT and more generally for life-style-related diseases and diseases associated with aging including cancer and heart disease. Large studies of HRT have demonstrated clear risks of endometrial cancer and venous thromboembolism, probable risks of breast cancer and gallbladder disease, clear protective effects against osteoporosis, and as yet uncertain effects on heart disease, colorectal cancer, and cognitive dysfunction.[3] IFs, on the other hand, may provide many of the same benefits of HRT with considerably fewer risks. However, many unknown factors remain including appropriate doses for various health outcomes, effective forms and sources of IFs, duration of intervention, and effects in different populations.

Isoflavonoids are divided into seven categories: isoflavone, isoflavane, isoflavanone, coumestane, pterocarpane, rotenoid, and coumaronochromone (Figure 5.1). The IF coumesterol was first identified as a potent phytoestrogen when it was discovered to be the cause of infertility in Australian sheep that were consuming large amounts of clover, which is rich in IFs. The IFs that naturally occur in red clover are biochanin A (which is a precursor of genistein) and formonetin (which is a precursor of daidzein). In beans, IFs usually take the glycoside or malonyl glycoside form (Figure 5.2). The major IFs in soybeans, such as genistein, daidzein, and glycitein, are present in the form of 7-O-glycosides and further esterified between malonic acid and the 6 position of glucose. Raw soybeans are

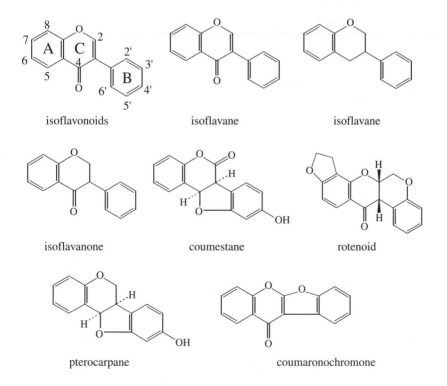

isoflavonoids          isoflavane          isoflavane

isoflavanone          coumestane          rotenoid

pterocarpane          coumaronochromone

**FIGURE 5.1** Basic structure of the isoflavone family.

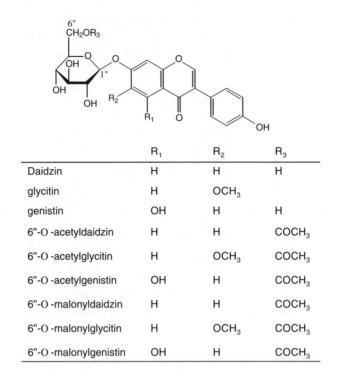

| | R₁ | R₂ | R₃ |
|---|---|---|---|
| Daidzin | H | H | H |
| glycitin | H | OCH₃ | |
| genistin | OH | H | H |
| 6"-O -acetyldaidzin | H | H | COCH₃ |
| 6"-O -acetylglycitin | H | OCH₃ | COCH₃ |
| 6"-O -acetylgenistin | OH | H | COCH₃ |
| 6"-O -malonyldaidzin | H | H | COCH₃ |
| 6"-O -malonylglycitin | H | OCH₃ | COCH₃ |
| 6"-O -malonylgenistin | OH | H | COCH₃ |

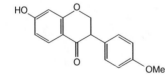

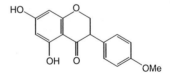

formononetin                          Biochanin A

**FIGURE 5.2**  Isoflavones in the soybean.

rich in malonyl glycosides, and acetyl glycosides increase by decarboxylation of malonyl residues during roasting.

Soybeans are well known to be rich in genistein and daidzein. After ingestion, plant precursors are converted to daidzein, genistein, and relevant aglycone forms. Glycitin and its malonyl derivatives are only present in the hypocotyls (soybean germ). Coumestrol is synthesized from daidzein, but it is only detected in sprouts. The physiological function of IF in plants is believed to be related to node formation, but antistress molecules, phytoalexin of soyabean glyceollin I, glyceollin II, and glyceollin III, are also produced from daidzein. Thus, the source of IF for supplements is important for evaluating their physiological activities.

In the human intestine, bacterial enzymes convert glycated IFs to aglycones and conjugate with glucuronides or sulfides. Some IF metabolites such as equol are considered to be animal IFs, as they are not found in plants and require metabolism by bacterial enzymes.

IFs, because of their estrogenic properties, were hypothesized to be the active components in lowering the risk of cancer.[2] However, subsequent research has shown that the relationship between soy and health is not that simple.[1] Genistein exerts many effects that are not mediated through estrogen receptors (e.g., tyrosine kinase inhibitors). Soy protein (without IFs) has also been shown to exhibit beneficial health effects, and these may be mediated through short-chain peptides, lecithin, saponin, and so on.

In order to understand the health effects of IFs and to optimize supplementation and interventions, an understanding of the metabolism of IF precursors by humans and the effects of IFs and metabolites on myriad metabolic pathways is necessary. To more precisely characterize the various health effects and limitations of clinical intervention studies carried out to date, we performed a systematic review of studies using extracted IF supplements in humans.

The conflicting and nonsignificant results most likely result from data and study design limitations, and thus we propose a set of minimum requirements and guidelines for future research to enable comparison between studies and meta-analysis of future results.

## 5.2 MATERIALS AND METHODS

For study identification and selection, PubMed was searched using the query of "(isoflavone or equol or isoflavones) and (intervention or supplement) and Clinical Trial[ptyp] and Human[MeSH]" on 3 August 2004, which resulted in 64 articles. Twenty-two articles[4–25] were selected for systematic review after reading abstracts, as they met the criteria of being intervention studies using extracted IF supplements in humans.

## 5.3 RESULTS

### 5.3.1 STUDY DESIGN AND DIFFERENT SOURCES OF ISOFLAVONES

Characteristics of the 22 intervention studies that used extracted IF in humans are shown in Table 5.1. The studies used three sources of IF (red clover, subterranean clover, and soy) and reported a range of health outcomes. IF doses ranged from 20 to 160 mg, with variable IF and precursor content (Table 5.2). Nine studies used red clover IFs, one used subterranean clover,[13–15] six used soy protein IF, and three used IF derived from soy germ.[23–25] One study[7] was a nonrandomized controlled clinical trial, one study[25] used a clinical trial design, and all others were randomized controlled trials. The intervention periods ranged from 7 d to 12 months.

**TABLE 5.1**
**Characteristics of the 22 Intervention Studies Using Pure Isoflavones in Humans**

| Reporter | Year | Ref. | Subject[a] | Study Design[b] | IF Source | IFs, mg/d | Outcome[c] |
|---|---|---|---|---|---|---|---|
| Baber et al. | 1999 | 4 | n = 51 (MW) | RCT, CO, PC, 31 weeks | Red clover | 40 | Menopausal symptom |
| Nestel et al. | 2004 | 5 | n = 80 (46 men, 34 MW; FL) | RCT, P, CO, DB, PC, 15 weeks | Red clover | 40 | Lipid |
| Atkinson et al. | 2004 | 6 | n = 205 (women) | RCT, P, DB, PC, 1 year | Red clover | 43.5 | Bone density |
| Teede et al. | 2003 | 7 | n = 80 (46 men, 34 MW; H) | RCT, P, CO, DB, PC, 15 weeks | Red clover | 80 | Vascular effects |
| Campbell et al. | 2004 | 8 | n = 23 (16 PW, 7 MW; H) | RCT, CO, PC, DB, 4 months | Red clover | 86 | IGF, lipid, antioxidant |
| Blakesmith et al. | 2003 | 9 | n = 25 (PW; H) | RCT, P, DB, PC, 4 months | Red clover | 86 | Lipid, insulin resistance |
| van de Weijer et al. | 2002 | 10 | n = 30 (MW) | RCT, P, SB, PC, 12 weeks | Red clover | 80 | Hot flashes |
| Tice et al. | 2003 | 11 | n = 252 (MW) | RCT, P, DB, PC, 12 weeks | Red clover | 82 or 57 | Hot flashes |
| Jarred et al. | 2002 | 12 | n = 20 (men; prostate cancer) | CCT, CO, NB, HMC, 7–54 d | Red clover | 160 | Prostate apoptosis |
| Hodgson et al.[d] | 1999 | 13 | n = 59 (46 men, 13 women) | RCT, P, DB, PC, 8 weeks | Subterranean clover | 55 | Blood pressure |
| Hodgson et al.[d] | 1998 | 14 | n = 59 (46 men, 13 MW; H) | RCT, P, DB, PC, 8 weeks | Subterranean clover | 55 | Lipid |
| Hodgson et al.[d] | 1999 | 15 | n = 59 (46 men, 13 women) | RCT, P, DB, PC, 8 weeks | Subterranean clover | 55 | Lipid peroxidation |
| Mitchell et al. | 2001 | 16 | n = 15 (men) | CT, CO, 2 months | Soy | 40 | Reproductive health *(continued)* |

| Author | Year | Ref | n | Design | Intervention | Dose | Outcome |
|---|---|---|---|---|---|---|---|
| Duffy et al. | 2003 | 17 | n = 33 (MW) | RCT, P, DB, PC, 12 weeks | Soy | 60 | Cognitive function |
| Penotti et al. | 2003 | 18 | n = 62 (MW, H) | RCT, P, DB, PC, 6 months | Soy | 72 | Hot flashes, ET, PI |
| Kritz-Silverstein et al. | 2003 | 19 | n = 56 (MW; H) | RCT, P, DB, PC, 6 months | Soy | 110 | Cognitive function |
| Maskarinec et al. | 2002 | 20 | n = 34 (PW) | RCT, P, DB, PC, 1 year | Soy | 100 | Ovulatory cycle |
| Maskarinec et al. | 2003 | 21 | n = 30 (PW) | RCT, P, DB, PC, 1 year | Soy | 100 | Mammographic density |
| Dewell et al. | 2002 | 22 | n = 36 (MW; MH) | RCT, P, PC, 6 months | Soy | 150 | Lipid |
| Watanabe et al. | 2000 | 23 | n = 38 (PW) | RCT, PC, 1 months | Soy germ tea | 15 | Lipid peroxides, DNA adduct |
| Watanabe et al. | 2001 | 24 | n = 40 (PW) | RCT, CO, 1 month | Soy germ tab | 20 or 40 | Hormonal states |
| Uesugi et al. | 2004 | 25 | n = 58 (women) | RCT, CO, DB, PC, 8 weeks | Soy germ tab | 40 | Bone, climacteric symptoms |

[a] PW, premenopausal women; MW, menopausal women; FL, free-living; H, healthy; MH, moderately hypercholesterolemic.

[b] RCT, randomized controlled trial; CCT, nonrandomized controlled clinical trial; CT, clinical trial; P, parallel; CO, crossover; DB, double-blind; SD, single blind; NB, nonblinded; PC, placebo-controlled; HMC, historically matched controls.

[c] IGF, insulin-like growth factor; ET, endometrial thickness; PI, pulsatility index of the uterine and cerebral arteries.

[d] Hodgson's reports[13-15] were based upon the same study.

**TABLE 5.2**
**Supplementation with Constituents of Pure Isoflavones
in 22 Intervention Studies**

| Reference | Isoflavone Contituents per Day |
|---|---|
| 4 | Genistein, daidzein, and their methylated precursors, biochanin and formononetin |
| 5 | B: formononetin in a ratio of 3.5:1 with 4% genistein and <1% daidzein or F: biochanin in a ratio of 4.9:1 with <1% genistein and daidzein |
| 6 | 26 mg biochanin A, 16 mg formononetin, 1 mg genistein, and 0.5 mg daidzein |
| 7 | B: formononetin in a ratio of 3.5:1 with 4% genistein and <1% daidzein or F: formononetin:biochanin in a ratio of 4.9:1 with <1% genistein and daidzein |
| 8 | 50 mg biochanin, 16 mg formononetin, 8 mg genistein, and 10 mg daidzein |
| 9 | 51.4 mg biochanin A, 8.6 mg genistein, 18.6 mg formononetin and 7.4 mg daidzein |
| 10 | Formononetin, daidzein, biochanin and genistein in active aglycone forms total 80 mg |
| 11 | Promensil: higher proportion of biochanin A and genistein or Rimostil: higher proportion of formononetin and daidzein |
| 12 | Aglycone, predomninantly formononetin and biochanin A with smaller amounts of genistein and daidzein in a ratio of biochanin A + genistein:formononetin + daidzein of 2:1 |
| 13 | 16 mg biochanin A, 30 mg genistein, 8 mg formononetin, and 1 mg daidzein |
| 14 | 16 mg biochanin A, 30 mg genistein, 8 mg formononetin, and 1 mg daidzein |
| 15 | 16 mg biochanin A, 30 mg genistein, 8 mg formononetin, and 1 mg daidzein |
| 16 | Genistein, daidzein, and glycitein |
| 17 | Genistein, daidzein, and glycitein |
| 18 | 11 mg genistein/genistine, 36 mg daidzein/daidzine, 25 mg glycitein/glycitine, and 96 mg soy saponine; the aglycate:glycate ratio was 3:2 |
| 19 | 60 mg total isoflavone equivalents |
| 20 | Equivalent to 76 mg aglycone; 51% daidzein, 44% genistein, and 5% glycitein; 1% aglycones, 91% glucosides, 5% malonylglucosides, 3% acetylglucosides |
| 21 | Equivalent to 76 mg aglycone |
| 22 | 90 mg aglycones and 60 mg glycosides; aglycones: 40 mg genistein, 50 mg daidzein and glycitein |
| 23 | daidzein 13 mg, genistein 1.9 mg, and glycitein 7.6 mg/L |
| 24 | daidzein 43.5 mg, genistein 6 mg, and glycitein 24 mg/g tablets |
| 25 | 20.46 mg daidzein, 5.46 mg genistein, and 16.2 mg glycitein |

Formonetin (daidzein precursor), biochanin A (genistein precursor).

## 5.3.2 HEALTH OUTCOMES

### 5.3.2.1 Breast Cancer

High concentrations of insulin-like growth factor-1 (IGF-1) in serum are associated with an increased risk of premenopausal breast cancer (RR = 7.28).[26] For premenopausal subjects, the change in IGF-1, IGF-BP1, and IGF-BP3 assessed at different points of the menstrual cycle did not differ between the

IF and placebo phase. However, the change in IGF-1, when examined pre- and postsupplementation, was nonsignificantly reduced ($P = 0.06$) on the IF supplement compared to placebo. For postmenopausal subjects, the change in IGF-1, IGF-BP1, and IGFBP-3 concentrations over the supplementation period did not differ between the IF or placebo phase. This study showed that 1-month supplementation with red clover IFs had at most a small effect on IGF status in premenopausal and no effect in postmenopausal subjects. Further studies are required to ascertain the role these dietary compounds may have to play in breast cancer prevention. Maskarinec et al.[21] reported no significant changes in mammographic densities (a predictor of breast cancer risk) after a 1-year IF intervention.

### 5.3.2.2 Prostate Cancer

One report suggested that dietary IFs might halt the progression of prostate cancer by inducing apoptosis in low- to moderate-grade tumors.[12] There were no significant differences between pre- and posttreatment, serum prostate-specific antigen (PSA, a proliferative risk parameter that is implicated in prostate cancer promotion), Gleason score, serum testosterone, or biochemical factors in the treated patients ($P > 0.05$). Apoptosis in radical prostatectomy specimens from treated patients was significantly higher than in control subjects ($P = 0.0018$), specifically in regions of low- to moderate-grade cancer (Gleason grade 1 to 3). No adverse events related to the treatment were reported.

### 5.3.2.3 Cardiovascular Disease

One study showed a decrease in blood pressure, one study showed a decrease in arterial stiffness and total vascular resistance, and another study found no significant differences.[7,13,25] IF intervention significantly reduced arterial stiffness with improved systemic arterial compliance ($P = 0.04$; repeated-measures ANOVA, Bonferroni correction) attributable to a reduction in total peripheral resistance ($P = 0.03$) and a corresponding reduction in central pulse wave velocity ($P = 0.02$) compared with placebo. IF from subterranean clover did not affect blood pressure or flow-mediated vasodilation. Improvements seemed limited to formononetin-enriched IFs (adjusted $P = 0.06$). Formononetin treatment also reduced circulating vascular adhesion cell molecule-1 ($P < 0.01$). These data suggest that red clover IFs enriched in formononetin reduce arterial stiffness and total vascular resistance but have no effect on blood pressure in normotensive men and postmenopausal women.[7] There was no significant difference between groups, after adjustment for baseline values, in postintervention clinic supine blood pressure, clinic erect blood pressure, or 24-h ambulatory blood pressure. Adjustment for age, gender, and weight change did not alter the results.[13] Systolic and diastolic blood pressure of hypertensive participants decreased significantly after 40 mg/d soy germ IF treatment compared with baseline and the placebo treatment.[25]

### 5.3.2.4  Bone Metabolism

Effects of IF on bone seem to be relatively robust among the studies reviewed here. Loss of lumbar spine bone mineral content and bone mineral density was significantly ($P = 0.04$ and $P = 0.03$, respectively) lower in women taking the IF supplement than in those taking the placebo.[6] There were no significant treatment effects on hip bone mineral content or bone mineral density and markers of bone resorption, but bone formation markers were significantly increased ($P = 0.04$ and $P = 0.01$ for bone-specific alkaline phosphatase and $N$-propeptide of collagen type I, respectively) in the intervention group compared with placebo in post-menopausal women. These data suggest that through attenuation of bone loss, IFs have a potentially protective effect on the lumbar spine in women.

Urinary deoxypyridinoline, a marker of bone resorption, decreased significantly with 40 mg/d IF treatment.[25] This tendency was remarkable among equol producers. Plasma osteocalcin and bone mineral density did not change after 4 weeks of treatment. Osteocalcin increased after 4 months and bone mineral density improved after 1 year.[1]

### 5.3.2.5  Effects on Lipids

Individual studies showed no significant effects of IF on lipids. The difference between placebo and biochanin effects on LDL-C was 9.5%. No other lipid was affected, and women failed to respond significantly to treatment.[5] IFs increased HDL in postmenopausal women compared to placebo ($P = 0.02$) but did not alter either cholesterol or triacylglycerol concentrations.[8] There were no significant effects on TC, LDL- and HDL-cholesterol, HDL subfractions, triacylglycerol, or lipoprotein(a).[9] The results (mean ± SEM for the placebo and the PE groups, respectively) indicated no significant differences in total triacylglycerol (1.3 ± 0.2 vs. 1.2 ± 0.2 mmol/l), TC (6.4 ± 0.4 vs. 6.5 ± 0.2 mmol/l), or HDL cholesterol (1.0 ± 0.1 vs. 1.0 ± 0.1 mmol/l) after 2 months of treatment. Moreover, total triacylglycerol and cholesterol remained unchanged after 6 months.[22] After adjustment for baseline values, no significant differences in postintervention serum lipid and lipoprotein (a) concentrations between groups were identified. Further adjustment for age, gender, and weight change did not alter the results.[14] There were no significant differences in plasma lipid (TC, LDL-C, HDL-C, and TG) between 40 mg/d IF treatment with baseline and placebo treatment.[25]

### 5.3.2.6  Antioxidant Status

Effects of antioxidant status varied by IF source. Red clover–derived IF supplementation had no effect on blood antioxidant status.[8] After adjustment for baseline values, there was no significant difference between groups in creatinine adjusted postintervention F2-isoprostane (currently the best available marker of *in vivo* lipid peroxidation) concentrations ($P = 0.74$).[15] Soy germ IF showed decreased phophatidylcholine hydroperoxide and 8ohdG, which was a marker of DNA damage.[23]

### 5.3.2.7  Symptoms of Menopause

Effects of IF on vasomotor symptoms are mixed. Two of five studies showed a decrease in hot flashes, but three studies showed no significant effects. In comparison with the placebo group, 41% of participants in the Promensil (82 mg of total IFs per day) group showed a reduction of hot flashes, but 34% did in the Rimostil (57 mg of total IFs per day) group. Neither supplement had a clinically important effect on quality-of-life improvements or adverse events.[11] The daily administration of 72 mg of soy-derived IFs was no more effective than placebo in reducing hot flashes in postmenopausal women. It also had no effect on endometrial thickness or the pulsatility index (PI) of the uterine and cerebral arteries.[18] The frequency of hot flashes significantly decreased by 44% in the 80-mg IF group ($P < 0.01$), and the Greene score decreased in the active group by 13%.[10] There was no significant difference between active and placebo groups in the reduction in hot flashes between start and finish time-points. Analysis performed on interim data time-points revealed a substantially greater reduction in hot flashes in the active group than the placebo at 4 and 8 weeks after commencement of treatment, but this was not statistically significant. There were no significant differences between groups for Greene scores or transvaginal ultrasound data of endometrial thickness.[4] Hot flashes decreased significantly after 40 mg/d soy germ IF supplementation.[25]

### 5.3.2.8  Menstrual Cycle and Hypothalamo–Pituitary– Gonadal (HPG) Hormone

Results are mixed but suggest that IF can exert effects on menstrual cycle length and hormones of the HPG axis. Menstrual cycle length did not change significantly during 100 mg/d of soy IF for 1 year. No significant changes in hormone levels were observed in the treatment group.[20] Administration of 20 mg/d or 40 mg/d soy germ IF caused a prolonged menstruation in 60% of young women, shortened menstruation in 20% of young women, no change in 17%, and irregular menstruation in 3%.[24] The higher dose tended to lengthen menstrual periods, but 17 β-estradiol levels in both follicular and luteal phages were not different between 20 mg and 40 mg IF intake. Equol excreters tended to show low plasma progesterone levels in the luteal phase. Detailed hormonal analysis of three test subjects by a crossover study design showed decreased levels of 17 β-estradiol throughout the menstruation cycle.[23] SHBG significantly increased about 10% in all three. DEAS, androstenedione, and testosterone showed different responses according to the follicular or luteal phase. T3 and T4 increased as a result of IF tablet administration in the follicular phase but decreased in the luteal phase. These changes suggest that IFs influence not only estrogen receptor–related functions but also the HPG axis.[23] The value of E2 and progesterone concentration tended to increase among the postmenopausal group following IF treatment. Luteinizing hormone (LH) and follicle stimulating hormone (FSH) did not show any change among postmenopausal women. SHBG in the plasma was lower among postmenopausal women following soy germ IF treatment.[25]

### 5.3.2.9  Reproductive Health in Normal Males

There was no effect on blood gonadotrophin and reproductive hormone levels, testicular volume, or semen quality (ejaculate volume, sperm concentration, total sperm count, sperm motility, and sperm morphology) over the study period.[16]

### 5.3.2.10  Cognitive Function

Those receiving 12 weeks of soy IF supplementation showed significantly greater improvements in a recall of pictures and in a sustained attention task.[19] The groups did not differ in their ability to learn rules, but the IF supplement group showed significantly greater improvements in learning rule reversals. They also showed significantly greater improvement in a planning task. Treatment had no effect on menopausal symptoms, self-ratings of mood, bodily symptoms, or sleepiness. Thus, significant cognitive improvements in postmenopausal women can be gained from 12 weeks of consumption of a supplement containing soy IFs that are independent of any changes in menopausal symptoms, mood, or sleepiness[17] Comparisons of percentage change in cognitive function between baseline and follow-up showed greater improvement in category fluency for women on active treatment as compared with those on placebo ($P = 0.02$). These results suggest that IF supplementation has a favorable effect on cognitive function, particularly verbal memory, in postmenopausal women.

### 5.3.2.11  Insulin Resistance

Serum concentration of insulin and glucose, and homeostasis model assessment insulin resistance index (HOMA-IR) were unaffected by IF supplementation.[9]

## 5.4  DISCUSSION

Populations consuming high levels of soy have documented low levels of reproductive-related cancers.[27] Soybeans are consumed in many Asian countries, and they are the major source of IFs.[28] Japanese intake of IFs ranges from 20 to 50 mg/d.[29,30] From a public health perspective, soy contains many other factors besides IFs that may be protective against disease.[1] The U.S. Food and Drug Administration has proposed allowing some soy products to carry a label indicating that they may reduce heart-disease risk by taking 25 g/d of soy protein as a source of 60 mg of soy phytoestrogens. The average Japanese consumes about 30 mg of IFs per day; yet for the purpose of interventions and marketing of commercial supplements, identifying the major components and standardizing them is necessary.

Our systematic review of the current state of research on the health effects of extracted IF supplementation unfortunately reveals that to date, results and research designs have been so variable as to render comparison difficult at best. However, these limitations can be addressed, and we believe that incorporating eight recommendations will greatly improve the quality of research in this field and facilitate meta-analyses that are needed to make definitive assessments (Table 5.3).

**TABLE 5.3**
**Minimum Requirements for Future Research Design**
**and Reporting of Results**

1. Subject selection and characteristics
2. Characterization of equol producer status
3. IF source (red clover, subterranean clover, soy seed, soy germ)
4. Dietary sources of IFs (in order to assess true intake)
5. IF dose (ideally expressed in molar equivalents)
6. IF form (precursors, aglycone forms, etc.); presence of soy protein
7. Blood or urinary levels of IFs (measured at specified time after ingestion of supplement)
8. Intervention duration
9. End point

For example, although individual studies often have insufficient statistical power to detect significant differences following IF supplement intervention, our recent meta-analysis of the effects of IFs on LDL-cholesterol demonstrates that meta-analysis can be an effective tool when studies report necessary data and have comparable protocols.[31]

### 5.4.1 Subject Selection and Characteristics

Depending on the health outcome of interest, populations need to be selected carefully and characterized fully in all reports to allow appropriate comparisons. For example, comparing the effects of IF supplementation on cholesterol in pre- and postmenopausal women, given the changes in cholesterol levels and metabolism that occur after menopause, may not be appropriate. Since much of the epidemiological data on soy intake and reproductive cancers derives from Asian populations, other factors such as genetics and life-style (e.g., diet) must be considered, and future studies should not only identify the ethnic backgrounds of study participants but also characterize life-style factors such as dietary intake.[25,32]

### 5.4.1.1 Equol Producer Status

Although the initial research and epidemiological focus was on daidzein and genistein, recently the metabolite equol has moved into the spotlight.[33] Equol is more estrogenic than its precursor daidzein, as well as genistein, and is believed to be responsible for many of the observed health effects of IFs. Most animals, such as rats, mice, and monkeys, metabolize almost 100% of daidzein into equol, while humans vary considerably in their ability produce equol.[34] The ability to produce equol derives from intestinal microflora, not from endogenous enzymes. So far, several bacteria have been isolated that convert daidzein to equol, including *Streptococcus intermedius* ssp., *Bacteroides ovatus* ssp., and *Ruminococcus products* ssp.[35]

Thus, equol-producing ability may change over an individual's lifetime. Not all individuals harbor the necessary microflora, and the percentage of equol producers in a given population varies from 20% (low in Americans, young Japanese) to 50% (highest in older Japanese). In studies in which populations are divided into equol producers and nonproducers, significant effects of IF supplementation are often seen in the producer subpopulations, while slight or no effects are observed in the nonproducer populations. Given that the epidemiological data on the protective effects of IFs derive mostly from Asian populations, yet many of the intervention studies have been carried out in Western populations, differences in equol production capability (in addition to genetics, life-style factors, daily diet, etc.) may partly explain the lack of consistent or significant results.

To accurately assess equol producer status, challenge tests should be administered in which participants consume a known quantity of IFs followed by measurement of blood or urinary samples drawn at a specified time after ingestion. Because equol-producing capability may change, measurement of equol and IFs in blood or urine at baseline, midpoint in the intervention study, and after the intervention period is recommended.

## 5.4.2 IF SOURCE

IFs derived from soy are generally produced either from the seed or from the germ. Seed-derived supplements generally have a daidzein:genistein ratio of 1:1.1, while germ-derived supplements generally have a 5:1 ratio.[36] This is an important distinction, given the hypothesized primary role of equol in most health effects of IFs. Germ-derived supplements will provide potential equol producers with five times as much substrate, and thus for health outcomes with linear dose–response relationships potentially five times the beneficial effect compared to seed-derived supplements. Many IF supplements use red clover, which contains 26 mg biochanin A (genistein precursor), 16 mg formonetin (daidzein precursor), 1 mg genistein, and 0.5 mg daidzein.[6] The higher ratio of genistein and its precursors to daidzein and its precursors mean that equol precursors are relatively low in red clover IF supplements compared to seed-derived soy IF supplements and considerably lower than those derived from soy germ. Only comparing total amounts of IFs between studies is inadequate given the variability in individual IF content and the implications for metabolite (equol) concentrations. In order to perform meta-analyses and investigate dose–response relationships, data need to be presented for all individual IFs (ideally in molar equivalents as opposed to weight), particularly for daidzein and genistein and their precursors.

### 5.4.2.1 Dietary Sources of IFs

Baber et al.[4] suggest that the apparent placebo effect in many studies of menopausal symptoms may be attributable to dietary sources of isoflavones, thereby demonstrating the importance of accounting for (or controlling for) dietary intake of IFs, preferably by using dietary records during the intervention period or using food frequency questionnaires.[30,39]

### 5.4.3  IF DOSE AND FORM

Traditional Japanese women ingest about 100 g of soy and soy products daily, which include about 30 mg of isoflavones per day.[29] Total daily consumption of IFs was estimated to be 32 to 35 mg/d, ranging from almost null to 1000 mg. In a Shanghai study, daily consumption of IFs was calculated to be 100.6 mg (median), 36.8 mg (25th percentile), and 238.2 mg (75th percentile).[37]

The minimum IF amount needed to observe effects may depend on the health outcome of interest. However, the maximum safe dose may also vary for different populations, for example, pre- vs. postmenopausal women vs. men with different amounts of endogenous estrogen. Again, to facilitate comparisons between studies, researchers should report molar equivalents, not just weights, if possible.

Additionally, to facilitate comparisons between studies, aglycone-equivalent amounts should be reported. Contents of IFs in commercial supplements are variable.[38] In the case of soy, it is important to distinguish between studies performed with or without soy protein, as other components of soy, such as peptides, saponin, and other minor components, may also be very important and possibly have greater effects than IFs on some health outcomes.

### 5.4.4  BLOOD OR URINARY LEVELS OF IFS

Absorption of IF in the alimentary tract occurs mostly in the form of agly-cones.[40,41] It has been suggested that bacterial hydrolysis of the glycosidic link of the glycosidic forms of isoflavonoids must occur before absorption from the intestinal tract. Three different locations of absorption are considered according to the conjugate form of IF: stomach, small intestine, and large intestine.

In humans, about 95% of IF is in the glucuronide form, and only about 5% is in the active free or sulfated form.[41] Some IFs may also become bound to plasma proteins, like SHBG. The plasma half-life of daidzein was 6.31 h, and that of genistein was 8.95 h.[40] King and Bursill[42] also showed the same values. Genistein seems to be more efficiently absorbed from the intestinal tract and to remain in circulation longer. With daily ingestion, chronic IF levels will increase gradually. Since blood is usually drawn in the morning for most studies, timing of supplement ingestion is also important to consider. Morning ingestion will result in low levels, while night ingestion (before bedtime) will result in the highest levels.

### 5.4.5  INTERVENTION DURATION

Depending on the health outcome of interest, minimum time periods required to observe significant effects will vary. Obviously for bone mineral density, a longer time is required to observe significant changes, but for markers of bone turnover shorter periods may be adequate.[39]

## 5.4.6 END POINTS

### 5.4.6.1 Clinical Symptoms

While several weeks or months may be adequate to observe changes in climacteric symptoms, there may also be a large placebo effect, so it is important to have appropriate controls. Many menopausal IF supplements are derived from clover, not soy, and thus are lower in precursors of equol, which may have the strongest effect on menopausal symptoms.

Cancer preventive effects of soy foods have been well accepted.[44–46] In the case of cancer and other chronic disease prevention by intervention study, 10 or more years are necessary, so proper selection of biomarkers should be necessary. Sometimes, a transgeneration study would be necessary.[47]

### 5.4.6.2 Biomarkers

Serum biochemisty could be easily available. Soy protein (without IFs) has been shown to have positive effects on lipid profiles. Thus, it is important to identify the sources of IFs and other components of the supplement that may be involved. It is also important to distinguish between subjects with hyperlipidemia and those with normal values, as due to homeostatic control, great changes may not occur in the latter population.

More specified biomarkers are widely accepted. Antioxidant activity has been measured by reduction of free radicals and other peroxides.[22,48]

## 5.5 SUMMARY AND RECOMMENDATIONS

Due to financial and logistic constraints, intervention studies generally have much smaller sample sizes than epidemiological studies, and thus, the power to observe significant effects during short time periods is often low. Meta-analysis techniques permit combining many smaller studies to increase statistical power, and in the case of IF interventions often demonstrate significant effects.[43] For this review, we initially performed meta-analyses on TC, LDL cholesterol (LDL-C), HDL cholesterol (HDL-C), and triglycerides/ triacylglycerol (TG). However, no significant differences were observed. Our recent meta-analysis of IFs in which soy protein intake was controlled demonstrated significant lowering of LDL-cholesterol,[31] suggesting that the lack of significance observed in the current meta-analyses may not be due to a true lack of effect of IF on lipids, but rather to limitations of the studies. In order to facilitate meta-analysis of IF intervention results, future studies should report the following data: subject selection and characteristics, equol producer status, IF source, IF dose, IF intervention duration, blood levels of IFs, and dietary sources of IFs.

## ABBREVIATIONS

IF, isoflavone; TC, total cholesterol; LDL-C, LDL cholesterol; HDL-C, HDL cholesterol; TG, triglycerides/triacylglycerol.

## REFERENCES

1. Watanabe, S., Uesugi, S., and Kikuchi, Y., Isoflavones for prevention of cancer, cardiovascular diseases, gynecological problems and possible immune potentiation, *Biomed. Pharmacother.,* 56(6), 302–312, 2002.
2. Adlercreutz, C.H., Goldin, B.R., Gorbach, S.L., Hockerstedt, K.A., Watanabe, S., Hamalainen, E.K., Markkanen, M.H., Makela, T.H., Wahala, K.T., and Adlercreutz, T., Soybean phytoestrogen intake and cancer risk, *J. Nutr.,* 125(3 Suppl.), 757S–770S, 1995.
3. Manson, J. and Martin K., Postmenopausal hormone replacement therapy. *New Engl. J. Med.,* 344(1), 34–40, 2001.
4. Baber, R.J., Templeman, C., Morton, T., Kelly, G.E., and West, L., Randomized placebo-controlled trial of an isoflavone supplement and menopausal symptoms in women, *Climacteric,* 2(2), 85–92, 1999.
5. Nestel, P., Cehun, M., Chronopoulos, A., DaSilva, L., Teede, H., and McGrath, B., A biochanin-enriched isoflavone from red clover lowers LDL cholesterol in men, *Eur. J. Clin. Nutr.,* 58(3), 403–408, 2004.
6. Atkinson, C., Compston, J.E., Day, N.E., Dowsett, M., and Bingham, S.A., The effects of phytoestrogen isoflavones on bone density in women: a double-blind, randomized, placebo-controlled trial, *Am. J. Clin. Nutr.,* 79(2), 326–333, 2004.
7. Teede, H.J., McGrath, B.P., DeSilva, L., Cehun, M., Fassoulakis, A., and Nestel, P.J., Isoflavones reduce arterial stiffness: a placebo-controlled study in men and postmenopausal women, *Arterioscler. Thromb. Vasc. Biol.,* 23(6), 1066–1071, 2003.
8. Campbell, M.J., Woodside, J.V., Honour, J.W., Morton, M.S., and Leathem, A.J., Effect of red clover-derived isoflavone supplementation on insulin-like growth factor, lipid and antioxidant status in healthy female volunteers: a pilot study, *Eur. J. Clin. Nutr.,* 58(1), 173–179, 2004.
9. Blakesmith, S.J., Lyons-Wall, P.M., George, C., Joannou, G.E., Petocz, P., and Samman, S., Effects of supplementation with purified red clover (*Trifolium pratense*) isoflavones on plasma lipids and insulin resistance in healthy premenopausal women, *Br. J. Nutr.,* 89(4), 467–674, 2003.
10. van de Weijer, P.H. and Barentsen, R., Isoflavones from red clover (Promensil) significantly reduce menopausal hot flush symptoms compared with placebo, *Maturitas,* 42(3), 187–193, 2002.
11. Tice, J.A., Ettinger, B., Ensrud, K., Wallace, R., Blackwell, T., and Cummings, S.R., Phytoestrogen supplements for the treatment of hot flashes: the Isoflavone Clover Extract (ICE) Study: a randomized controlled trial, *JAMA,* 290(2), 207–214, 2003.
12. Jarred, R.A., Keikha, M., Dowling, C., McPherson, S.J., Clare, A.M., Husband, A.J., Pedersen, J.S., Frydenberg, M., and Risbridger, G.P., Induction of apoptosis in low to moderate-grade human prostate carcinoma by red clover-derived dietary isoflavones, *Cancer Epidemiol. Biomarkers Prev.,* 11(12), 1689–1696, 2002.

13. Hodgson, J.M., Puddey, I.B., Beilin, L.J., Mori, T.A., Burke, V., Croft, K.D., and Rogers, P.B., Effects of isoflavonoids on blood pressure in subjects with high-normal ambulatory blood pressure levels: a randomized controlled trial, *Am. J. Hypertens.*, 12(1 Pt 1), 47–53, 1999.

14. Hodgson, J.M., Puddey, I.B., Beilin, L.J., Mori, T.A., and Croft, K.D., Supplementation with isoflavonoid phytoestrogens does not alter serum lipid concentrations: a randomized controlled trial in humans, *J. Nutr.*, 128(4), 728–732, 1998.

15. Hodgson, J.M., Puddey, I.B., Croft, K.D., Mori, T.A., Rivera, J., and Beilin, L.J., Isoflavonoids do not inhibit *in vivo* lipid peroxidation in subjects with high-normal blood pressure, *Atherosclerosis*, 145(1), 167–172, 1999.

16. Mitchell, J.H., Cawood, E., Kinniburgh, D., Provan, A., Collins, A.R., and Irvine, D.S., Effect of a phytoestrogen food supplement on reproductive health in normal males, *Clin. Sci. (London)*, 100(6), 613–618, 2001.

17. Duffy, R., Wiseman, H., and File, S.E., Improved cognitive function in postmenopausal women after 12 weeks of consumption of a soya extract containing isoflavones, *Pharmacol. Biochem. Behav.*, 75(3), 721–729, 2003.

18. Penotti, M., Fabio, E., Modena, A.B., Rinaldi, M., Omodei, U., and Vigano, P., Effect of soy-derived isoflavones on hot flushes, endometrial thickness, and the pulsatility index of the uterine and cerebral arteries, *Fertil. Steril.*, 79(5), 1112–1117, 2003.

19. Kritz-Silverstein, D., Von Muhlen, D., Barrett-Connor, E., and Bressel, M.A., Isoflavones and cognitive function in older women: the SOy and Postmenopausal Health In Aging (SOPHIA) Study, *Menopause*, 10(3), 196–202, 2003.

20. Maskarinec, G., Williams, A.E., Inouye, J.S., Stanczyk, F.Z., and Franke, A.A., A randomized isoflavone intervention among premenopausal women, *Cancer Epidemiol. Biomarkers Prev.*, 11(2), 195–201, 2002.

21. Maskarinec, G., Williams, A.E., and Carlin, L., Mammographic densities in a one-year isoflavone intervention, *Eur. J. Cancer Prev.*, 12(2), 165–169, 2003.

22. Dewell, A., Hollenbeck, C.B., and Bruce, B., The effects of soy-derived phytoestrogens on serum lipids and lipoproteins in moderately hypercholesterolemic postmenopausal women, *J. Clin. Endocrinol. Metab.*, 87(1), 118–121, 2002.

23. Watanabe, S., Haba, R., Terashima, K., Arai, Y., Miura, T., Chiba, H., and Takamatsu, K., Antioxidant activity of soya hypocotyls tea in humans, *BioFactors*, 12(1–4), 227–232, 2000.

24. Watanabe, S., Terashima, K., Sato, Y., Arai, S., and Eboshida, A., Effects of isoflavone supplement on healthy women, *Biofactors*, 12(1–4), 233–241, 2000.

25. Uesugi, S., Watanabe, S., Ishiwata, N., Uehara, M., and Ouchi, K., Effects of isoflavone supplements on bone metabolic markers and climacteric symptoms in Japanese women, *BioFactors*, 22(1–4), 221–228, 2004.

26. Hankinson, S.E., Willett, W.C., Colditz, G.A., Hunter, D.J., Michaud, D.S., Deroo, B., Rosner, B., Speizer, F.E., and Pollak, M., Circulating concentrations of insulin-like growth factor-I and risk of breast cancer, *Lancet*, 351(9113), 1393–1396, 1998.

27. Watanabe S. and Koessel, S., Colon cancer: approach from molecular epidemiology, *J. Epidemiol.*, 3, 47–61, 1993.

28. Watanabe, S., Uesugi, S., and Haba, R., Chemical analysis and health benefits of isoflavones, in *Bioprocesses and Biotechnology for Functional Foods and Nutraceuticals*, Neeser, J.R. and German, J.B., Eds., Marcel Dekker, New York, 2003, pp. 207–224.

29. Kimira, M., Arai, Y., Shimoi, K., and Watanabe, S., Japanese intake of flavonoids and isoflavonoids from foods, *J. Epidemiol.,* 8, 168–175, 1998.

30. Yamamoto, S., Sobue, T., Sakasi, S., Kobayashi, M., Arai, Y., Uehara, M., Adlercreutz, H., Watanabe, S., Takahashi, T., Iitoi, Y., Iwase, Y., Akabane, M., and Tsugane, S., Validity and reproducibility of a self-administered food-frequency questionnaire to assess isoflavone intake in a Japanese population in comparison with dietary records and blood and urine isoflavones, *J. Nutr.,* 131, 2741–2747, 2001.

31. Zhuo, X.G., Melby, M.K., and Watanabe, S., Soy isoflavone intake lowers serum LDL cholesterol: a meta-analysis of 8 randomized controlled trials in humans, *J. Nutr.,* 134, 2395–2400, 2004.

32. Tsugane, S., Gotlieb, S.L., Laurenti, R., Souza, J.M., and Watanabe, S., Mortality and cause of death among first-generation Japanese in Sao Paulo, Brazil, *Int. J. Epidemiol.,* 18, 647–651, 1989.

33. Duncan, A.M., Merz-Demolow, B.E., Xu, X., Phipps, W.R., and Kurzer, M.S., Premenopausal equol excretors show plasma hormone profiles associated with lowered risk of breast cancer, *Cancer Epidemiol. Biomarkers Prev.,* 9, 581–586, 2000.

34. Haba, R., Watanabe, S., Arai, Y., Chiba, H., and Miura, T., Suppression of lipid-hydroperoxide and DNA-adduct formation by isoflavone-containing soy hypocotyls tea in rats. *Environ. Health Prev. Med.,* 7, 64–73, 2002.

35. Xu, X., Harris, K.S., Wang, H.J., Murphy, P.A., and Hendrich, S., Bioavailability of soybean isoflavones depends upon gut microflora in women, *J. Nutr.,* 125, 2307–2315, 1995.

36. Tsukamoto, C., Shimada, S., Igita, K., Kudou, S., Kokubun, M., Ohubo, K., and Kitamura, K., Factors affecting isoflavone content in soybean seeds. Changes in isoflavones, saponins, and composition of fatty acids at different temperatures during seed development, *J. Agric. Food Chem.,* 43, 1184–1192, 1995.

37. Xu, W.H., Zheng, W., Xiang, Y.B., Ruan, Z.X., Cheng, J.R., Dai, Q., Gao, Y.T., and Shu, X.O., Soya food intake and risk of endometrial cancer among Chinese women in Shanghai: population-based case-control study, *Br. Med. J.,* 328, 1285, 2004.

38. Setchell, K.D., Brown, N.M., Desai, P., Zimmer-Nechemias, L., Wolfe, B.E., Brashear, W.T., Kirschner, A.S., Cassidy, A., and Heubi, J.E., Bioavailability of pure isoflavones in healthy humans and analysis of commercial soy isoflavone supplements, *J. Nutr.,* 131(Suppl. 4), 1362S–1375S, 2001.

39. Kritz-Silverstein, D. and Goodman-Gruen, D.L., Usual dietary isoflavone intake, bone mineral density, and bone metabolism in postmenopausal women, *J. Womens Health Gend. Based Med.,* 11(1), 69–78, 2002.

40. Watanabe, S., Yamaguchi, M., Sobue, T., Takahashi, T., Miura, T., Arai, Y., Mazur, W., Wahala, K., and Adlercreutz, H., Pharmacokinetics of soybean isoflavones in plasma, urine and feces of men after ingestion of 60 g baked soybean powder (kinako), *J. Nutr.,* 128, 1710–1715, 1998.

41. Adlercreutz, H., Markkanen, H., and Watanabe, S., Plasma concentrations of phytooestrogens in Japanese men, *Lancet,* 342, 1209–1210, 1993.

42. King, R.A. and Bursill, D.B., Plasma and urinary kinetics of the isoflavones aidzein and genistein after a single soy meal in humans, *Am. J. Clin. Nutr.,* 67, 867–872, 1998.

43. Weggemans, R.M. and Trautwein, E.A., Relation between soy-associated isoflavones and LDL and HDL cholesterol concentrations in humans: a meta-analysis, *Eur. J. Clin. Nutr.,* 57(8), 940–946, 2003.

44. Kumar, N.B., Cantor, A., Allen, K., Riccardi, D., Besterman-Dahan, K., Seigne, J., Helal, M., Salup, R., and Pow-Sang, J., The specific role of isoflavones in reducing prostate cancer risk, *Prostate,* 59(2), 141–147, 2004.

45. Ingram, D., Sanders, K., Kolybaba, M., and Lopez, D., Case-control study of phyto-oestrogens and breast cancer, *Lancet,* 350, 990–994, 1997.

46. Scheiber, M.D., Liu, J.H., Subbiah, M.T., Rebar, R.W., and Setchell, K.D., Dietary inclusion of whole soy foods results in significant reductions in clinical risk factors for osteoporosis and cardiovascular disease in normal postmenopausal women, *Menopause,* 8, 384–392, 2001.

47. Adlercreutz, H., Yamada, T., Wahala, K., and Watanabe, S., Maternal and neonatal phytoestrogens in Japanese women during birth, *Am. J. Obstet. Gynecol.,* 180, 737–743, 1999.

48. Djuric, Z., Chen, G., Doerge, D.R., Heilbrun, L.K., and Kucuk, O., Effect of soy isoflavone supplementation on markers of oxidative stress in men and women, *Cancer Lett.,* 172(1), 1–6, 2001.

# 6 Soy for "Health for All": Message from WHO CARDIAC Study and Dietary Intervention Studies

*Yukio Yamori*

## CONTENTS

## 6.1 INTRODUCTION

Soy and soy products, traditionally eaten in Asian countries, are now being proved to contribute to the health of mankind worldwide, particularly of the Japanese, who are enjoying nearly the longest life expectancy in the world. The average life expectancies of Japanese men and women have reached over 78 and 85, respectively. As will be described in detail below, aging in humans depends on the aging process of blood vessels. We believe soy intakes may affect the aging process because we found experimentally that soy intake can prevent stroke, the most common age-related cerebrovascular disease.

In this review, the effect of soy diets on stroke prevention first proven in rat models of hypertension and stroke is briefly introduced. Second, a World Health Organization (WHO)-coordinated worldwide study of nutrition and cardiovascular diseases (CVDs), which was based on the experimental studies in rat models, is summarized with a special emphasis on the major findings on CVD risk factors and their gender differences. Third, we discuss the geographic differences in the menopausal increase of CVD risk factors, suggestive of the importance of soy intakes in women's health. Fourth, we describe the epidemiology of soy intakes in relation to CVD risk factors in China and Japan as well as in Okinawan immigrants. Fifth, the implication of dietary soy and phytoestrogen intakes are reviewed in association with health and are highlighted in the relationship of 24-h urinary isoflavone excretions with differences in CVD and cancer mortalities in worldwide populations. Finally, our ongoing dietary intervention studies by the supplementation of soy protein and isoflavones are summarized to demonstrate the prospectives of daily soy intakes for CVD and life-style-related disease prevention.

## 6.2 EXPERIMENTAL EVIDENCE FOR CVD PREVENTION BY SOY INTAKES

I dedicated myself to pathology in the early days of my research life and succeeded establishing a unique rat model for strokes, stroke-prone spontaneously hypertensive rats (SHRSPs)[1,2] with my mentor, the late Professor Kozo Okamoto, from spontaneously hypertensive rats (SHRs).[3] SHRSPs develop cerebral hemorrhage or infarction genetically, without exception. Since SHRSPs develop severe hypertension and stroke genetically, they are the best models so far for the analyses of genes related to hypertension and stroke.[4–6] Various loci are related to hypertension, and some genes are involved in environmental factor–induced hypertension such as stress-sensitive and salt-sensitive genes on chromosomes 1[7] and 10,[6] respectively. Therefore, there is hope for us to prevent hypertension by controlling environmental factors, particularly nutrition.

We learned much from our extensive nutritional experiments about how stroke could be prevented by nutrition.[8–10] Among extensive experimental studies in SHRSP previously reviewed,[11] one series of experiments on the preventive effect of nutrition is summarized here. The survival rates of SHRSP were the worst and they all died before 100 d of age when fed an excess-salt diet, 1% salt in drinking water. Their survival rates were much improved due to the prevention of stroke by feeding them diets such as soy-protein-, Ca-, or Mg-fortified diets. The average life spans were up to twice as long, and the diets supplemented with all combined nutrients allowed these rats to survive for four or five times longer than the average survival period of SHRSP on the control excess-salt diet.

## 6.3  MAJOR CVD RISK FACTORS AND GENDER DIFFERENCES

Our worldwide epidemiological study called the WHO CARDIAC (Cardiovascular Diseases and Alimentary Comparison) Study[12,13] has been carried out successfully in 60 populations in 25 countries (Figure 6.1) since I proposed this study to WHO in 1983 by organizing international meetings in Kyoto and Izumo.[14,15]

The aim of this study is to analyze biological markers of diets in various populations in the world on their relationship with blood pressure (BP) and CVD mortalities in "core" and "complete" studies, respectively.[16] About 100 males and 100 females aged 46 to 58 were randomly selected from each population, for weight and height measurements, and BP was taken by an automated system. Blood tests, 24-h urine collection, and medical history interviews including dietary

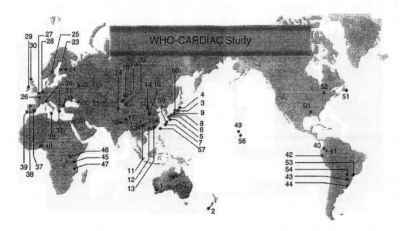

**FIGURE 6.1** Study sites of the WHO CARDIAC Study. The first surveys were carried out in 1985–1995. The underlined populations were followed-up after 1997 as MONALISA (MONEO ALIMENTATIONIS SANAE = Reminding Healthy Nutrition Study). 1. Australia (Perth), 2. New Zealand (Dunedine), 3. Japan (Toyama), 4. Japan (Hirosaki), 5. Japan (Beppu), 6. Japan (Kurume), 7. Japan (Naha), 8. Japan (Hiroshima), 9. Japan (Ohda), 10. China (Urumqi), 11. China (Guiyang), 12. China (Guangzhou), 13. China (Guanzhou), 14. China (Beijing), 15. China (Shanghai), 16. China (Shijiazhuang), 17. China (Lhasa), 18. China (Altai), 19. China (Heitan), 20. China (Tulufan), 21. Georgia (Tbilisi), 22. Russia (Moscow), 23. Finland (Kuopio), 24. Finland (Kuopio), 25. Sweden (Goetheborg), 26. France (Orleans), 27. Belgium (Leuven), 28. Belgium (Ghent), 29. U.K. (Belfast), 30. United Kingdom (Stornoway), 31. Bulgaria (Sofia, urban), 32. Bulgaria (Sofia, rural), 33. Greece (Athens), 34. Italy (Milan), 35. Italy (Palermo), 36. Israel (Tel Aviv), 37. Spain (Navas), 38. Spain (Madrid), 39. Portugal (Lisbon), 40. Ecuador (Quito), 41. Ecuador (Vircavamba), 42. Ecuador (Manta), 43. Brazil (Uruguaiana), 44. Brazil (Baje), 45. Tanzania (Handeni), 46. Tanzania (Shinya), 47. Tanzania (Dar es Salaam), 48. Nigeria (Ibadan), 49. United States (Honolulu), 50. United States (Jackson), 51. Canada (St. John), 52. Canada (Montreal), 53. Brazil (Sao Paulo), 54. Brazil (Campo Grande), 55. Nepal (Namche Bazar), 56. United States (Hilo), 57. China (Taipei), 58. China (Huaxi), 59. Japan (Nago), 60. Japan (Amino).

habits were conducted of over 14,000 participants over the past 18 years. We are now re-examining the populations for the second survey over 10 years after the first survey.

Our worldwide health examination and the follow-up examination are now confirming that obesity is a common expanding health problem even in developing countries. Obese people are increasing in number and ratio, such as in Dar es Salaam, the urbanized capital of Tanzania. We revisited Dar es Salaam to monitor CVD risks and found that obesity had increased to over 50% of women in their fifties during the period from the fist survey in 1987 to the second survey in 1998, and hypertension had concomitantly increased to over 50%.[17] The CARDIAC Study demonstrated that obesity was the major risk factor of hypertension, both in males and females. Body mass index was significantly positively related to both systolic and diastolic BP.[16,18]

In contrast, among the nomadic population of Masai living in Tanzania, there were apparently no obese men, and our first health survey of them in 1987 demonstrated that the prevalence of hypertension was very low. BP was examined by an automated system introduced into the CARDIAC Study. They used no salt at the time of the first survey in 1987, but started to use salt by the second survey in 1998, and the prevalence of hypertension increased up to 12% for those aged 48 to 56, still lower than the world average of 20%.[17]

For our worldwide study, we successfully collected 24-h urine by using a special urine container, called an Aliquot cup to sample one fortieth of all voided urine.[19,20] Dietary intake of salt confirmed by 24-h Na excretion was very high, for example, in Tibet, where our health examination in 1986 confirmed their high daily salt intake of 17 g on average and their high prevalence of hypertension (over 40%).

The WHO CARDIAC Study confirmed that both systolic and diastolic BP is positively related to Na excretion in 24-h urine.[16] Therefore, the mortality rates from stroke were significantly positively related with 24-h urinary salt excretion and with urinary Na/K ratios.[16] These data support that the reduction of daily salt intake down to 6 g, as recommended by WHO, or 7 g as recommended by the Japanese Hypertension Society should greatly contribute to the prevention of stroke. By decreasing our present salt intake about 12 g/d in Japan to as low as 6 or 7 g/d we would be able to reduce stroke mortality to nearly 0 and the morbidity of dementia and bed-ridden disability by nearly a half, because stroke is estimated to cause half of these diseases in Japan.

We noted also a gender difference in the relationship between stroke mortality and 24-h urinary salt excretion. As indicated in Figure 6.2, the adverse effect of excess salt intake is greater in men than in women, indicating protective effects of female sex hormones on stroke mortality.

Unfortunately, urbanization increases salt intake and elevates serum cholesterol levels worldwide. Age-adjusted mortality rates from coronary heart diseases (CHD) are strongly positively related with serum total cholesterol levels.[16] If we look carefully at the relation between serum cholesterol levels and CHD mortality rates, the rate of French people (examined in Orleans) was very low despite their high cholesterol level: 230 mg/dl on average. In contrast, Scottish and Irish people with relatively lower serum cholesterol levels, 210 mg/dl, close to the upper level

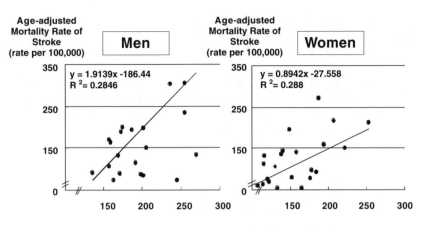

**FIGURE 6.2** Gender difference in the association between age-adjusted mortality rates from stroke and 24-h urinary sodium (Na) excretion. Men are more salt-sensitive than women.

of the Japanese, suffer from CHD in a high prevalence as indicated by their nearly highest mortality rates in Europe.[21] This discrepancy is called the French paradox and is often ascribed to the beneficial effect of polyphenols in red wine, but we noted that Frence people get more antioxidants, not only from red wine but also from vegetables and fruits, than Scottish people.

We further noted marked gender differences in the association of cholesterol levels with the mortality rates from CHD, as shown in Figure 6.3.[16] The risk is

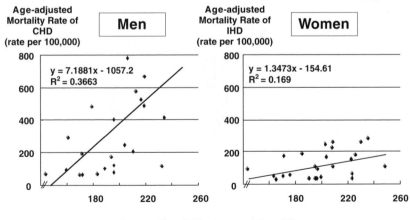

**FIGURE 6.3** Gender difference in the association between coronary heart diseases (CHD) and serum total cholesterol. Men are more vulnerable to CHD than women even when serum cholesterol levels are similar.

far greater in males than in females. The level of 220 mg/dl is the cut point for hypercholesterolemia in Japan, and this level corresponds to the CHD mortality rate of 600/100,000 in males, four times greater than the mortality rate of 150/100,000 in females.

Therefore, in our CARDIAC Study populations, there were big gender differences in CHD mortality rates. The rates in females were about 30 to 40% of those in males in various countries examined, with the highest rate in Scotland and the lowest in Japan.[16] This indicates that female sex hormones may be protective against atherosclerosis, the major cause of CHD.

## 6.4  WOMEN'S HEALTH AND SOY ISOFLAVONES WITH ESTROGENIC ACTIVITY

Since our study populations include both pre- and postmenopausal women, we noted that changes in CVD risks such as blood pressure during menopause were not significant in populations in Japan and China, where soybeans are commonly consumed, in contrast to other populations, where soybeans are not eaten (Figure 6.4). Therefore, we became interested in soybean isoflavones, typical diet-derived phytoestrogens. The Japanese get 18 mg of isoflavones a day from tofu, bean card, fermented soybeans, and other soy products (Figure 6.5). In order to test the effect of isoflavones, we first observed that BP increase after ovariectomy was attenuated by soybean– or isoflavone (daidzein)–supplemented diets in SHRSP.[22] Since acetylcholine-induced endothelium-dependent vasodilatation was

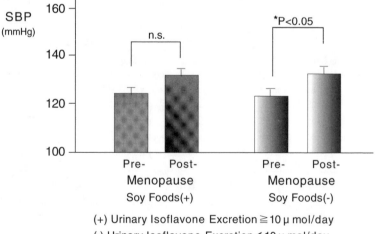

(+) Urinary Isoflavone Excretion $\geqq 10\,\mu$ mol/day
(-) Urinary Isoflavone Excretion $< 10\,\mu$ mol/day

**FIGURE 6.4** Menopausal changes in systolic blood pressure (SBP) of CARDIAC Study population where soy food is common (+) or not (−). Whether soy food is common or not is defined according to 24-h urinary isoflavone excretion more than (or equal to) 10 μ moles or less. SBP rises significantly at menopause where soy food is not common.

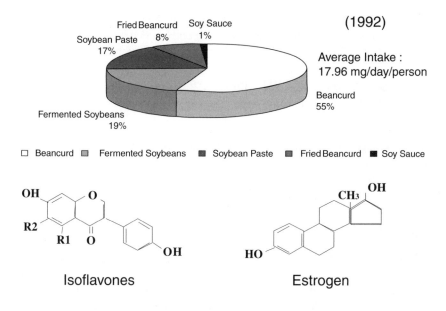

**FIGURE 6.5** Food sources of isoflavones and the average daily isoflavone intake of the Japanese (1992) and chemical structure of isoflavones compared with estrogen. The Japanese get about 18 mg of isoflavones per day in average from bean curd, fermented soy bean, soy bean paste, etc.

improved by feeding daidzein-supplemented diets in the aortic ring of ovariecto-mized SHRSP,[23] we assayed the metabolites of nitro-oxide (NO), which were maintained high by daidzein supplementation at the level of sham-operated rats or became even higher by soybean feeding, although the marked reduction was noted in ovariectomized rats.[23]

We further demonstrated that NO synthesis was accelerated by detecting the increased mRNA expression of the NO synthase (NOS) gene in the aorta from daidzein-treated SHRSP compared with the controls, indicating that dietary isofla-vones like estrogen upregulate NO synthesis through gene expression. We further observed by counting cell numbers, as well as by checking tritiated thimidine incorporation into DNA, that the aglycones of isoflavones such as genistein, daidzein, and glycitein decreased the proliferation of cultured vascular smooth muscle cells (VSMC) from SHRSP.[24] The growth inhibition of VSMC is supposed to be due to the inhibition of tyrosine phosphorylation or through NO production by isoflavones, and we can conclude that isoflavones affect blood vessels func-tionally by accelerating NO synthesis and structurally by attenuating VSMC proliferation for reducing CVD. Since NO is converted into peroxinitrile by oxygen radicals, antioxidants are important in increasing the bioavailability of NO in vascular walls.

As for soy isoflavone and protein effects on cholesterol metabolism reviewed[25] so far, soy protein interrupts intestinal absorption of bile acids and dietary cholesterol in animal experiments, and soy isoflavones may activate low-density lipoprotein (LDL) receptor mRNA expression, thus decreasing LDL levels in the blood and resulting in the regression or prevention of atherogenic vascular lesions.

## 6.5 SOY DIETS AND CVD RISKS IN IMMIGRANT STUDIES

Our WHO CARDIAC Study has shown that eating soybeans or soy products daily is related to the longevity of the Japanese, particularly Okinawans, who enjoy the longest life spans in Japan and thus in the world. Their traditional diet includes eating tofu, a typical soy product, daily together with vegetables containing antioxidants. Okinawans eat low salt diets and low fat pork together with a lot of seaweed, which is good for reducing cholesterol.[26]

The effect of Westernization on Japanese longevity can be demonstrated by our immigrant studies on Okinawans living in Okinawa, Hawaii, and Brazil. Although Okinawans enjoyed the longest life expectancy in 1990s, people of Okinawan descent in Brazil lived 17 years less on average. In contrast, Okinawans living in Hawaii reached the longest life expectancy of today's Japanese.

The CARDIAC Study has confirmed that Okinawans living in Hawaii still eat a lot of soy products and traditional Okinawan vegetables rich in antioxidants, fish, and seaweed. Since their salt intake was reduced to 6 g/d in the elderly, stroke mortality as well as dementia were decreased in Hawaii, and these dietary customs appeared to contribute to their healthy long life. However, Japanese immigrants living in Brazil have been strongly influenced by Western dietary customs like eating a lot of beef, called *chulasco*, with excessive rock salt on it. CVD risk factors such as hypertension, hypercholesterolemia, obesity, and diabetes, the "deadly quartet," were higher in Japanese immigrants in Brazil than in Japanese living in Japan resulting in the 17-year difference in life span.

Moreover, the rate of diabetes, shown by high glycohemoglobin levels, was markedly increased in Japanese immigrants in Brazil. One out of four or five showed high glycohemoglobin levels, while the prevalences of hyperglycemia based on the same criteria were still low in Okinawa and Hawaii, less than 10% in males and females, indicating that the Japanese are vulnerable to diabetes because of the extreme Westernization of dietary custom.

The differences in soy and fish intakes were demonstrated in Japanese immigrants, particularly in Brazil, by measuring 24-h urinary isoflavone or taurine excretions as the biomarkers of the dietary intake of soy products or fish and measuring the percentage of n-3 fatty acids in plasma phospholipids as the marker of fish consumption. They eat fish once every 2 weeks in Campo Grande but four and two times a week in Okinawa and Hawaii, respectively. n-3 fatty acids in plasma phospholipids were concomitantly decreased with the reduction in fish intake, less than 3% in Campo Grande, Brazil, compared to over 6% in Japanese living in Japan.

The CARDIAC Study first demonstrated worldwide that CHD mortality rates were inversely related to n-3 fatty acid ratios in plasma phospholipids, indicating the preventive effect of fish oil on CHD.[16]

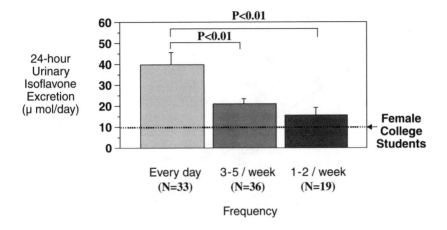

**FIGURE 6.6** Twenty-four-hour urinary isoflavone excretion in relation to the frequency of soy product intake in the Japanese. The average of 250 Japanese female college students, 10 μ mol/d indicates that young Japanese females eat soy products less than one or two times a week.

Although abundant soybeans are produced in Brazil, soy products are mainly used for feeding cattle. Correspondingly, isoflavone excretion of 24-h urine was remarkably decreased, less than 10 μ mol/d in Brazilian descendants of Okinawans in their fifties, far less than 30 to 40 μ mol/d in Okinawans living in Okinawa.

As shown in Figure 6.6, the frequency of soy product intake is closely related to 24-h urinary excretion of isoflavones, indicating that Okinawans in Okinawa eat soy products almost every day, but Japanese immigrants in Brazil eat soy products less than one or two times a week on average.

## 6.6 CORRELATION BETWEEN SOY ISOFLAVONES AND CVD AND LIFE-STYLE-RELATED DISEASES

The age-adjusted mortality rates from CHD were proven by the WHO-CARDIAC Study to be significantly inversely related with 24-h urinary isoflavone excretion (Figure 6.7).[26] The lower CHD mortality in the Japanese and Chinese can therefore be ascribed to the high consumption of soybean products. Data analysis of urinary isoflavone excretion in relation to daily isoflavone intake suggests that a daily intake of 50 mg of isoflavone may be effective in maintaining urinary isoflavone levels enough for preventing CHD. This corresponds to the amount in 100 g of tofu, 50 g of fermented soybeans, or 20 g of soy powder. In contrast, Scottish and Irish people, who do not eat soybeans, show the lowest isoflavone excretion and the highest CHD mortality.

The benefit of soybean intake is not limited to the reduction of CHD risks. Although genetic factors are involved in CHD and other life-style-related diseases

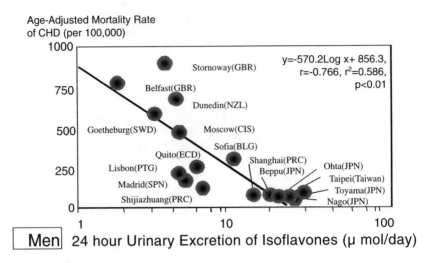

**FIGURE 6.7** Association between age-adjusted coronary heart disease (CHD) mortality and 24-h urinary excretion of isoflavones. The CHD mortality rates are low in Japan and China, where soybean products are commonly eaten and urinary isoflavone excretion exceeds 10 μ mol/d.

such as osteoporosis and some types of cancers, nutritional influence has been observed epidemiologically and experimentally in relation to soybean intakes.

The beneficial effect of isoflavones on bone metabolism was confirmed since significant reductions in urinary pyridinoline and deoxypyridinoline excretions, the markers of bone resorption were observed concomitantly with increased urinary isoflavone excretion in Japanese immigrants in Brazil given isoflavone during the intervention study.[27] The beneficial metabolic effect of isoflavone intake was further confirmed in menopausal Japanese women.[28,29] Daily administration of the higher doses of isoflavones (100 mg/d for 6 months) not only suppressed bone resorption but increased bone density detected by DEXA.[30] Isoflavone excretion in 24-h urine was positively related with bone density corresponding to calcium content in Japanese women over 70 years old in Hilo, Hawaii, indicating that the weak estrogen-like activity of isoflavones improved Ca metabolism of the bones in postmenopausal women.[31] These data indicate that soy isoflavones can prevent osteoporosis by reducing bone resorption in menopausal women.

The Western life-style is related to increases in mortality from prostate and breast cancers, which used to be very low in Japan but are now increasing. They are also increasing in Japanese immigrants in the United States. The CARDIAC Study demonstrated a significant inverse relationship between urinary isoflavone excretion and the age-adjusted mortality rates from prostate cancer, high in Western countries but very low in Asian countries.[26] Isoflavones with weak estrogenic activity have an inhibitory effect on the excessive proliferation of prostate cancer.

A similar inverse relationship was observed between urinary isoflavone excretion and age-adjusted mortality rates from breast cancer.[26] The mortality rate is the lowest in Okinawa, where a lot of tofu is consumed daily and urinary isoflavone excretion is the highest in women so far examined worldwide. The beneficial effect of isoflavones on breast cancer can be explained by the estrogen receptor occupancy with isoflavones, which blocks the strong effect of estrogen causing breast cancer. The similar blocking action of isoflavones is being observed in cultured human breast cancer cells exposed to endocrine disrupters, which accelerate the growth of cancer cells.[32]

Therefore, isoflavones may have inhibitory effects on the growth of cancers at all sites because of a significant inverse relationship between urinary isoflavone excretion and the age-adjusted mortality rates from cancers at all sites.[26] This beneficial effect of isoflavones can be explained by their inhibitory effect on angiogenesis, which is essential for the growth and metastasis of cancer cells.[33]

Isoflavone excretion in 24-h urine is a reliable biomarker of soybean intake, since the frequency of soy product intake is associated with the excretion. We divided our participants of the WHO CARDIAC health survey into soybean eaters and noneaters by the level of 10 μ moles isoflavone excretion in 24-h urine. The results clearly indicate that soybean eaters have lower CVD risks such as obesity, and hypertension and hypercholesterolemia in males.[18] In addition, the worldwide CARDIAC Study populations were divided into fish eaters and noneaters by the level of 1000 and 800 μ mole taurine excretion in 24-h urine samples in males and females, respectively. The results indicate fish eaters have lower CVD risks such as obesity, hypertension, and hypercholesterolemia.[18] Since fish and soybean eaters are usually rice eaters like the Japanese and Chinese, CVD risk factors such as obesity and hypercholesterolemia and the mortality rates from CHD are definitely lower in rice eaters.

## 6.7 NUTRITIONAL INTERVENTION BY SOY PROTEIN AND ISOFLAVONES

The WHO CARDIAC Study indicated the beneficial effect of dietary soy protein and isoflavones on CVD, osteoporosis, prostate, and breast and other cancers; and the intake of soy nutrients was confirmed to be very low in Western countries, particularly in Scotland, where soybeans are not customarily eaten.

In order to help Scottish people eat soy and fish, we asked a local bakery to bake four kinds of special breads, one containing 2 g of docosahexaenoic acid (DHA) rich in fish oil, another containing 25 g of soy protein, the third containing both, and the forth containing none as a placebo. Then we carried out an intervention study for 260 Scottish men and women initially with slightly high risks of CHD by giving them these breads for 4 weeks. When their average urinary isoflavone excretion increased up to two times, their BP as well as LDL cholesterol levels were significantly reduced in the isoflavone group.[21] We carried out a similar intervention study of Japanese immigrants living in Campo Grande, Brazil, where the prevalence of hypertension and hypercholesterolemia were further increased compared with the first survey in 1992.

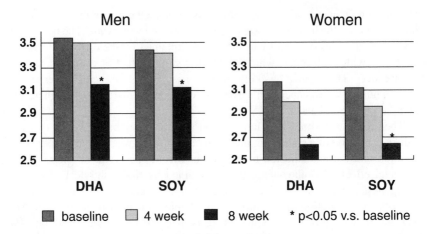

FIGURE 6.8 Effect of daily intake of DHA (2 g) and soy protein (25 g) in breads on atherogenic index (AI). AI is calculated as the ratio of non-HDL cholesterol (total cholesterol − HDL cholesterol) divided by HDL cholesterol, high in men, reduced down to the lower women's level after an 8-week intervention.

Since the U.S. Food and Drug Administration approved the health claim of soy protein intake over 25 g/d being beneficial for reducing CHD risks in October 1999, in 2000 we started an intervention study of Japanese men and women aged 45 to 59 with relatively higher risks of CHD. We offered special breads containing 25 g of soy protein or 2 g of DHA daily for 4 to 8 weeks. We noted significant reductions in BP, both in males and females.[34] Moreover, atherogenic indices, the ratio of LDL to high-density lipoprotein (HDL) cholesterol, decreased in males and females, indicating that regular fish and soybean intake may prevent CHD (Figure 6.8).

Gender difference in average life spans, nearly 7 years longer in females than in males in Japan, is supposed to be due to the difference in the higher initial atherogenic indices in males than in females. A definite reduction of the atherogenic index (AI) in males down to the level in females as a result of taking soybean protein and fish oil for 8 weeks may correspond to the 7-year prolongation of average life expectancy if soy protein or DHA supplementation is continued life long.

All our epidemiological and intervention studies in humans have indicated that genetic–environmental interaction is important in the development of common life-style-related diseases including some types of cancers. We further confirmed that Japanese lunches containing less salt, more vegetables, more fish, and more soybean products were effective in Japanese workers with relatively higher risks of CVD. These healthy lunches eaten daily for 4 weeks significantly decreased the AI and LDL to HDL cholesterol ratios, indicating the important role food companies have in the production of easily available healthy food to promote health for all in the world.

## 6.8 CONCLUSIONS

Our experimental and epidemiological studies, particularly intervention studies in animal models and humans, clearly indicated the importance of soy nutrients in the prevention of stroke and CHD, and probably all types of cancers, since nutritional factors such as isoflavones can modify gene expression as demonstrated by our animal experiments. Hypertension and hypercholesterolemia are the major risks for stroke, including vascular dementia, and CHD, respecively. Excess intakes of salt, cholesterol, and animal fat and obesity are nutrition-related risk factors. In contrast, there are also protective nutritional factors such as K, Ca, Mg, dietary fibers, protein, amino acids such as taurine, and fatty acids such as DHA-3 and antioxidants. Our recent study as reported here indicates that isoflavones and soybeans functionally and structurally affect blood vessels, inhibit thrombosis, and improve lipid metabolism, thus contributing to CVD prevention. Isoflavones may also contribute to the prevention of osteoporosis, prostate and breast cancers, and other types of cancer and may improve quality of life in the elderly for realizing healthy longevity.

## REFERENCES

1. Okamoto, K., Yamori, Y., and Nagaoka, A., Establishment of the stroke-prone spontaneously hypertensive rat (SHR), *Circ. Res.,* 34/35(Suppl.1), 143–153, 1974.
2. Yamori, Y., The stroke-prone spontaneously hypertensive rat: contribution to risk factor analysis and prevention of hypertensive diseases, in *Handbook of Hypertension,* Vol. 4, *Experimental and Genetic Models of Hypertension,* De Jong, W., Ed., Elsevier, Amsterdam, 1984, pp. 99, 240–255.
3. Okamoto, K. and Aoki, K., Development of a strain of spontaneously hypertensive rats, *Jpn. Circ. J.,* 27, 282–293, 1963.
4. Nara, Y., Nabika, T., Ikeda, K., Sawamura, M., Endo, J., and Yamori, Y., Blood pressure cosegregates with a microsatellite of anagiotensin coverting enzyme (ACE) in F2 generation from a cross between original normotensive Wistar-Kyoto rats (WKY) and stroke-prone spontaneously hypertensive rats (SHRSP), *Biochem. Biophys. Res. Commun.,* 181, 941–946, 1991.
5. Hilbert, P., Lindpainter, K., Beckmann, J.S., Serizawa, T., Soubrier, F., Dubay, C., Cartwright, P., De-Gouyon, B., Julier, C., and Takahasi, S., Chromosomal mapping of two genetic loci associated with blood pressure regulation in hereditary hypertensive rats, *Nature,* 353, 521–528, 1991.
6. Jacob, H., Lindpainter, J., Lincolin, S.E., Kusumi, K., Bunker, R.K., Mao, Y.P., Ganten, D., Dzau, VJ., and Lander, E.S., Genetic mapping of a gene casing hypertension in the stroke-prone spontaneously hypertensive rat, *Cell,* 27, 213–224, 1991.
7. Cui, Z.H., Ikeda, K., Kawakami, K., Gonda, T., Masuda, J., and Nabika, T., Exaggerated response to cold stress in a congenic strain for the quantitive trait locus for blood pressure, *J. Hypertens.,* 22, 2103–2109, 2004.
8. Yamori, Y., Horie, R., Ikeda, K., Nara, Y., and Lovenberg, W., Prophylactic effect of dietary protein on stroke and its mechanisms, in *Prophylactic Approach to Hypertensive Diseases,* Yamori, Y., Lovenberg, W., and Freis, E.D., Eds., Raven Press, New York, 1979, pp. 497–504.

9. Yamori, Y., Environmental influence on the development of hypertensive vascular diseases in SHR and related models and their relation to human diseases, in *New Trends in Arterial Hypertension,* ISERM Symposium No.17, Worcel, M., Bonvalct, J.P., Langer, S.A., Menard, J., and Sasard, J., Eds., Elsevier/North-Holland Biochemical Press, Amsterdam, 1981, pp. 305–320.
10. Yamori, Y., Horie, R., and Nara, Y., Pathogenesis and dietary prevention of cerebrovascular diseases in animal models and epidemiological evidence for the applicability in man, in *Prevention of Cardiovascular Diseases: An Approach to Active Long Life,* Yamori, Y. and Lenfant, C., Eds., Elsevier, Amsterdam, 1987, pp. 163–177.
11. Yamori, Y., Predictive and preventive pathology of cardiovascular diseases, *Acta. Pathol. Jpn.,* 36, 683–705, 1989.
12. WHO Collaborating Center on Primary Prevention of Cardiovascular Diseases, Izumo, Japan and Cardiovascular Diseases Unit. *CARDIAC (Cardiovascular Diseases and Alimentary Comparison) Study Protocol and Manual of Operations,* WHO, Geneva, 1986.
13. Yamori, Y., Nara, Y., Mizushima, S. et al., International cooperative study on the relationship between dietary factors and blood pressure: a report from the cardiovascular diseases and alimentary comparison study, *J. Cardiovasc. Pharmacol.,* 16, S43–S47, 1990.
14. Lovenberg, W. and Yamori, Y., Eds., *Nutritional Prevention of Cardiovascular Disease,* Academic Press, Orlando, 1984.
15. Yamori, Y. and Lenfant, C., Eds., *Prevention of Cardiovascular Diseases: An Approach to Active Long Life,* Excerpta Medica, Amsterdam, 1987.
16. Yamori, Y., Mizushima, S., Sawamura, M., and Nara, Y., Nutritional factors for hypertension and major cardiovascular diseases: international cooperative studies for dietary prevention, *Dtsch. Med. Wochenschr.,* 15, 1825–1841, 1994 (in Japanese).
17. Njelekela, M., Negishi., H., Nara, Y., Miki, T., Kuga, S., Noguchi, T., Kanda, T., Yamori, M, Mashalla, Y., Liu L., Mtabaji, J., Ikeda, K., and Yamori., Y., Cardiovascular risk factors in Tanzania, *Acta Trop.,* 79, 231–239, 2001.
18. Yamori Y., World-wide epidemic of obesity: hope for Japanese diets, *Clin. Exp. Pharmacol. Physiol.,* in press.
19. Yamori, Y., Nara, Y., Kihara, M., Mano, M., and Horie, R., Simple method for sampling consecutive 24-hour urine for epidemiological and clinical studies., *Clin. Exp. Hypertens.,* 1161–1167, 1984.
20. Nara, Y., Kihara, M., Mano, W., Horie, R., and Yamori, Y., 'Aliquot Cups': simple method for collecting consecutive 24-hour urine samples for epidemiological and clinical studies, in *Nutritional Prevention of Cardiovascular Disease,* Lovenberg, W. and Yamori, Y., Eds., Academic Press, Orlando, 1984.
21. Sagara, M., Kanda, T., Njelekela, M. et al., Effects of dietary intake of soy protein and isoflavones on cardiovascular diseases risk factors in high risk, middle-aged men in Scotland: cardiovascular risk reduction by soy, *J. Am. Coll. Nutr.,* 23, 85–91, 2003.
22. Teramoto, T., Fukui, Y., Ikeda, K., and Yamori, Y., Soy isoflavones attenuate ovariectomy-induced bone loss in stroke-prone spontaneously hypertensive rats (SHRSP). *J. Clin. Biochem. Nutr.,* 28, 15–20, 2000.
23. Xing, A.S., Pan, W., Ikeda, K., Takebe, M., Noguchi, T., and Yamori, Y., Effect of fermented soy bean extract on blood pressure in SHRSP rat. 10th International Symposium on SHR and Molecular Medicine, Berlin-Buch, May 2–4, 2001.

24. Pan, W., Ikeda, K., Takebe M., and Yamori, Y., Genistein, daidzein and glycitein inhibit growth and DNA synthesis of aortic smooth muscle cells from stroke-prone spontaneously hypertensive rats, *J. Nutr.,* 131, 1154–1158, 2001.
25. Potter, S.M., Soy protein and cardiovascular disease: the impact of bioactive components in soy, *Nutr. Rev.,* 56, 231–235, 1998.
26. Yamori, Y., Miura, A., and Taira, K., Implication from and for food cultures for cardiovascular diseases: Japanese food, particularly Okinawan diets, *Asia Pac. J. Clin. Nutr.,* 10, 144–145, 2001.
27. Yamori, Y., Moriguchi, E., Teramoto, T., Miura, A., Fukui, Y., Honda, K., Fukui, M., Nara, Y., Taira, K., and Moriguchi, Y., Soybean isoflavones reduce postmenopausal bone resorption in female Japanese immigrants in Brazil: a ten-week study, *J. Am. Coll. Nutr.,* 21, 560–563, 2002.
28. Uesugi, T., Fukui, Y., and Yamori, Y., Beneficial effects of soybean isoflavone supplementation on bone metabolism and serum lipids in postmenopausal Japanese women: a four-week study, *J. Am. Coll. Nutr.,* 21, 97–102, 2002.
29. Mori, M., Aizawa, T., Tokoro, M., Miki, T., and Yamori, Y., Soy isoflavone tablets reduce osteoporosis risk factors and obesity in middle-aged Japanese women, in press.
30. Mori, M., Sagara, M., Ikeda, K., Miki, T., and Yamori, Y., Soy isoflavones improve bone metabolism in postmenopausal Japanese women, in press.
31. Yamori, Y., Soy beans for health in the world: lessons from Okinawan diets and health longevity by WHO-CARDIAC and immigrants study, in *Proceedings from the Third International Soybean Processing and Utilization Conference, Ibaraki, Japan, Oct. 15–20,* 2000, pp. 196–198.
32. Yoshida, H., Teramoto, T., Ikeda, K., and Yamori, Y., Supressive effect of isoflavones on proliferation of breast cancer cells induced by nonylphenol and bisphenol A, *Proceedings of the Third International Soybean Processing and Utilization Conference, Ibaraki, Japan, Oct. 15–20, 2000,* pp. 177–178.
33. Fotsis, T., Pepper, M., Adlercreutz, H., Fleischmann, G., Hase, T., Montesano, R., and Schweigerer, L., Genistein, a dietary derived inhibitor of *in vitro* angiogenesis, *Proc. Natl. Acad. Sci. USA,* 90, 2690–2694, 1993.
34. Kanda, T., Sagara, M., Hirao, S., Liu, L., Negishi, H., Akazawa, T., Yoshida, H., Honda, K., Ikeda, K., and Yamori, Y., Soy bean diets decrease cardiovascular risk factors in Japanese immigrants living in Hawaii, in *Proceedings of the Third International Soybean Processing and Utilization Conference, Ibaraki, Japan, Oct. 15–20,* 2000, pp. 199–200.

# 7 Soy Allergy

*Tadashi Ogawa*

## CONTENTS

## 7.1 INTRODUCTION

Food allergy is an abnormal response of the body's immune system to food components. The proportion of patients with food allergies is considered to be increasing to about 10% in the general population in the developed countries. Eggs, milk, legumes (e.g., soybean and peanut), cereals (e.g., wheat and rice), and fish are common allergenic foods. Among them, the prevalence of soybean allergy in Japan is probably around 3% for the general population. However, allergy to soybean is more common in food-allergic children younger than 3 years of age. In countries of the European Union adverse reactions caused by soybean formulas are seen in 14 to 35% of cow's milk–allergic infants. In food-allergic subjects with atopic dermatitis, milk, egg, soybean, peanut, and wheat account for almost 90%

of allergic reactions. Symptoms of food allergies range from a mild response such as atopic dermatitis, gastrointestinal, and respiratory reactions to rare life-threatening reactions such as severe systemic anaphylaxis. Soybean proteins are used, with almost no limits, in food processing as ingredients in processed meats, hamburgers, sausages, infant food, bakery products, pastries, pasta flour, yogurts, and sauces and as flavor enhancers because of their high nutritional quality, processing functionality, and economy. Therefore, it is very difficult for soybean-allergic patients to find safe foods free from allergens in commercially available processed foods.

The allergenicity of soybean resides in the protein fractions, not in soybean oil itself,[1] whereas oxidized soybean oil has been shown to enhance the immunoglobulin E (IgE)-binding ability against soybean or other food proteins.[2] Soybean allergen is mainly protein; therefore, fermented soybean products in which protein constituents are highly hydrolyzed, such as miso (soybean paste), natto (fermented soybean), and shoyu (soy sauce), are considered to be potentially less allergenic than raw soybeans.

Currently, a strict elimination of offending foodstuffs from dishes is generally recommended as a conventional and effective treatment of food allergies. The avoidance of nutritionally fundamental or essential foods in the long term, however, may lead to malnutrition for young patients. There is, therefore, an urgent demand on food scientists to identify the protein components eliciting the allergic manifestation to reduce the allergenicity of soybean products.

In 1934, Duke[3] first pointed out soybean as a possible important source of a food allergy among people taking soymilk formula as a milk substitute. In 1980, a soybean allergen was first demonstrated by Moroz and Yang,[4] using a serum of a worker in laboratory who might be sensitized through the airway. The allergen was isolated and identified as Kunitz type soybean trypsin inhibitor (KSTI). Shibasaki et al.[5] also reported that various allergenic protein components occurred in soybean protein fractions and the IgE antibodies in sera of the soybean-allergic patients showed the cross-reactivity among the 2S-, 7S-, and 11S-globulin fractions by the radioallergo solvent test (RAST) inhibition analyses. However, this method could not characterize the individual protein component responsible for allergic reactions. Shibasaki et al. demonstrated that the most allergenic fractions were the 2S-, 7S-, and 11S- globulin fractions, in this order. Several investigators described the features of soybean allergens, but no detailed information was presented until 1985.

## 7.2 SOYBEAN ALLERGY

### 7.2.1 PREVALENCE, SYMPTOMS, AND THRESHOLD OF SOYBEAN ALLERGY

The prevalence of soybean allergy in the general population has been reported from 1,397 unselected Swedish adults to be about 2% determined by the RAST method.[6] Prevalence increases in patients allergic to egg, milk, fish, wheat, peanuts, and rice to about 10% to 50% in developed countries such as Japan, Poland, Germany, and the United States.[7] In the United States, 28% of food-allergic patients with atopic dermatitis were reported to be soybean positive by a double-blind, placebo-controlled food challenge (DBPCFC) test.[8] About 17% of cow milk–sensitive children are reported to be soybean sensitive as screened by clinical history in Thailand.[9] In Japan, when 86 patients randomly selected according to their case histories (25% of 361 patients diagnosed with food allergies with atopic dermatitis) were examined by RAST, using various allergen discs, the incidence of the positive responses to individual food disks was estimated as follows: egg white (26.7%), soybean (14.0%), wheat (12.7%), milk (11.6%), and rice (8.1%).[10] Regarding the threshold for elicitation of symptoms, Sicherer et al.[11] reported that in about 16% of 196 food-allergic children with atopic dermatitis, the amounts of soybean-inducing symptoms could be estimated at about 500 mg or less under DBPCFC, or 1 g to 8 g of soybean (estimated protein content of 0.3 g to 2.7 g for soybean-allergic children under the DBPFC examination). Sensitization to soybean allergens is known to mainly occur not only through the gastrointestinal tract after ingestion of foods but, in rare cases, through the airway (inhalation and bronchospasm as an occupational or environmental allergy to soybean dust in Barcelona[12]) and skin (occupational contact dermatitis).[13]

### 7.2.2 SOYBEAN ALLERGENS

#### 7.2.2.1 Gly m Bd 30K

The soybean allergenic protein Gly m Bd 30K,[10] which is most strongly and frequently recognized by the IgE antibodies in the sera of soybean-sensitive patients with atopic dermatitis, has been isolated and characterized to be a soybean seed 34-kDa oil-body–associated protein.[14] This protein was first identified by Kalinski et al. from the fractionated soybean oil body membrane, whereas the cDNA was isolated and cloned as a vacuolar storage protein P34 with close homology to thiol proteases classified into a group of the papain superfamily.[15] The primary structure of Gly m Bd 30K has about 30% homology or 54% similarity with Der p 1, a house dust mite allergen that is a thiol protease found in the feces of *Dermatophagoides preronyssius*.[16] The mature P34 vacuolar protein consists of 257 amino acid residues (see Figure 7.1) and is derived by removing part of the N-terminal 122–amino acid residues from a precursor protein with a molecular weight of about 47,000 during maturation in a vacuole.[15] The glycosylation site of Gly m Bd 30K is on the $Asn^{170}$ residue of a mature protein,[17] which consists of mannose, $N$-acetylglucosamine, xylose, and fucose in a molar ratio of 3:2:1:1, respectively, indicating a typical plant asparagine N-linked oligo mannose type glycans with a xylose and fucose branch. The localization of Gly m Bd 30K (P34) in vacuoles of soybean cotyledons was confirmed by an electron microscopic immunostaining technique.[18]

Recently, Helm et al. investigated IgE binding sites (B-cell epitopes) located on Gly m Bd 30K using synthetic peptides and showed that the epitope sites are located on the 3 to 12, 100 to 110, 229 to 238, 299 to 308, and 331 to 340 amino acid residues.[19] All the epitope sites recognized by human IgE antibodies are quite different from those found on a house dust mite allergen, Der p 1 (Figure 7.1). Gly m Bd 30K is specifically associated with a subunit of β-conglycinin through a disulfide linkage. These properties will provide important information

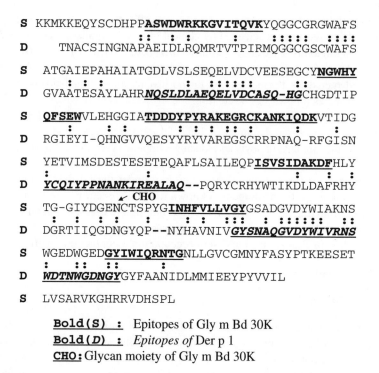

```
S   KKMKKEQYSCDHPPASWDWRKKGVITQVKYQGGCGRGWAFS
              ::    : :        :       :::::  ::::
D      TNACSINGNAPAEIDLRQMRTVTPIRMQGGCGSCWAFS

S   ATGAIEPAHAIATGDLVSLSEQELVDCVEESEGCYNGWHY
         :  :  :            :   ::::::        ::
D   GVAATESAYLAHRNQSLDLAEQELVDCASQ-HGCHGDTIP

S   QFSEWVLEHGGIATDDDYPYRAKEGRCKANKIQDKVTIDG
        :     : : :: :  : :    :
D   RGIEYI-QHNGVVQESYYRYVAREGSCRRPNAQ-RFGISN

S   YETVIMSDESTESETEQAFLSAILEQPISVSIDAKDFHLY
        :                       :    :  :  :
D   YCQIYPPNANKIREALAQ--PQRYCRHYWTIKDLDAFRHY
                    ↙ CHO
S   TG-GIYDGENCTSPYGINHFVLLVGYGSADGVDYWIAKNS
        :  :  : :  :         : :  ::: :  ::::::  ::
D   DGRTIIQGDNGYQP--NYHAVNIVGYSNAQGVDYWIVRNS

S   WGEDWGEDGYIWIQRNTGNLLGVCGMNYFASYPTKEESET
    :    ::    ::        :
D   WDTNWGDNGYGYFAANIDLMMIEEYPYVVIL

S   LVSARVKGHRRVDHSPL
```

**Bold(S) :** Epitopes of Gly m Bd 30K
**Bold(D) :** *Epitopes of* Der p 1
**CHO:** Glycan moiety of Gly m Bd 30K

**FIGURE 7.1** Amino acid sequence alignment between Gly m Bd 30K and Der p 1 and their IgE epitopes.

for developing a hypoallergenic soybean protein isolate (SPI) by biotechnological methods. Furthermore, there are no soybean varieties that lack Gly m Bd 30K in their stock culture. The cDNA was cloned and the recombinant allergen without glycan moiety was prepared from *Escherichia coli*, which could be recognized by sera of soybean-sensitive patients, suggesting that rGly m Bd 30K may be applicable for diagnostic use as an allergen standard of RAST.[20] In addition, the distribution of Gly m Bd 30K as the index of a soybean allergenicity in soybean varieties or soybean products can be selectively determined by the use of monoclonal antibodies (e.g., F5).[21] Okinaka et al. showed that Gly m Bd 30K, namely, P34, is a receptor of syringolide, which is an elicitor produced by *Pseudomonas syringe*, and the P34-elicitor complex probably induces a hypersensitive response through the inhibition of peroxisomal NADH-dependent hydroxypyruvate reductase,[22] suggesting that Gly m Bd 30K might be related to the pathogenesis-related proteins known as plant defense systems.

### 7.2.2.2 Gly m Bd 28K

One of major allergens, Gly m Bd 28K, is a minor protein component in soybean recognized by soybean-sensitive patients with about 25% incidence. It was isolated and purified from 7S-globulin fraction prepared from defatted soybean flakes.[23] The purified allergen is a glycoprotein with the molecular mass of 26 kDa and isoelectric point of 6.1. An Asn-N linked glycan moiety with the same sugar composition as Gly m Bd 30K was identified on the Asn20 residue of Gly m Bd 28K. The N-terminal amino acid sequence analysis gave a result of FHDDEGGDKKSPKSLFMSDSTRVFK-, and no homologous proteins (peptides) could be found in a database of soybean proteins.[23]

In 2001, Tsuji et al.[24] isolated a cDNA clone encoding Gly m Bd 28K. The open reading frame encoded a polypeptide composed of 473 amino acids, and the N-terminal region of this peptide contained the same amino acid sequence as the N-terminal peptide of Gly m Bd 28K with the preceding 21 amino acids. The polypeptide for the cDNA exhibits high homology with the MP27/MP32 proteins in pumpkin seeds and the carrot globulin-like protein, indicating that the protein deduced from this cDNA clone might be converted to Gly m Bd 28K and 23 kDa protein fragment during the development of soybean cotyledonous proteins. In addition, a nucleotide sequence deduced from the N-terminal amino acid sequence[23] was shown to completely coincide with a part of the sequence of a cDNA clone reported from *Glycine max* (GenBank accession no. AI416520), which was assumed to encode a vicilin-like protein similar to that reported for peanuts.[25] When the soybean varieties lacking this 28-kDa allergen were screened in the Japanese stock cultures and imported soybean seeds, about 80% of varieties examined were shown to lack the allergen Gly m Bd 28K. The commercial SPI prepared from defatted soybean flakes, however, was shown to contain this allergenic protein, and the processed foods with SPIs as ingredients also contained Gly m Bd 28K as well as Gly m Bd 30K.[26]

### 7.2.2.3  Gly m Bd 60K (α Subunit of β-Conglycinin)

The other major allergenic protein, which was recognized by about 25% of sera from soybean-sensitive patients with atopic dermatitis, was identified as the α subunit of β-conglycinin.[27] The IgE antibodies recognizing the α subunit showed no cross-reactivity against either the α′ or α subunit of β-conglycinin, which is known to be highly homologous to α subunit. The α subunit of β-conglycinin is a glycoprotein with a molecular weight of 57,000, and with the isoelectric point (pI) of 4.90.[28] The amino acid sequence of the precursor deduced from the cDNA consisted of 543 amino acid residues.[29] The B-cell epitope of patient IgE antibodies was located on the peptide of the 232-383 residue from the N-terminal, which is highly homologous to the peptide sequence of the α subunit of phaseolin, a storage protein of *Phaseolus vulgaris*.[27]

### 7.2.2.4  Other Allergenic Proteins

Soybean low-molecular-weight proteins that Rodrigo et al.[12] identified as allergens eliciting Barcelona asthma by were named Gly m 1.0101 (Gly m 1A) and Gly m 1.0102 (Gly m 1B), which are isoforms with molecular weights of 7500 and 7000, respectively.[30] Their amino acid sequences are well matching to a part of the hydrophobic protein, first reported by Odani et al.,[31] which is synthesized in endocarp on the inner ovary wall and is deposited on the seed surface during development of the soybean.[32] Patients with Barcelona asthma have specific IgE antibodies recognizing these unique glycoproteins distributed in soybean hull. Gly m 2 is an allergen in hull that also elicits a Barcelona asthma, with molecular weight 8000 and pI 6.0, which is homologous to a storage protein from cotyledons of *Vigna radiata* (cow pea) and to a disease response protein from *Pisum sativum* (green pea).[33] However, the cross-reactivity among them is not clear.

Soybean profilin was also identified as an allergen (Gly m 3) with a molecular weight of 14,000 and pI of 4.4, which is homologous to Bet v 2, a birch pollen allergen, with a sequence identity of 73%, and 11 other plant profilins with 69% to 88% identity.[34] These three allergens are recognized as inhalant allergens eliciting Barcelona asthma when the soybean grains are unloaded from cargo ships, because the allergenic proteins are located in hulls of the grain surface. There are several reports on glycinin as allergens, and acidic subunits A1a, A1b, A2, A3, and A4 have been suggested to be allergenic.[35]

The IgE epitope on the acidic chain of glycinin G1 is located on the 192 to 306 amino acid residue.[36] KSTI was first identified as a soybean allergen by using sera of patients with asthma working in a laboratory and sensitized through the airway by working with a fine powder of KSTI as a reagent,[4] as well as by using sera of bakers.[37,38] We examined sera of the patients and found that few of them had IgE against KSTI (frequency of sensitization about 1.5% in the soybean-sensitive patients with atopic dermatitis).[10]

Mittag et al.[39] demonstrated that patients with allergic reactions to a dietary product containing SPI had a specific IgE that reacted to Gly m 4, which shows about 50% homology to Bet v 1-related pathogenesis-related protein 10 (PR-10) (Figure 7.2). They reported that Gly m 4 content in several soy products ranged between 0 and 70 mg/kg, which depends on the degree of food processing. Gu et al.[40] have shown the presence of IgE-binding proteins in soy lecithin, which is widely used as an emulsifier in processed foods, pharmaceuticals, and cosmetics. The sera of soybean-sensitive patients reacted with protein bands with 7, 12, 20, 39, and 57 kDa on SDS-PAGE. The analysis of the N-terminal amino acid sequence of these proteins revealed that a 12-kDa protein was a methionine-rich protein and a member of the 2S albumin class of proteins, that the 20-kDa band was KSTI, and that the 39-kDa was a soy protein with unknown function. Lin et al.[41] suggested that soybean 2S albumin storage proteins, AL1 and AL3, play a role in food allergy similar to other plant allergens, which are stable to heat and chemical treatments.

### 7.2.2.5 Carbohydrate Determinants as a Common Cross-Reactive Antigenic Site

Hiemori et al. demonstrated the occurrence of a specific IgE-recognizing glycan moiety common to plant glycoproteins in sera of soybean-sensitive patients.[42] In

```
          10        20        30        40        50
S  MGVFTFEDEINSPVAPATLYKALVTDADNVIPK-ALDSFKSVENVEGNGGPGTIKKITFL
   ::::..:.:  .: .   : :.::..  ..:..::: :  ....::::.::::::::::::::
B  GVFNYESETTSVIPAARLFKAFILEGDTLIPKVAPQAISSVENIEGNGGPGTIKKITFP
          10        20        30        40        50
    60        70        80        90       100       110
S  EDGETKFVLHKIESIDEANLGYSYSVVGGAALPDTAEKITFDSKLVAGPNGGSAGKLTVK
   :  .  :.:  ....  .:.::.  ::::::.. :.:: :: ::: . :.:: :.::: :.. :
B  EGSPFKYVKERVDEVDHANFKYSYSMIEGGALGDTLEKICNEIKIVATPDGGSILKISNK
    60        70        80        90       100       110
   120       130       140       150
S  YETHGDAEPNQDELKTGKAKADALFKAIEAYLLAHPD-YN
   :.::::: :  . ...:. : :..::..:.:.::::: : ::
B  YHTKGDQEMKAEHMKAIKEKGEALLRAVESYLLAHSDAYN
   120       130       140       150
```

        **S:** Soybean (Gly m 4)
        **B:** Bet v 1 (Birch pollen allergen)

**FIGURE 7.2** Amino acid sequence alignment between Gly m 4 and Bet v 1.

the cases of Gly m Bd 30k and 28K, both the allergenic proteins have a typical asparagine-N-conjugated oligo mannose type glycan moiety of Man3GlcNac2 with the β1-2 xylose and α1-3 fucose branches (Figure 7.3). Therefore, sera of these soybean-sensitive patients recognize horseradish peroxidase, bromelain, and ascorbate oxidase, all of which carry asparagine-N-linked oligo mannose type glycan moiety with the β1-2 xylose or α1-3 fucose branches. The ratio of the IgE antibodies recognizing the peptide sequences of Gly m Bd 30K protein as an epitope to those recognizing the glycan moiety are estimated to be 1:4, indicating that about 80% of the IgE antibodies reacted with Gly m Bd 30K are carbohydrate-determinant specific and other glycoproteins with similar glycan moieties may react with IgE as a common cross-reactive carbohydrate determinant (CCD).[42] Batanero et al.[43] also reported that patients sensitive to olive pollen allergen, Ole e 1, recognized the N-linked glycan moiety of Ole e 1 and CCDs associated with the IgE-mediated clinical reactions. However, little is known about the clinical relevance of the CCD-directed IgE antibodies in soybean allergy.

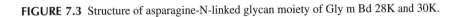

**Manα1-6**

**Manβ1– 4GlcNAcβ1– 4GlcNAcβ1– N.Asn**

**Manα1-3** **Xylβ1-2** **Fucα1-3**

**FIGURE 7.3** Structure of asparagine-N-linked glycan moiety of Gly m Bd 28K and 30K.

## 7.3 DEVELOPMENT OF HYPOALLERGENIC SOYBEAN AND SOYBEAN PRODUCTS

### 7.3.1 DETERMINATION OF ALLERGENICITY

It is important to establish a convenient, selective, and semiquantitative method for determination or evaluation of the allergenicity of soybean and soybean products. The immunoblotting method (Western blot) is a useful technique to detect very small amounts of allergens, but it is not a quantitative way to evaluate and compare the allergenicity (amounts of allergens) during the course of reduction processing. The most suitable method for selective and quantitative analysis of allergens is considered to be the enzyme-linked immunosorbent assay (ELISA) using allergen-specific antibodies. In the case of the measurement of allergenicity of soybean, Gly m Bd 30K is the target allergen to be determined, because about two thirds of soybean-sensitive patients examined have IgE antibodies binding to the Gly m Bd 30K. Furthermore, Gly m Bd 30K is a suitable index allergen molecule because of its wide distribution in processed foods.

The monoclonal antibody F5 was prepared from the hybridoma of spleen cells of Balb/c mice immunized with a reductively carboxymethylated allergen.[22] Immunoblot of Gly m Bd 30K by F5 mAb was carried out in various soybean products. The allergen was hardly detected in fermented products, such as soybean paste (miso) and fermented soybean (natto).[44] The positive bands were clearly observed in blots of meatballs, beef croquettes, and fried chicken, while no bands showed in hamburger and fish sausage containing plant proteins, indicating that the former three products contained soybean protein isolate and the latter two contained wheat gluten. Gly m Bd 30K was shown to be a good index of soybean allergens for evaluating the allergenicity of soybean products, with additional support given by Yaklich et al. from the results of an analysis of distribution of Gly m Bd 30K in core collections of *Glycine max* accessions.[45]

### 7.3.2 MOLECULAR BREEDING

The target molecular species to be removed are three major allergens, such as Gly m Bd 60K, 30K, and 28K. Among them, a new soybean line (*Glycine max* Tohoku 124) lacking both the $\alpha$ and $\alpha'$ subunits of $\beta$-conglycinin (Gly m Bd 60K) was induced by irradiation with a 20-kR (1.0 kR/h) $\gamma$-ray to Karikei 434, with marked decrease in the level of the $\alpha$-, $\alpha'$-, and $\beta$-subunits of $\beta$-conglycinin, which was achieved by the cross hybridization.[46] Recently, it was confirmed that this mutant Tohoku 124 also lacks another major allergen, Gly m Bd 28K, together with the $\alpha$ subunit of $\beta$-conglycinin as a result of the immunoblotting analysis using a monoclonal antibody raised against Gly m Bd 28K, C5.[26] This indicates that an application of Tohoku 124 for processing of soybean products is beneficial for developing hypoallergenic soybean products because of the absence of the two major allergens, Gly m Bd 28K and 60K. In 2000, Tohoku 124 was registered as a new variety named "Yumeminori," which means "dream comes true" for soybean-allergic patients. During the screening of the major three allergenic proteins in soybean varieties, about 80% of edible varieties cultivated in Japan were shown to lack the Gly m Bd 28K allergen. However, a mutant lacking Gly m Bd 30K was hard to find, even by screening the soybean varieties and mutants available in the stock culture of the soybean breeding laboratory at the Tohoku National Agricultural Experiment Station.

### 7.3.3 REDUCTION OF GLY M BD 30K BY GENETIC MODIFICATION

Herman et al.[47] removed most of the immunodominant soybean allergen Gly m Bd 30K by using a genetic modification technique. Elimination of the undesirable protein components makes soybean products available to many sensitive patients allergic to soybean. Herman et al. developed a genetically modified soybean line by transgene-induced gene silencing of the Gly m Bd 30K gene.[47] The modified transgenic soybean seeds do not accumulate the Gly m Bd 30K allergenic protein and appear to be otherwise unchanged by the removal of this protein. The introduction of this transgenic technique into a hypoallergenic soybean variety of Yumeminori may provide a hypoallergenic product that can be safely accepted by patients.

### 7.3.4 PHYSICOCHEMICAL REDUCTION OF GLY M BD 30K

Heat treatment is a general method of food processing and induces the destruction of protein structures. Epitopes, that is IgE-binding sites of allergens, are, however, assumed to be sequential structures on a peptide chain (about ten amino acid residues), so that the reduction of allergenicity from heat denaturation of proteins (unfolding of polypeptide chains) would not be expected. It has been reported that the IgE-binding activity of Gly m Bd 30K is remarkably enhanced by an autoclave treatment of soybean grain during natto processing.[44] As a unique technique of the hypoallergenic process, the selective removal of Gly m Bd 30K from soymilk or defatted soymilk by centrifugation under a specified condition has been achieved. The selective removal of Gly m Bd 30K depended on the unique solubilities of the major storage proteins, glycinin and β-conglycinin. In the case of non-defatted soymilk, about 90% of Gly m Bd 30K could be removed into an oil pad layer formed by centrifugation in the presence of reducing agents.[48] In the case of defatted soymilk, about 97% of Gly m Bd 30K could be removed as a precipitate in the presence of reducing agents (10 m$M$ sodium bisulfite) under the specified condition (1 $M$ Na$_2$SO$_4$ in acidic pH of 4.5). The major storage soybean proteins, glycinin and β-conglycinin, remained in the supernatant after centrifugation.[49]

A small amount of Gly m Bd 30K, however, could not be removed from supernatant in the absence of reducing reagents. A possible disulfide linkage between Gly m Bd 30K and the α(α′) subunits of β-conglycinin formed.[49] This hypothesis was proved by the following fact. By using a mutant soybean Tohoku 124 lacking the α and α′ subunits, the removal ratio of Gly m Bd 30K from defatted soymilk was improved (97.0% to 99.8%) without the addition of reducing agents for reductive cleavage of the disulfide linkage between Gly m Bd 30K and the α and α′ subunits of β-conglycinin.[50] Accordingly, as a result of the combination of an application of Tohoku 124 and a physicochemical procedure, the substantially complete removal of the three major allergenic proteins (Gly m Bd 30K, α subunit of β-conglycinin, and Gly m Bd 28K) from defatted soymilk and SPI was attained.[50] The average removal rate of the three allergens was almost 99.9%. Since these procedures for reducing allergenicity do not include the methods for modifying protein structures and, especially, enzymatic digestion, the processing functionality of soybean storage proteins could be retained for making the traditional soybean products, for example, tofu (soybean cake) and ganmodoki (cooked soybean cake).

### 7.3.5 ENZYMATIC DIGESTION OF ALLERGENS

An enzymatic treatment of whole soybean seeds effectively reduces allergenicity. Autoclaved soybean was treated by certain proteases from *Bacillus* sp. at 37°C for 20 h, which is the same condition required for fermentation natto with *Bacillus natto*.[51] The product has a natto-like texture but no natto-like flavor. When the residual allergens were examined by immunoblot and ELISA (inhibition ELISA), the product showed no binding activity against F5 mAb and patient sera, and all the proteins in the enzyme-treated soybean grains were hydrolyzed into the peptides with molecular weights of less than 10,000. Miso (fermented soybean paste) also showed no residual immunoreactivity against patient sera after fermentation for 3 months.[44] These facts indicate that fermented soybean products such as natto, miso (soy paste), and syoyu (soy sauce) are candidates for naturally occurring hypoallergenic soybean products. Obata et al.[52] reported the reduction of allergenicity of tofu (soybean curd) by an enzymatic digestion method. They also produced the hypoallergenic tofu-textured food by use of a coagulant (e.g., polysaccharide) and an enzyme-treated hypoallergenic soymilk.[52]

Recently, Tsumura et al.[53] reported a novel hydrolytic processing of soybean proteins. Under the limited hydrolytic conditions (pH and temperature), the selective digestion of β-conglycinin (but not glycinin) was attained. The key point of selective digestion is based on the different denaturation temperatures present in β-conglycinin and glycinin at neutral pH. The digestion of denatured soybean proteins could proceed more rapidly than that of native proteins with proteases at 70°C. Among *Bacillus* proteases used for the treatment, Proleather FG-F (Amano Enzymes Co.) was found to be effective for the selective hydrolysis of Gly m Bd 30K as well as β-conglycinin. As a result of the treatment with proteases under optimum conditions, the three major allergens could be digested. The product containing glycinin showed that the processing functionality remained intact, such as gelation to produce tofu and emulsification activity.[53]

### 7.3.6 CHEMICAL MODIFICATION OF ALLERGENS

An attempt to mask the allergenic sites (epitopes) of soybean proteins using the Maillard-type polysaccharide conjugation was examined. Acid-precipitated soybean proteins (APP or SPI) and galactomannan mixed in weight ratio of 1:5 were dissolved in water at 10% (W/V) and freeze-dried. The Maillard reaction was then induced at 60°C under 79% relative humidity in a desiccator for several days.

The allergenic potential of APP was shown to be reduced by the conjugation of galactomannan molecules to the lysine residues of APP,[54] which was confirmed by dot blotting of treated APP with F5 mAb, patient sera, and inhibition ELISA.

### 7.3.7 EXTRUSION COOKING

Ohishi et al.[55] reported that the antigenicity of soybean meal against calf sera was reduced to 0.1% of the original activity by extrusion cooking with screws containing kneading-disc elements and die-end temperatures exceeding 66°C. SDS-PAGE analysis of the cooked meal indicated that the reduction of antigenicity was due to destruction or modification of protein molecules. Frank et al.[56] reported that texturized soy proteins, produced by a process that includes heating, mechanical pressure, and acid treatment (pH 4.5) led to the disappearance of the major allergen Gly m Bd 30K, whereas a 38-kDa allergenic band corresponding to the glycinin fragment remained intact. However, they suggested that further studies of texturized soy protein could lead to the development of modified technologies using a complementary enzymatic treatment[56] in order to obtain more hypoallergenic products.

### 7.3.8 EVALUATION OF HYPOALLERGENICITY

Hypoallergenic soybean products have been developed and evaluated by physicians and dieticians. *In vitro* examination of IgE-binding activity was done with immunoblot and ELISA techniques. In the case of *in vivo* examination of allergenicity, a single-blind food challenge test or open challenge test are practical in evaluating the processed foods. However, the products used in challenge tests are served to patients on a strict elimination diet of soybean and soybean products for about 3 weeks under the control of physicians. A challenge test is carried out after symptoms disappear from the patients by the elimination of a causative diet. As a standard case, for the first 5 d the patients received the hypoallergenic soybean products. If no symptomatic change was observed during this period, they received the control (allergen-containing) diets for an additional 5 d. If some adverse reactions appeared, the challenge test was stopped. By the preliminary challenge trial it was confirmed that at least 80% of the soybean-allergic patients could eat the hypoallergenic products without any adverse reactions. In addition, further information on soybean allergens, sensitization to soybean allergens, persistence and symptoms of soybean allergy, and diagnostic features are available in a data collection of the Internet Symposium on Food Allergens.[7]

## REFERENCES

1. Bush, R.K. and Taylor, S.L., Soybean oil is not allergenic to soybean-sensitive individuals, *J. Allergy Clin. Immunol.*, 76, 242–245, 1985.
2. Doke, S., Nakamura, R., and Torii, S., Allergenicity of food proteins interacted with oxidized lipids in soybean-sensitive individuals, *Agric. Biol.Chem.*, 53, 1231–1235, 1989.

3. Duke, W.W., Soybean as a possible important source of allergy, *J. Allergy,* 5, 300–305, 1934.

4. Moroz, L.A. and Yang, W.H., Kunitz soybean trypsin inhibitor: a specific allergen in food anaphylaxis, *New Engl. J. Med.,* 302, 1126–1128, 1980.

5. Shibasaki, M., Suzuki, S., Tajima, S., Nemoto, H., and Kuroume, T., Allergenicity of major component proteins of soybean, *Int. Arch. Allergy Appl. Immunol.,* 1, 441–448, 1980.

6. Bjornsson, E., Janson, C., Plaschke, P., Norman, E., and Sjoberg, O., Prevalence of sensitization to food allergens in adult Swedes, *Ann. Allergy Asthma Immunol.,* 77(4), 327–332, 1996.

7. Besler, M., Helm, R.M., and Ogawa, T., Allergen Data Base Collection: update: Soybean (*Glycine max*), *Internet Symp. Food Allergens,* 2(Suppl. 3), 1–37, available athttp://www.food-allergens.de.

8. Sampson, H.A. and Ho, D.G., Relationship between food-specific IgE concentrations and the risk of positive food challenges in children and adolescents, *J. Allergy Clin. Immunol.,* 100(4), 444–451, 1997.

9. Harikul, S., Haruehasavasin, Y., Varavithya, W., and Chaicumpa, W., Cow milk protein allergy during the first year of life: a 12-year experience at the children's hospital, Bangkok, *Asian Pac. J. Allergy Immunol.,* 13(2), 107–111, 1995.

10. Ogawa, T., Bando, N., Tsuji, H., Okajima, H., Nishikawa, K., and Sasaoka, K., Investigation of the IgE-binding proteins in soybeans by immunoblotting with the sera of the soybean-sensitive patients with atopic dermatitis, *J. Nutr. Sci. Vitaminol.,* 37, 555–565.

11. Sicherer, S.H., Morrow, E.H., and Sampson, H.A., Dose-response in double-blind, placebo-controled oral food challenge in children with atopic dermatitis, *J. Allergy Clin. Immunol.,* 105, 582–586, 2000.

12. Rodrigo, M.J., Morell, F., Helm, R.M., Swanson, M., Greif, A., Antonio, J.M., Sunyer, J., and Reed, C.E., Identification and partial characterization of the soybean-dust allergens involved in the Barcelona asthma epidemic, *J. Allergy Clin. Immunol.,* 5, 778–784, 1990.

13. Ikeda, I., Ogawa, T., and Ono, T., Tofu induced urticarial contact dermatitis, *Arch. Dermatol.,* 136, 127–128, 2000.

14. Ogawa, T., Bando, N., Tsuji, H., Nishikawa, K., and Kitamura, K., Identification of soybean allergenic protein, Gly m Bd 30K, with the soybean seed 34-kDa oil-body-associated protein, *Biosci. Biotechnol. Biochem.,* 57, 1030–1033, 1995.

15. Kalinski, A., Weisemann, J.M., Matthews, B.F., and Herman, E.M., Molecular cloning of a protein associated with soybean seed oil bodies that is similar to thiol proteinases of the papain family, *J. Biol. Chem.,* 265, 13843–13848, 1990.

16. Chua, K.Y., Stewart, G.A., Thomas, W.R., Simpson, R.J., Dilworth, R.J., Plozza, T.M., and Turner, K.J., Sequence analysis of cDNA coding of a major house dust mite allergen, Der p 1: homology with cystein proteases, *J. Exp. Med.,* 57, 175–182, 1988.

17. Bando, N., Tsuji, H., Yamanishi, R., Nio, N., and Ogawa, T., Identification of glycosylation site of a major soybean allergen, Gly m Bd 30k, *Biosci. Biotechnol. Biochem.,* 60, 347–348, 1996.

18. Kalinski, A., Melroy, D.L., Dwivedi, R.S., and Herman, E.M., A soybean vacuolar protein (P34) related to thiol prtoeases is synthesized as a glycoprotein precursor during seed maturation, *J. Biol. Chem.,* 267, 1992.

19. Helm, R.M., Cockrell, G., Herman, E., Burks, A.W., Sampson, H.A., and Bannon, G.A., Cellular and molecular characterization of a major soybean allergen, *Int. Arch. Allergy Immunol.,* 117, 29–37, 1998.

20. Babiker, E.E., Azakami, H., Ogawa, T., and Koto, A., Immunological characterization of recombinant soy protein allergen produced by *Esherichia coli* expression system, *J. Agric. Food Chem.*, 48, 571–575, 2000.

21. Tsuji, H., Bando, N., Kimoto, M., Okada, N., and Ogawa, T., Preparation and application of monoclonal antibodies for a sandwich enzyme-linked immunosorbent assay for the major soybean allergen, Gly m Bd 30K, *J. Nutr. Sci. Vitaminol.*, 39, 389–397, 1993.

22. Okinaka, Y., Yang, C.H., Herman, E., Kinney, A., and Keen, N.T., The P34 syringolide elicitor receptor interacts with a soybean photorespiration enzyme, NADH-dependent hydroxypyruvate reductase, *Mol. Plant Microbe Interact.*, 15, 1213–1218, 2002.

23. Tsuji, H., Bando, N., Hiemori, M., Yamanishi, R., Kimoto, M., and Ogawa, T., Purification and characterization of soybean allergen Gly m Bd 28K, *Biosci. Biotechnol. Biochem.*, 61, 942–947, 1997.

24. Tsuji, H., Hiemori, M., Kimoto, M., Yamashita, H., Kobatake, R., Adachi, M., Fukuda, T., Bando, N., Okita, M., and Utsumi, S., Cloning of cDNA encoding a soybean allergen, Gly m bd 28K, *Biochim. Biophys. Acta.*, 1518, 178–182, 2001.

25. Burks, A.W., Shin, D., Cockrell, G., Stanley, J.S., Helm, R.M., and Bannon, G.A., Mapping and mutational analysis of the IgE-binding epitopes on Ara h 1, a legume vicilin protein and a major allergen in peanut hypersensitivity, *Eur. J. Biochem.*, 245, 334–339, 1997.

26. Bando, N., Tsuji, H., Hiemori, M., Yoshizumi, K., Yamanishi, R., Kimoto, M., and Ogawa, T., Quantitative analysis of Gly m Bd 28K in soybean products by a sandwich enzyme-linked immunosorbent assay, *J. Nutr. Sci. Vitaminol.*, 44, 655–774, 1998.

27. Ogawa, T., Bando, N., Tsuji, H., Nishikawa, K., and Kitamura, K., Alpha subunit of beta-conglycinin, an allergenic protein recognized by IgE antibodies of soybean-sensitive patients with atopic dermatitis, *Biosci. Biotechnol. Biochem.*, 59, 831–833, 1995.

28. Thanh, V.H. and Shibasaki, K., Beta-conglycinin from soybean proteins isolation and immunological and physicochemical properties of the monomeric forms, *Biochim. Biophys. Acta.*, 490, 370–384, 1977.

29. Sebastiani, F.L., Schmit, E.S., and Beachy, R.N., Complete sequence of a cDNA of alpha subunit of beta-conglycinin, *Plant Mol. Biol.*, 15, 197–201, 1985.

30. Gonzalez, R., Polo, F., Zapatero, L., Caravaca, F., and Carreira, J., Purification and characterization of major inhalant allergens from soybean hulls, *Clin. Exp. Allergy,* 22, 748–755, 1992.

31. Odani, S., Koide, T., Ono, T., Seto, Y., and Tanaka, T., Soybean hydrophobic protein. Isolation, partial characterization and the complete primary structure, *Eur. J. Biochem.*, 162, 485–491, 1987.

32. Gijzen, M., Miller, S.S., Kufku, K., Buzzelul, R.I., and Miki, B.L., Hydrophobic protein synthesized in the pod endocarp adheres to the seed surface, *Plant Physiol.*, 120, 951–959, 1999.

33. Codina, R., Lockey, R.F., Fernandez-Caldas, E., and Rama, R., Purification and characterization of a soybean hull allergen responsible for the Barcelona asthma outbreaks. II. Purification and sequencing of the Gly m 2 allergen, *Clin. Exp. Allergy,* 27, 424–430, 1997.

34. Rihs, H.P., Chen, Z., Rueff, F., Petersen, A., Royznek, R., Heimann, H., and Baur, X., IgE binding of the recombinant allergen soybean profilin (rGly m 3) is mediated by conformational epitopes, *J. Allergy Clin. Immunol.*, 104, 1293–1301, 1999.

35. Djurtoft, R., Pedersen, H.S., Aabin, B., and Barkholt, V., Studies of a soybean allergens: soybean and egg proteins, *Adv. Exp. Med. Biol.,* 289, 281–293, 1991.

36. Zeece, M.G., Beardslee, T.A., Markwell, J.P., and Sarath, G., Identification of an IgE-binding region in soybean acidic Glycinin G1, *Food Agric. Immunol.,* 11, 83–90, 1999.

37. Baur, X., Pau, M., Czuppon, A., and Fruhmann, G., Characerization of soybean allergens causing sensitization on occupationally exposed bakers, *Allergy,* 51, 326–330, 1996.

38. Quirce, S., Fernandez-Nieto, M., Polo, F., and Sastre, J., Soybean trypsin inhibitor is an occupational inhalant allergen, *J. Allergy Clin. Immunol.,* 109(1), 178, 2002.

39. Mittag, D., Vieths, S., Vogel, L., Becker, W.M., Rihs, H.P., Helbling, A., Wuthrich, B., and Ballmer-Weber, B.K., Soybean allergy in patients allergic to birch pollen: clinical investigation and molecular characterization of allergens, *J. Allergy Clin. Immunol.,* 113(1), 148–154, 2004.

40. Gu, X., Beardslee, T., Zeece, M., Sarath, G., and Markwell, J., Identification of IgE-binding proteins in soy lecithin, *Int. Arch. Allergy Immunol.,* 126(3), 218–225, 2001.

41. Lin, J., Fido, R., Shewry, P., Archer, D.B., and Alcocer, M.J., The expression and processing of two recombinant 2S albumin from soybean (*Glycine max*) in the yeast *Pichia pastoris, Biochim. Biophys. Acta.,* 1698(2), 203–212, 2004.

42. Hiemori, M., Bando, N., Ogawa, T., Shimada, H., Tsuji, H., Yamanishi, R., and Terao, J., Occurrence of IgE antibody recognizing N-linked glycan moiety of Gly m Bd 28K of soybean allergen, *Int. Arch. Allergy Immunol.,* 122, 238–245, 2000.

43. Batanero, E., Crespo, J.F., Monsalve, R., Martin-Esteban, M., Villalba, M., and Rodriguez, R., IgE-binding and histamine-release capabilities of the main carbohydrate component isolated from the major allergen of olive tree pollen, Ole e 1, *J. Allergy Clin. Immunol.,* 103, 147–153, 1999.

44. Yamanishi, R., Huang, T., Tsuji, H., Bando, N., and Ogawa, T., Reduction of the soybean allergenicity by the fermentation with *Bacillus natto, Food Sci. Technol. Int.,* 1, 14–17, 1995.

45. Yaklich, R.W., Helm, R.M., Cockrell, G., and Herman, E.M., Analysis of the distribution of the major soybean seed allergens in a core collection of *Glycine max* accessions, *Crop Sci.,* 39, 1444–1447, 1999.

46. Takahashi, K., Banba, H., Kikuchi, A., Ito, M., and Nakamura, S., An induced mutant line lacking the alpha subunit of beta-conglycinin in soybean (*Glycine max* (L) Merrill), *Breed. Sci.,* 44, 65–66, 1994.

47. Herman, E.M., Helm, R.M., Jung, R., and Kinney, A.J., Genetic modification removes an immunodominant allergen from soybean, *Plant Physiol.,* 132, 36–43, 2003.

48. Hosoyama, H., Obata, A., Hamano, M., and Ogawa, T., Development of hypoallergenic processed foods, *Shokuhin Kagaku,* 38(11), 39–48, 1996 (in Japanese).

49. Samoto, M., Miyazaki, C., Akasaka, T., Mori, H., and Kawamura, Y., Specific binding of allergenic soybean protein Gly m Bd 30K with alpha and alpha' subunit of beta-conglycinin in soy milk, *Biosci. Biotechnol. Biochem.,* 60, 1006–1010, 1996.

50. Samoto, M., Takahashi, K., Fukuda, Y., Nakamura, S., and Kawamura, Y., Substantially complete removal of the 34 kDa allergenic soybean protein, Gly m Bd 30K from soy milk of a mutant lacking alpha and alpha' subunits of conglycinin, *Biosci. Biotechnol. Biochem.,* 60, 1911–1913, 1996.

51. Yamanishi, R., Tsuji, H., Bando, N., Yamada, Y., Nadaoka, Y., Huang, T., Nishikawa, K., Emoto, S., and Ogawa, T., Reduction of the allergenicity of soybean by treatment with proteases, *J. Nutr. Sci. Vitaminol.*, 42, 581–587, 1997.
52. Obata, A., Hosoyama, H., and Ogawa, T., Development of Tofu-like product from soy milk for soybean-sensitive patients, *Shokuhin Kogyo*, 41, 39–48, 1998 (in Japanese).
53. Tsumura, K., Kugimiya, W., Bando, N., Hiemori, M., and Ogawa, T., Preparation of hypoallergenic soybean protein with processing functionality by selective enzymatic hydrolysis, *Food Sci. Technol. Res.*, 5, 171–175, 1999.
54. Babikwer, E.E., Hiroyuki, A., Matsudomi, N., Iwata, H., Ogawa, T., Bando, N., and Kato, A., Effect of polysaccharide conjugation or transglutaminase treatment on the allergenicity and functional properties of soybean protein, *J. Agric. Food Chem.*, 46, 866–871, 1998.
55. Ohishi, A., Watanabe, K., Urushibata, M., Utsuno, K., Ikuta, K., Sugimoto, K., and Harada, H., Detection of soybean antigenicity and reduction by twin-screw extrusion, *J. Am. Oil Chem.*, 71, 1391–1396, 1994.
56. Frank, P., Vautrin, D.A.M., Dousset, B., Kanny, G., Nabet, P., Guenard-Bilbaut, L., and Parisot, L., The allergenicity of soybean-based products is modified by food technologies, *Int. Arch. Allergy Immunol.*, 128, 212–219, 2002.

# 8 Longevity and Age-Related Disease

*Yoshiaki Fujita and Yuko Araki*

## CONTENTS

## 8.1 INTRODUCTION

In Japan, for hundreds, perhaps thousands, of years, rice, fish, soybean products, and green vegetables made up the traditional diet. However, after World War II, Western habits penetrated Japanese life to an enormous extent, bringing about important changes in dietary and eating practices. In particular, consumption of rice as a staple food declined sharply. By contrast, intake of animal foods, such as meat, eggs, milk, and dairy products, has markedly increased, resulting in a relatively expanded intake of animal protein and fats and total fats. This change has greatly improved the nutritional status of the Japanese people.

Results from the recent National Nutrition Survey[1] showed that in comparison to the recommended dietary allowances (RDAs), the nation's mean nutrient intake comes close to expectations and nutritional status has been satisfactory, excluding calcium intake. The proportions of energy derived from protein, fats, and carbohydrates in a conventional Japanese diet are 15%, 25%, and 60%, respectively, of total energy. This ratio is almost satisfactory. However, it should be noted that the average value encompasses large deviations, from under- to overconsumption.

## 8.2 LONGEVITY

### 8.2.1 CHANGES IN DIETARY HABITS AND DISEASE STRUCTURE

Changes in dietary and eating habits in Japan have greatly improved the nutritional status of the nation, resulting in decreased incidence in undernutrition-related communicable infectious diseases, such as pneumonia and tuberculosis. However, subsequent changes in the nation's life-style, in particular, the relative increase of energy intake caused by decreases in physical activities in daily living and working has increased the incidence of obesity, resulting in an increased incidence of degenerative diseases such as cancer, heart disease, and cerebrovascular diseases, because obesity is one of the risk factors for these diseases. These diseases are listed as the leading causes of death in Japan.[2] However, it is important to note that age-adjusted mortality rates, in which the population composition is expressed on an equalized age distribution, show that the number of those suffering from chronic degenerative diseases has remained almost constant during the past three decades. This indicates that the rise in crude mortality rates from these diseases is mainly due to increases in the actual numbers of elderly persons, rather than to westernizing effects on dietary habits. That is, a moderate westernizing of dietary habits prolonged the mean life expectancy of the nation through improved nutritional status, resulting in an increased elderly population.

### 8.2.2 PROLONGED LIFE EXPECTANCY

Japan is moving toward an advanced-age society at a very high speed. In 2003, mean life expectancy of the Japanese was 78.36 years for males and 85.33 years for females. Nineteen percent of the population is over 65 years old, and statistical data indicate that by 2020 one out of every four Japanese will be at over 65 years old. This prolongation of mean life expectancy has been greatly contributed to not only by developments in medical technology and environmental sanitation but also by improved dietary and eating habits, as described above.

The leading causes of death in Japan are malignant neoplasm, heart disease, and cerebrovascular disease, followed by suicide and accidents for the middle-aged but followed by malnutrition-related infectious diseases for older persons. In elderly Japanese, not only overnutrition but also undernutrition has started to become a serious nutritional problem. The existence of these discrepant nutritional groups in elderly people is closely related to the traditional and consistent eating habits, dietary customs, characteristic food preferences, and individual differences in socioeconomic background, chronological and physiological ages, and lowered daily physical activity.

### 8.2.3 FOOD PREFERENCES IN THE ELDERLY

Table 8.1 summarizes several reports on food preferences of the elderly. As a group, the elderly, in contrast to younger Japanese, prefer traditional dishes over Western foods. Moreover, they prefer dishes made with the best natural, fresh ingredients rather than highly processed foods. The National Nutrition Survey[1] shows that mean daily intake of potatoes, legumes, fruits, and green vegetables increased with the age, whereas daily intake of fat and oil, milk and dairy products, meats, and precooked foods decreased.

There is no conclusive evidence on whether characteristic food preferences of older Japanese result from physiological changes, a desire to return to familiar foods, or an adaptation to changes in their living environments. Suyama et al.[3] examined 422 elderly men and women (69 years to 71 years old) living in an urban area and found that the three leading factors determining the number and variety of foods consumed were the level of education, the level of the activity of daily living (ADL), and for males the type of living arrangements and level of education but for females the level of the ADL and business experience. These findings suggest that characteristic food preferences and eating habits among elderly persons depend strongly on changes in their socioeconomic environment rather than on age-related changes in their physiological functioning.

### 8.2.4 ACTIVITIES OF DAILY LIVING IN THE ELDERLY

Among aged persons, the "dynamic elder," who takes an active part in his or her community or household, generally has good nutritional status.[4] In contrast,

**TABLE 8.1**
**Food Preferences of Elderly Japanese**

| Prefer | Rather than |
|---|---|
| Fish and shellfish | Meats |
| Boiled rice and noodles | Bread |
| Native vegetables | Imported vegetables |
| Animal foods | Vegetable foods |
| Seasoned by soy sauce | Seasoned by milk |
|   Soy paste |   Butter |
|   Vinegar |   Ketchup |
| Boiled foods | Fried |
| Stewed foods | Frizzled |

housebound and bedridden elderly persons are often deficient in quality protein, vitamin A, riboflavin, iron, and calcium.[5] Nutritional status in the elderly seems to be closely related to levels of ADL rather than to chronological age. We[6] examined the intensity of daily physical activity in institutionalized Japanese elderly women (n: 113, aged 79.5 ± 7.0 years) who habitually spent many hours a day either sitting or lying in homes. When daily physical activity was expressed on the basis of a physical activity index (total/basal energy expenditure), the values ranged from 1.01 to 1.57, and the mean value was calculated as to be 1.26 ± 0.14. More than 64% of the subjects examined had a value below 1.30 of the physical activity index, that is, the lowest value shown in the current RDAs in Japan[7] This suggests that increasing daily physical activity can improve the nutritional status of the elderly.

## 8.3  EXERCISE

### 8.3.1  BENEFITS OF LIGHT EXERCISE

Laboratory rats are usually confined to cages that markedly restrict their physical activity and are provided with food *ad libitum*. In laboratory rats housed in cages, basal metabolism accounts for about 90% of their daily energy expenditure, and daily physical activities for the remaining 10%.[8] This profile of daily energy expenditure is similar to that of bedridden or housebound elderly persons.[9]

Goodrick showed that in aging rats, voluntary wheel running prolonged survival, as compared with sedentary rats in cages.[10] Another report showed that exercise and daily physical activity had a favorable effect on physiological and metabolic functions.[11] However, most such investigations involved moderate or heavy exercise with a higher consumption of oxygen over a shorter period of time. Few studies have examined the beneficial effects of long-term, light exercise throughout life, which is almost equivalent to regular physical activity in day-to-day life in humans, on age-related changes in physiological and metabolic functions.

As a model of light exercise virtually equivalent to normal physical activity in day-to-day life in humans, we[12] loaded 3000 m/d of running exercise on rats throughout their lives. Male Wistar rats were fed a 20% casein diet *ad libitum* until maturity (100 d old) and then were divided them into two groups. The rats in one group (the RS group) received 10 g/d of a 20% casein diet, which is about 60% of the daily food consumption of rats fed *ad libitum*, and were maintained under sedentary conditions until 900 d old. Those in the other group (the RE group) were fed 11 g/d of the same diet and simultaneously underwent running exercise (3000 m daily). From a preliminary study, the energy expenditure for this exercise loading was determined to be equivalent to about 1.0 g/d of the 20% casein diet. The RE rats were housed individually in a structure that consisted of a housing area, a running wheel, and an automatic feeding device interlocked electrically with the running wheel. The animals received a constant amount of food and exercise throughout the test period. As compared with the sedentary group, long-term, light exercise significantly increased body nitrogen retention and serum protein levels,

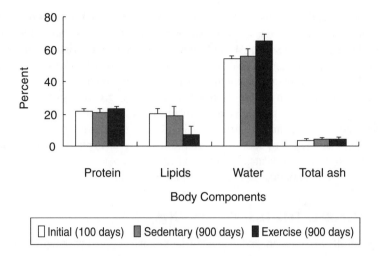

**FIGURE 8.1** Effects of long-term, light exercise under restricted feeding on body compositions at 900 d of age in male Wistar rats. Rats were fed a 20% casein diet *ad libitum* until 100 d of age and were then divided into two groups. The sedentary group (n: 12) received 10 g/d of the 20% casein diet and were kept under sedentary conditions in cages until 900 d of age. The exercise group (n: 11) was given 11 g/d of the same diet, with 3000 m/d of running-wheel exercise. Values are mean ± standard deviation (SD).

decreased body fat and plasma insulin levels, prevented age-related decline in the basal metabolic rate, and reduced age-associated histopathological changes in some visceral organs, particularly the kidneys and liver (Figure 8.1). Compared with sedentary daily living, long-term, light exercise further enhanced the benefits of restricted feeding on age-related deterioration of physiological and metabolic variables and improved body composition but did not prolong survival at 900 days of age.

## 8.3.2 INTERACTION OF NUTRITION AND EXERCISE

Adequate physical activity not only makes you feel refreshed but also stimulates your appetite, resulting in an increased intake of food. Therefore, through exercise, elderly people can more easily obtain essential nutrients without becoming overweight, and thus have an improved nutritional status. Exercise increases a person's requirement for energy and vitamins that relate to energy metabolism, such as thiamine and riboflavin. However, exercise itself does not increase the need for dietary protein, because adequate and appropriate exercise does not significantly increase the total amount of nitrogen and urea excreted in the urine.[13] Nonetheless, it seems that the effect of exercise on physical fitness is accelerated by supplementation with a balanced diet consisting of adequate amounts of essential nutrients (including amino acids) rather than by foods containing energy sources alone.

Meredith and colleagues have examined the effects of additional food on gains in strength and muscle mass during heavy training by elderly men.[14] During the 12 weeks of knee extensor and flexor training, group S was given a daily supplement of 560 kcal/d consisting of a balanced diet, whereas group U received no supplement. The exercise resulted in midthigh muscle hypertrophy, which was significantly greater in group S than in group U. However, group S showed increased body weight, skin fold thickness, and subcutaneous midthigh fat. Results of other studies demonstrated that in elderly people, plasma glycerol levels during exercise significantly decreased by 50%, despite a normal increase in plasma norepinephrine (noradrenalin). This indicates an impaired lipolytic response of fat cells to catecholamine stimulation and to exercise in elderly people.[15]

## 8.4  AGE-RELATED DISEASES IN HUMANS

It is generally accepted that adequate nutrient intake coupled with regular physical activity reduces the risk of degenerative diseases, such as coronary heart disease, diabetes, hypertension, and osteoporosis, through increased muscle mass and improved physiological and metabolic functions. Chronic obstructive pulmonary disease (COPD) is a serious chronic disease in the elderly, and most COPD patients have suffered from protein and energy malnutrition. Malnourished elderly COPD patients could improve through not only supplementation of energy intake but also sufficient protein intake.[16] Furthermore, appropriate exercise plays an important part in the rehabilitation programs for patients with such diseases, as do drug therapy and nutritional control. Australian Aborigines, after making the transition from a traditional life-style (characterized by a high level of physical activity and a diet low in fat and high in fiber) to a Western life-style (characterized by reduced physical activity and a diet high in refined carbohydrates and fat) develop a high prevalence of these kinds of degenerative diseases.[17]

### 8.4.1  Osteoporosis

Osteoporosis is associated with genetic background, life-style, nutritional environment, and aging. Bone fracture is a leading cause of disability and subsequent confinement to bed, especially in postmenopausal women. Bone mass and mineral density increase with age in early life until about 20 years of age, and then start to decrease progressively. This age-related decline in bone mineral density, given similar genetic backgrounds, life-style and nutritional conditions, and the same gender, is primarily associated with age-related decreases in serum levels of estrogen and vitamin $D_3$ (cholecalciferol) and an increase in parathyroid hormone levels. Such changes in hormone levels seem to be physiological rather than pathological. Therefore, the best way to maintain a sufficient level of bone mineral density in later life is to reserve as much bone mineral as possible during early life by ensuring adequate nutritional intake, particularly of calcium and protein.

Results from the recent Japanese National Nutrition Survey[1] show that calcium is the sole nutrient for which the national mean daily intake failed to meet the current RDA (600 mg/d, or 10 mg/kg body weight, for adults). Actual dietary calcium intake of the survey population was found to range from 7 to 10 mg/kg body weight.[18,19] The calcium allowance for elderly persons is the same as that for young adults. However, there are reports[20,21] that the daily intake necessary for the elderly to maintain calcium balance ranges from 10 to 18 mg/kg body weight per day. Although it is true that intake of animal foods has increased greatly in Japan over the past four decades, among the animal foods, milk and dairy products are the most efficient and convenient sources of calcium. By comparison with meats and eggs, milk and dairy products do not merge well into traditional Japanese dishes, and older Japanese prefer the traditional Japanese foods to Western dishes that are much richer in calcium.

It has been reported that an insufficient intake of calcium is one cause of osteoporosis, a typical age-related disorder. Calcium intake has gradually increased among the Japanese in the past four decades; however, in 2002, the mean calcium intake of the population as a whole was only 546 mg/d, or about 60 to 70% of that in Western countries.[22]

However, the incidence of femoral neck fracture is significantly lower in Japanese females[23,24] than in women in Western countries,[25,26] irrespective of age. In cross-cultural studies, there is no consistent evidence for a causal relationship among dietary calcium intake, osteoporosis, and bone fractures.

In Western countries, about 70 to 80% of dietary calcium is provided by milk and dairy products, as compared to only 25% in Japan.[1] This indicates that the appearance and development of osteoporosis and the incidence of bone fractures may be closely related not only to differences in dietary calcium intake, genetic background, and life-style, but also to differences in the variety of dietary calcium sources and food patterns.

### 8.4.2 CARDIOVASCULAR DISEASE

Adequate nutrient intake coupled with adequate and regular physical activity is essential to reduce the risk of cardiovascular diseases such as coronary heart disease. The best choice to prevent cardiovascular diseases is to practice such dietary habits as lowering blood pressure, maintaining serum cholesterol and triglycerides at the normal levels, and preventing obesity. However, dietary protein sources are also closely related to reducing the risk of cardiovascular disease. Kanda et al.[27] showed that soy protein ingestion of over 25 g/d containing over 50 mg/d of isoflavones in elderly women can prevent cardiovascular diseases through lowering blood pressure and serum total and low-density lipoprotein (LDL) cholesterol.

### 8.4.3 DIABETES MELLITUS

Changes in life-style including dietary and eating habits and stressful daily living have progressively increased the number of cases of diabetes mellitus. Insulin-dependent diabetes mellitus (Type I diabetes) is more common in younger people than in adults and elderly people. Since this type of diabetes is primarily caused by poor excretion of insulin, exogenous insulin administration is essential. If this treatment is accompanied by appropriate dietary control and a physical exercise program, the efficiency of insulin treatment is further accelerated.[28]

Non-insulin-dependent diabetes mellitus (Type II diabetes) is associated with insulin resistance, hyperinsulinemia, diminished islet β-cell function, and glucose intolerance. These effects have been closely associated with the aging process, and nearly 50% of patients with this type of diabetes are over 65. Oral administration of hypoglycemic agents such as sulfonylureas is a useful treatment in patients with Type II diabetes. However, since oral hypoglycemic agents have no direct effect on the level of plasma glucose, individuals for whom plasma glucose levels cannot be controlled with diet and exercise must be treated with insulin. Moreover, in elderly patients, since administration of these drugs can produce marked hypoglycemia, especially when the therapy is a combination of insulin with oral hypoglycemic agents, caution must be exercised.

In contrast, controlled and appropriate exercise loading accompanied by an adequate dietary treatment produces mild beneficial effects on blood glucose levels of elderly people. Hughes and colleagues trained glucose-intolerant 64-year-old people at 50 to 75% of their maximum heart rate for 12 weeks and then examined oral glucose tolerance and insulin action.[29] After training, glucose tolerance and plasma glucose concentration were significantly improved, although the plasma insulin response remained unchanged. Long-term exercise training, without changes in body composition, improved peripheral insulin action in participants with impaired glucose tolerance. However, in glucose-intolerant individuals, aerobic exercise training without dietary control does not appear to decrease lipoprotein cholesterol and triglyceride levels in the serum.[30]

### 8.4.4 INTERACTION OF NUTRITION AND DRUGS

In Japan, medical expenditures continue to increase. The proportion of pharmaceutical expense to total medical expenditure is over 30%. Use of prescription drugs for chronic diseases is more common and continuous in elderly persons, as compared with younger generations. However, certain prescription drugs cause malabsorption of some nutrients, particularly vitamins and minerals, and an abnormal metabolism and utilization of certain nutrients may impair the functioning of some organs, resulting in malnutrition in spite of adequate dietary nutrient intakes.[31] To ensure nutritional well-being in the elderly, it is very important to consider what sorts of drugs each person normally uses.

## 8.5 ANIMAL STUDIES

### 8.5.1 DIETARY RESTRICTION AND LONGEVITY

Many investigators have shown that compared with rats fed diets rich in energy and protein such as commercial stock diet *ad libitum*, animals on restricted diets show reductions in the prevalence and the progression of age-related diseases, as well as reductions in age-related declines in physiological and metabolic functions, resulting in prolonged survival.[32–35]

We[34] examined the effect of dietary restriction from the weanling period on longevity. Weanling rats were divided into three groups of 12 rats each. One group received food *ad libitum* throughout life (group A), and the two other groups received 80% (group 80) and 50% (group 50) of the amount consumed by group A. Until day 600 of life, the animals received a commercial stock diet *ad libitum*, and then the diet was changed to a 20% casein diet, and the daily food intakes of groups 80 and 50 were fixed at 14.0 g and 8.7 g, respectively, calculated from the feed consumption of group A, which remained constant between day 400 and 500. Survival was greater in the groups with restricted food intakes. The first death occurred on day 615 in group A, day 645 in group 80, and day 710 in group 50, and the 50% survival times of these groups were 719, 951, and 1004 d, respectively. When the last rat in group A died at 879 d of age, 75% of the rats in group 50 were still alive. As indicated by many investigators,[36–38] survival of rats under restricted-feeding conditions was better than that of animals fed *ad libitum*. The life span was longest in group 50, followed by groups 80 and A. Then the life spans were related to the severity of tumor or renal diseases as indicated by Berg and Simms[36] and Yu et al.[33]

## 8.5.2 KIDNEY FUNCTION AND DIETARY PROTEIN

The kidney loses more than 30% of its weight between the third and ninth decades; simultaneously, the glomerular filtration rate (GFR) and renal blood flow decrease to about 50%. Although the creatinine clearance falls by about 30% between the second and eighth decades, the serum concentration of nonprotein nitrogen (NPN) does not always increase in the elderly. A possible explanation for this is that age-related decline in body cell mass, particularly of muscle, results in decreased release of creatinine and that daily protein intake decreases with age. Therefore, when the elderly with deteriorated renal function continue to ingest a large amount of dietary protein for long periods, an abnormal elevation in serum NPN is inevitable. Kountz et al.[39] showed that the serum NPN of elderly subjects increased with increases in protein intake, and the serum NPN of subjects fed 1.5 g/kg BW (body weight) of protein for 75 d increased to about 40 mg N/100 ml. In addition, the elevation of serum NPN with increasing protein intake was more accelerated by animal foods than vegetable foods.[40]

## 8.5.3 DIETARY RESTRICTION AND PROTEINURIA

In aging rats receiving a commercial stock diet rich in energy and protein *ad libitum*, renal disease, in particular, nephrosis, is more frequent than other diseases, appears at an earlier age, and is the principal cause of death. Adult rats with severe proteinuria under *ad libitum* feeding excreted about 350 mg/d of proteins, mainly albumin, and this amount was equal to about 20% of total nitrogen excreted daily in the urine.[34] This albumin loss in the urine was compensated by the increase of albumin synthesis by the liver.[30] The appearance and development of proteinuria in rats and mice are influenced not only by aging, sex, and genetic background but also by dietary factors.

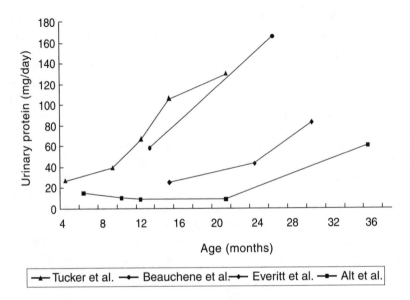

**FIGURE 8.2** Differences in the age of appearance and severity of proteinuria in male Wistar rats fed on different commercial stock diets. The major nutrient content in commercial stock diets differs slightly by manufacturer, but every product is adjusted to contain 20 to 25% protein. Nevertheless, the protein sources are probably different for each commercial stock diet on the market.

When male Wistar rats were fed 50% of the amount of food (20% casein diet) consumed by *ad libitum*–feeding rats from weanling or young adult age (80 d of age), the appearance of proteinuria was completely prevented throughout life.[24] However, when rats were fed the same restricted amount (8.7 g/d) of a 40% casein diet instead of the 20% casein diet, there was no change in the daily excretion of urinary proteins, but the excreted protein became predominantly albumin, although the overall electrophoretic pattern differed from that of protein excreted by rats with proteinuria. Bras and Ross[41] indicated that a diet restricted in total energy was best for preventing proteinuria in aging rats, but Everitt et al.[42] found that even with energy restriction, high protein diets resulted in increased protein excretion and increased incidences of glomerular lesions. Discrepant results have been reported on the age of appearance and severity of proteinuria in aging male Wistar rats fed a commercial diet *ad libitum*, as shown in Figure 8.2. These different findings suggest that proteinuria in aging rats depends not only on the total amounts of ingested dietary energy and protein but also on other dietary factors, such as a protein source.

### 8.5.4 PROTEIN SOURCES AND PROTEINURIA

Rice, fish, soybean and soy products, and green vegetables make up the traditional Japanese diet. In particular, soybean and products such as tofu (soybean-curd cake) and natto (fermented soybeans) are high-quality, traditional vegetable protein sources in Japan. Soy protein isolate (SPI) is widely recognized as an ingredient in processed foods that is a nutritionally high-quality protein source and a food substance with certain physiological and metabolic functions.

An early morphological study showed that different dietary proteins result in different types of renal lesions in aging rats. Kaunitz and Johnson[43] reported that kidney lesions were more severe in rats that received a 30% casein diet than in those fed a 30% lactalbumin diet. Soy protein appears to be a useful vegetable protein for preventing age-related diseases, compared with other proteins. Iwasaki et al.[44] showed that in Fischer 344 rats, the ingestion of a soy protein diet throughout life significantly suppressed histopathological changes in various tissues with advancing age, resulting in prolonged survival. Williams and Walls[45] showed that compared with a casein diet, soy protein appears beneficial to the survival, proteinuria, and renal histological damage of nephrectomized rats. Similarly, Ikeda and colleagues[46,47] also found that compared with a 40% pork protein diet, a 40% soy protein diet decreased urinary albumin excretions and improved renal hemodynamics in adult diabetic rats (WBN/Kob). In addition, compared with a 35% casein diet, a 35% soy protein diet reduced the development of renal hypertrophy in streptozotocin-induced diabetic rats through renal insulin-like growth factor (IGF)-1 mRNA expression. Yagasaki et al.[48] reported that compared with a 20% casein diet, a 20% SPI diet significantly suppressed the stimulation of tumor necrosis factor (TNF) productivity in nephritic rats induced by injecting nephritic serum.

### 8.5.5 AMINO ACIDS AND PROTEINURIA

We[49] examined the effects of dietary protein sources (lactalbumin and SPI) and levels (5, 10, 15, 40, and 60% protein) on urinary protein excretions of adult rats and found that even under restricted dietary energy conditions, urinary protein excretion increased with dietary protein levels with both protein sources. However, the increasing rate was significantly suppressed in the SPI diet compared with the lactalbumin diet, as shown in Figure 8.3. In addition, rats with severe proteinuria showed significant increases in threonine, cystine, tyrosine, and arginine in the serum and in methionine and histidine in the kidney. These amino acid increases in the serum of proteinuria rats were well consistent with the amino acids reported previously by Newburgh and Marsh;[50] the intravenous injection of arginine, cystine, tyrosine, or histidine caused acute renal toxicity.

These findings strongly suggest that the appearance and development of proteinuria in aging rats is closely related to the contents of certain amino acids in proteins ingested. When the amino acid contents of SPI and lactalbumin, which cause more severe proteinuria, are compared, lactalbumin contains three times more cystine than does SPI. This suggests that an excess intake of dietary cystine is associated with the appearance and development of proteinuria in aging rats. We[51] examined the effects of dietary cystine levels on the incidence of renal disease based on urinary protein excretion, urinary $N$-acetyl-$\beta$-D-glucosaminidase

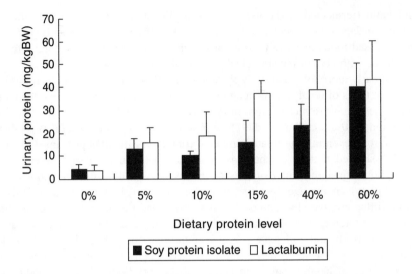

**FIGURE 8.3** Effects of dietary protein levels and sources on urinary protein excretion in adult rats. Male Wistar rats, aged 90 d old, were fed restricted amounts (8 g/d) of a diet containing graded levels of SPI and lactalbumin for 8 weeks. Values are means ± SD of five rats each.

(NAG) activity, which is one of the indices used to assess injury of the proximal tubules, and cathepsin B activity in the glomeruli, which is an index used to assess permeability in the glomerular basement membrane. Male Wistar rats (120 d of age) received 13 g of a 20% casein diet containing graded levels of L-cystine until 280 d of age. Increases in cystine intake significantly increased urinary protein excretions, urinary NAG activities, and cathepsin B activities in the glomeruli. The results suggest that increased cystine intake injures the glomerular basement membrane through the induction of cathepsin B activity and subsequently impairs the functions of the proximal tubules, resulting in increased protein excretions in the urine. In addition, our unpublished data suggest that well-controlled administration of dietary arginine results in beneficial effects on preventing proteinuria in aging rats. To elucidate the relation between the physiological and metabolic functions of individual amino acids and the appearance, development, and prevention of age-related diseases, further study is needed.

## REFERENCES

1. Ministry of Health, Labor and Welfare (Japan), The present nutritional status of Japanese: results of National Nutrition Survey, 2002. Tokyo, Dai-Ichi Shuppan Publishing, 2004 (in Japanese).
2. http://www.mhlw.go.jp/toukei/saikin/hw/life/life03/indexhtml. Accessed July 2004.
3. Suyama, Y., Shichida, K., and Haga, H., Food intake pattern and related factors in the community elderly, *Soc. Gerontol.,* 19, 58–66, 1984 (in Japanese).

4. Matsudaira, T., Okuda, T., Tamai, H., Shimoaragami, K., Miyoshi, H., Oi, Y., Koishi, H., Kitani, T., Nakata, M., Hara, K., and Fujita, D., Nutrition survey in community elderly persons: physique and nutrient intake, *J. Kyoto Med. Assoc.,* 34, 55–63, 1987 (in Japanese).

5. Hidari, A., Nakazato, H., Nakasato, F., and Takahara, J., The effect of the life environment and the health condition on the nutritional intake of the elderly, *Jpn. J. Publ. Health,* 31, 615–621, 1984 (in Japanese).

6. Ozeki, T., Ebisawa, H., Ichikawa, M., Nagasawa, N., Sato, F., and Fujita, Y., Physical activities and energy expenditures of institutionalized Japanese elderly women, *J. Nutr. Sci. Vitaminol.,* 46, 188–192, 2000.

7. Ministry of Health, Labor and Welfare, *Recommended Dietary Allowances and Dietary Reference Intake in Japan,* 6th rev., Tokyo, Dai-Ichi Shuppan Publishing, 1999.

8. Ichikawa, M. and Fujita, Y., Effects of nitrogen and energy metabolism on body weight in later life of male Wistar rats consuming a constant amount of food, *J. Nutr.,* 117, 1751–1758, 1987.

9. Fujita, Y. and Ohzeki, T., Energy requirements for frail elderly females, *Jpn. J. Geriatr.,* 30, 568–571, 1993 (in Japanese).

10. Goodrick, C.L., Effects of long-term voluntary wheel exercise on male and female Wistar rats, *Gerontology,* 26, 22–33, 1980.

11. Tobin, B.W. and Beard, J.L., Interaction of deficiency and exercise training to tissue norepinephrine turnover, triiodothyronine production and metabolic rate in rats, *J. Nutr.,* 120, 900–908, 1990.

12. Ichikawa, M., Fujita, Y., Ebisawa, H., and Ozeki, T., Effects of long-term, light exercise under restricted feeding on age-related changes in physiological and metabolic variables in male Wistar rats, *Mech. Ageing Dev.,* 113, 23–35, 2000.

13. Hickson, J.F., Pivarnik, J.M., and Wolinsky, I., Failure of weight training to affect urinary indices of protein metabolism in men, *Med. Sci. Sports Exerc.,* 18, 563, 1986.

14. Meredith, C.N., Frontera, W.R., O'Reilly, K.P., and Evans, W.J., Body composition in elderly men: effect of dietary modification during strength training, *J. Am. Geriatr. Soc.,* 40, 155–162, 1992.

15. Lonnqvist, F., Nyberg, B., Wahrenberg, H., and Arner, P., Catecholamine induced lipolysis in adipose tissue of the elderly, *J. Clin. Invest.,* 85, 1614–1621, 1990.

16. Ozeki, T., Fujita, Y., and Kida, K., Protein malnutrition in elderly patients with chronic obstructive pulmonary disease, *Geriatr. Gerontol. Int.,* 2, 131–137, 2002.

17. Voorrips, L.E., Lemmink, K.A., van-Heuvelen, M.J., Bult, P., and van-Stavere, W.A., The physical condition of elderly women differing in habitual physical activity, *Med. Sci. Sports Exerc.,* 25, 1152–1157, 1993.

18. Steggerda, F.R. and Mitchell, H.H., Further experiments on calcium requirement of adult man and utilization of calcium in milk, *J. Nutr.,* 21, 577–588, 1941.

19. Steggerda, F.R. and Mitchell, H.H., Variability in calcium metabolism and calcium requirements of adult human subjects, *J. Nutr.,* 31, 407–422, 1946.

20. Roberts, P.H., Kerr, C.H., and Ohlson, M.A., Nutritional status of older women: nitrogen, calcium, phosphorus retentions of nine women, *J. Am. Diet. Assoc.,* 24, 292–299, 1948.

21. Ackermann, P.G. and Toro, G., Calcium and phosphorus balance in elderly men, *J. Gerontol.,* 8, 289–300, 1953.

22. Nelson, M., Black, A.E., Morris, J.A., and Cole, T.J., Between- and within-subject variation in nutrient intake from infancy to old age: estimating the number of days

required to rank dietary intakes with desired precision, *Am. J. Clin. Nutr.*, 50, 155–167, 1989.

23. Kawashima, T., Epidemiology of the femoral neck fractures in 1985 Niigata, *Jpn. J. Bone Mineral Metab.*, 7, 46–54, 1989 (in Japanese).
24. Yoshikawa, T. and Norimatsu, H., Epidemiology of osteoporosis in Okinawa, *Jpn. J. Bone Mineral Metab.*, 9(Suppl.), 135–145, 1991 (in Japanese).
25. Gallagher, J.C., Melton, L.J., Riggs, B.L., and Bergstrath, E., Epidemiology of fractures of the proximal femur in Rochester, Minnesota, *Clin. Orthop.*, 150, 163–171, 1980.
26. Farmer, M.E., White, L.R., Brody, J.A., and Bailey, K.R., Race and sex differences in hip fracture incidence, *Am. J. Public Health*, 74, 374–380, 1984.
27. Kanda, T., Amano, M., Takamatsu, M., Sagara, M., and Yamori, Y., Effects of soy-protein-fortified foods on reducing risk factors for cardiovascular diseases in Japanese elderly women, *Soy Prot. Res. Jpn.*, 5, 138–143, 2002 (in Japanese, with English abstract).
28. Lyon, R.B. and Vinci, D.M., Nutrition management of insulin-dependent diabetes mellitus in adults: review by the Diabetes Care and Education Diabetic Practice Group, *J. Am. Diet. Assoc.*, 93, 309–314, 1993.
29. Hughes, V.A., Fiatarone, M.A., Fielding, R.A., Kahn, B.B., Ferrara, C.M., Shepherd, P., Fisher, E.C., Wolfe, R.R., Elahi, D., and Evans, W.J., Exercise increases muscle GLUT-4 levels and insulin action in subjects with impaired glucose tolerance, *Am. J. Physiol.*, 264 (6 Pt 1), E855–E862, 1993.
30. Hughes, V.A., Fistarone, M.A., Ferrara, C.M., McNamara, J.R., Charnley, J.M., and Evans, W.J., Lipoprotein response to exercise training and a low-fat diet in older subjects with glucose intolerance, *Am. J. Clin. Nutr.*, 59, 820–856, 1994.
31. Roe, D.A., Ed., *Drugs and Nutrition in the Geriatric Patient*, New York, Churchill Livingstone, 1984.
32. Ross, M.H., Length of life and nutrition in the rat, *J. Nutr.*, 75, 197–210, 1961.
33. Yu, B.P., Masoro, E.J., Murata, I., Bertrand, H.A., and Lynd, F.T., Life span study of SPF Fischer 344 male rats fed ad libitum or restricted diets: longevity, growth, lean body mass and disease, *J. Gerontol.*, 37, 130–141, 1982.
34. Fujita, Y., Ichikawa, M., Kurimoto, F., and Rikimaru, T., Effects of feed restriction and switching the diet on proteinuria in male Wistar rats, *J. Gerontol.*, 39, 531–537, 1984.
35. Herlihy, J.T. and Yu, B.P., Dietary manipulation of age-related decline in vascular smooth muscle function, *Am. J. Physiol.*, 238, H652–H655, 1980.
36. Berg, B.N. and Simms, H.S., Nutrition, onset of disease, and longevity in the rats, *Can. Med. Assoc. J.*, 93, 911–913, 1965.
37. Nolen, G.A., Effect of various restricted dietary regimens on the growth, health and longevity of albino rats, *J. Nutr.*, 102, 1477–1494, 1972.
38. Stuchlikova, E., Juricova-Horakova, M., and Deyl, Z., New aspects of the dietary effect of life prolongation in rodents. What is the role of obesity in aging? *Exp. Gerontol.*, 10, 141–144, 1975.
39. Kountz, W.B., Ackermann, P.G., Kheim, T., and Toro, G., Effects of increased protein intake in older people, *Geriatrics*, 8, 63–69, 1953.
40. Kountz, W.B., Hofstatter, L., and Ackermann, P.G., Nitrogen balance studies under prolonged high nitrogen intake levels in elderly individuals, *Geriatrics*, 3, 171–184, 1948.

41. Bras, G. and Ross, M.H., Kidney disease and nutrition in the rat, *Toxicol. Appl. Pharmacol.,* 6, 247–262, 1964.

42. Everitt, A.V., Porter, B.D., and Wyndham, J.R., Effects of caloric intake and dietary composition on the development of proteinuria, age-associated renal disease and longevity in the male rat, *Gerontology,* 28, 168–174, 1982.

43. Kaunitz, H. and Johnson, R.E., Dietary protein, fat, and minerals in nephrocalcinosis female rats, *Metabolism,* 25, 69–77, 1976.

44. Iwasaki, K., Gleiser, C.A., Masoro, E.J., McMahan, C.A., Seo, E., and Yu, B.P., The influence of dietary protein source on longevity and age-related disease processes of Fischer rats, *J. Gerontol. (Biol. Sci).,* 42, 5–12, 1988.

45. Williams, A.J. and Walls, J., Metabolic consequences of differing protein diets in experimental renal disease, *Eur. J. Clin. Invest.,* 17, 117–122, 1987.

46. Ikeda, Y. and Mori, Y., Effect of soy protein on renal hemodynamics and urinary albumin excretion in spontaneously developed diabetic WBN/Kob rats, *Rep. Soy Prot. Res. Com. Jpn.,* 15, 124–129, 1994 (in Japanese, with English abstract).

47. Utsunomiya, K. and Ikeda, Y., Influence of soy protein on renal hypertrophy and IGF-1 gene expression in diabetic rats, *Rep. Soy Prot. Res. Com. Jpn.,* 18, 87–91, 1997 (in Japanese, with English abstract).

48. Yagasaki, K., Nagata, J., and Miura, Y., Effects of dietary soy protein levels and amino acid supplement on cytokine productivity in macrophages from nephritic rats, *Soy Prot. Res. Jpn.,* 2, 106–111, 1999 (in Japanese, with English abstract).

49. Ebisawa, H., Ozeki, T., and Fujita, Y., Effect of soy protein isolate on proteinuria in adult rats, *Nutr. Sci. Soy Prot. Jpn.,* 8, 64–69, 1987 (in Japanese, with English abstract).

50. Newburgh, L.H. and Marsh, P.L., Renal injuries by amino-acids, *Arch. Intern. Med.,* 36, 682–711, 1926.

51. Ebisawa, H., Ichikawa, M., Ozeki, T., and Fujita, Y., Effect of cystine and methionine intake on incidence of proteinuria in adult rats, *Nutr. Sci. Soy Prot. Jpn.,* 12, 107–113, 1991 (in Japanese, with English abstract).

# 9 Soy Saponin

## Chigen Tsukamoto and Yumiko Yoshiki

## CONTENTS

## 9.1   INTRODUCTION

Daily intake of soybean processed foods appears to be one of the factors responsible for the health and longevity of the Japanese. Soybeans include various functional food components, among which isoflavones are a subject of increasing research interest. More recently, the health benefits of soybean saponins have also attracted attention.

The term *saponin* has the same origin as *soap*. During the production processes of tofu (bean curd), heating raw soymilk generates a lot of bubbles, in which saponin components can be detected in high concentrations. During ordinary cooking, these bubbles, which taste bitter, are skimmed off. However, they are not removed during the tofu production process in Japan; instead, an antifoamer is used. The result is that saponins are retained, so the conventional tofu production process may thus have contributed to our health and longer than average life span. Recently, an antifoamer-free technique that retains the saponin components in tofu curd has been developed.

About 1 million tons of food soybeans are consumed annually in the form of traditional soybean processed foods, including tofu, miso (fermented soybean paste), natto (fermented whole soybeans), nimame (boiled beans), and kinako (roasted soybean flour). Because soybeans include about 0.5% saponin components, 5000 tons of these components are included in the raw material of soybean processed foods annually. A rough calculation shows that the 126 million Japanese consume 5000 tons of saponins, so they each take in, on average, 100 mg or more of saponin components daily. Among these traditional foods, tofu (including the deep-fried version), for which half (about 500,000 tons) of food soybeans are used, are consumed the most, followed by 300,000 tons of miso, 100,000 tons of natto, and 100,000 tons of soybeans in other forms. These consumption figures have not changed much over the past decade, indicating that the total intake of soybean saponins in Japan is stable.

However, the composition and content of soybean saponins we take in do not necessarily reflect the volume of consumption of raw soybeans, since saponin levels may change markedly depending on how soybean foods are produced. For example, during the production of juten (filling) tofu about 70% of the saponins in the whole soybeans leach into the soymilk (the remaining 30% remain in the bean curd residue), whereas most of the saponins in soymilk are retained in tofu. If these bitter saponins were removed during the preparation of soymilk, the intake of saponins by Japanese people would be greatly reduced. In addition, saponins in whole soybeans undergo structural changes during the production of processed soybean foods. The state and degree of change vary depending on the process conditions. Moreover, the composition of soybean saponins shows genetic polymorphism depending on the strain; not all strains of soybeans have the same saponin composition. This diversity of the structure of saponins in processed soybean foods may be important for evaluating the functionality of saponins. However, few of the reports that have evaluated the physiological activity of soybean saponins specify which type of soybean saponin was used. Unclear correspondence to chemical structure based on genetic polymorphism may be one of the reasons for the delay in evaluating the functionality of soybean saponins compared to soybean isoflavones.

Due to recent advances in analysis and purification techniques, more reports have been published that evaluate the functionality of highly purified soybean saponins. This will, it is hoped, accelerate the evaluation of the functionality of each type of saponin and quantification of these components in foods. In this chapter, we first describe the basic concept essential for evaluating the functionality of soybean saponins; that is, the composition and content of soybean saponins are influenced by strain-specific and part-specific genetic polymorphism. Next, among studies on the physiological activity of soybean saponins, those using highly purified saponins and those describing the composition of saponin used in their experiments are reviewed and summarized.

## 9.2 SAPONIN COMPONENTS IN WHOLE SOYBEANS

Table 9.1 summarizes the reported soybean saponin components classified according to type of aglycon, the compounds at the C-22 position on the aglycon, and the carbohydrate sequences at the C-3 position on the aglycon.[1-3] Soybean saponins

## TABLE 9.1
## Composition and Nomenclature of Saponins Found in Soybean Seeds According to the Carbohydrate Sequences at the C-3 and the Compounds at the C-22 Positions of Soyasapogenols, A, B, and E

| | C-22 Position | | | | |
|---|---|---|---|---|---|
| | Soyasapogenol A | | Soyasapogenol B[a] | | Soyasapogenol E[a,b] |
| C-3 Position | AcXyl(1∇3)Ara- | AcGlc(1∇3)Ara- | -DDMP[c] | -OH | =O |
| Glc(1 → 2)Gal(1→ 2)GlcUA- | Aa [acetyl A4][e] | Ab [acetyl A1] | αg | Ba [V] | Bd |
| Rha(1 → 2)Gal(1 → 2)GlcUA-Gal(1 → 2) | (Au)[d] | Ac | βg | Bb [I] | Be |
| GlcUA- | Ae [acetyl A5] | Af [acetyl A2] | γg | Bb' [III] | Be' |
| Glc(1 → 2)Ara(1 → 2)GlcUA- | Ax | Ad | αa | Bx | Bf |
| Rha(1 → 2)Ara(1 → 2)GlcUA-Ara(1 → 2) | (Ay) | (Az) | βa | Bc [II] | Bg |
| GlcUA- | Ag [acetyl A6] | Ah [acetyl A3] | γa | Bc' [IV] | Bg' |

a No sugar chain is attached at the C-22 position of soyasapogenols B and E.
b Soyasapogenol E contains a ketone function at the C-22 position.
c DDMP: 2,3-dihydro-2,5-dihydroxy-6-methyl-4H-pyran-4-one.
d Unreported saponins are shown in parentheses.
e Kitagawa's nomenclature systems are shown in brackets.

can be divided into Group A and 2,3-dihydro-2,5-dihydroxy-6-methyl-4*H*-pyran-4-one (DDMP)-binding saponins according to their type of aglycon. Figure 9.1 shows the chemical structures of saponin Ab and saponin βg, representative of their respective groups. Group A saponins, which have soyasapogenol A as their aglycon, are typically bis-desmoside saponins with two carbohydrates at the C-3 and C-22 positions. DDMP saponins are composed of monodesmoside saponin with one carbohydrate at C-3 of soyasapogenol B as well as DDMP at C-22. The presence of a hydroxyl group at C-21 is what makes soyasapogenol A and B different from each other.

Compounds at C-22 of soyasapogenol A are two different carbohydrates. Arabinose binds to a hydroxyl group at C-22 on soyasapogenol A. Two types of sugar bind to a hydroxyl group on C-3 of the arabinose: one is 2,3,4-triacetyl-xylose and the other is 2,3,4,6-tetraacetyl-glucose. DDMP saponins are stable in whole beans but subject to enzymatic or oxidative degradation if their cells are destroyed. The DDMP moiety of the saponin is degraded into soyasapogenols B and E. For example, after saponin βg, a DDMP saponin, undergoes hydrolysis and oxidative degradation in the course of extraction or purification, no change will occur in the carbohydrate structure of C-3, but a structural change will occur in the DDMP binding site at C-22; saponin Bb with soyasapogenol B (with a hydroxyl group at C-22) as aglycon or saponin Be with soyasapogenol E (with a ketone function at C-22) as the aglycon is produced. The production ratio of saponins Bb and Be from degradation of saponin βg is approximately 2:1. Due to less controllability of the degradation rate of DDMP saponins, however, the proportion of each saponin component tends to be unstable in the saponin fractions prepared for evaluation of functionality. It should be remembered during evaluation that fractionated DDMP saponin components include by-products such as maltol that are produced during the degradation of DDMP saponins.

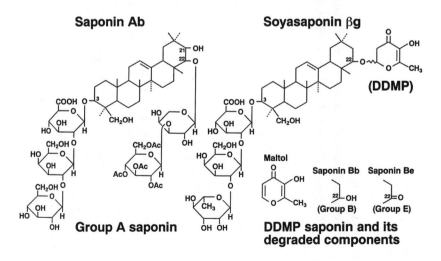

**FIGURE 9.1** Chemical structures of representative saponins found in soybean seeds.

Six carbohydrates have been found at C-3 on the aglycon. All these carbo-hydrates commonly have glucuronic acid as the first sugar binding site, via a glycosidic linkage, to C-3 on the aglycon. The next sugar binds to the hydroxyl group at C-2 of the glucuronic acid moiety via a glycosidic linkage can be divided into two types: arabinose and galactose. The third sugar is either glucose, rhamnose, or no sugar. Either of the former two sugars, glucose or rhamnose, binds to the hydroxyl group on C-2 of the second sugar, which is arabinose or galactose.

Therefore, there are a total of five carbohydrates — two different carbohydrates binding to soyasapogenol A, DDMP, and soyasapogenols B and E — at C-22 of the aglycon. Then, taking the above-mentioned six carbohydrates at the C-3 position into consideration, there are estimated to be 30 types of soybean saponin components. However, not all 30 saponin components can actually be detected from whole soybeans in a single assay. The genetic characteristics and localization in whole soybeans of each saponin component will now be described.

## 9.3 THE GENETICS OF SOYBEAN SAPONINS

The genetic localization of aglycons is as follows. Group A saponins (soyasapo-genol A) are produced only in the hypocotyl (including the plumule and radicle parts) of the seed.[1,4] This is probably because the gene producing soyasapogenol A expresses only at that location. Some mutants have also been found in which Group A saponin components, usually observed in the hypocotyl, cannot be detected.[5] One of them cannot produce soyasapogenol A.[6]

Next, we will discuss gene expression involved in carbohydrates at the C-22 position of soyasapogenol A. There are three types of sugar — xylose, glucose, or no sugar— that bind to the arabinose moiety at the C-22 position of Group A saponins, which are codominantly inherited,[7] as are human ABO blood types. However, the variant without a terminal sugar, corresponding to the O blood type, which has been found as a mutant, is not common.[8] Therefore, since soybean is an autogamous plant, if saponin components are prepared by using a single variant, Group A saponin components would include either of two series — saponin Aa (or the xylose type, including Aa and Ae) or Ab (or the glucose type, including Ab and Ac) — as shown in Table 9.1. Both types can be mixed only when variants Aa and Ab are mixed. A characteristic can be genetically controlled where the hydroxyl group of the terminal sugar (xylose or glucose) of carbohy-drates binding to the C-22 position can be fully acetylated.[4,9] Some mutants have been found at C-22 that cannot acetylate their terminal sugar.[2,5] The saponin components produced by these mutants are not included in the typical saponin components shown in Table 9.1.

Finally, we describe the characteristics of gene expression regarding carbo-hydrates at C-3. Saponin $\alpha_g$ is produced only in the hypocotyl. This is probably because the gene adding glucose to the terminal sugar at C-3 expresses only at that location.[6] Saponin $\beta_a$, however, is detected generally in the cotyledon, but

TABLE 9.2
**Saponin Components Detected in the Cotyledon and the Hypocotyl
of Soybean Seeds with Respective Genotypes[a]**

| Genotype | Cotyledon[b]<br>DDMP Saponins | Hypocotyl<br>Group A Saponins[c] | DDMP Saponins |
|---|---|---|---|
| Aa | βg, γg, βa, γa | Aa, Ae | αg, βg, γg |
| Ab | βg, γg, βa, γa | Ab, Ac, Af | αg, βg, γg |
| AaBc | βg, γg, βa, γa | Aa, Ae, Ax | αg, βg, γg, αa, βa, γa |
| AbBc | βg, γg, βa, γa | Ab, Ac, Af, Ad | αg, βg, γg, αa, βa, γa |

[a] Groups B and E saponin components, which are the derivatives of the corresponding DDMP saponins, are not listed here.
[b] Group A saponins are not detected in the cotyledon of the seeds.
[c] Minor components such as saponin Ag and Ah are barely detected in the normal soybean seeds.

not usually in the hypocotyl. However, there are several cultivars that produce this saponin in the hypocotyl.[10] In rare varieties such as these, saponin Ax or Ad, or saponin αa, which cannot be detected in normal soybean varieties, can be detected concomitantly with normal saponin components.[2] This can be interpreted as resulting from the expression of the gene in the hypocotyl that binds arabinose to carbohydrates at C-3, leading to complementary action of this gene with one added glucose that expresses in the hypocotyl.

In summary, of the demonstrated genetic characteristics related to polymorphism of soybean saponin composition, saponins in general soybean varieties can be roughly divided into four types. Table 9.2 shows the saponin components that each soybean variety, with respective genotype, produces in the cotyledon and the hypocotyl. Therefore, since not all of the reported soybean saponin components would be produced simultaneously, an appropriate variant must be selected in consideration of the genetic characteristics of candidate variants when we use soybean saponin components.

## 9.4 FUNCTIONALITY OF SOYBEAN SAPONINS

### 9.4.1 BIOTRANSFORMATION

Although the absorption of soybean saponins has been investigated since the 1960s, there are no definitive reports showing that soybean saponins are absorbed. Gestetner et al. investigated the absorption of soybean saponins into the blood and gastrointestinal tract based on the relationship between saponins and hemolytic activity by feeding chicken, rats, and mice a soybean saponin diet.[11] They detected saponins from the small intestine and the sapogenin, or aglycon, from the cecum and colon, but neither saponins nor sapogenin were detected in the blood, providing no evidence of absorption. Although a large amount of sapogenin was detected in the feces, the amount of aglycon in the feces was 60 to 65% of fed soybean saponins, suggesting that saponins are decomposed by enteric bacteria and absorbed. Yoshikoshi et al. investigated the content of saponins in the urine, feces, blood, and liver of rats fed with a hypocotyl diet and, as reported by Gestetner, demonstrated that there were no saponins detected in other than the feces.[12] DDMP-binding saponins and aglycons were detected in the feces, suggesting that most soybean saponins are either hydrolyzed by enteric bacteria into aglycons or excreted intact.

Although there are no definitive reports showing that soybean saponins are absorbed, various functionalities, such as increases in calcium content in bone components, alkaline phosphatase activity, and DNA content, have been reported in rats fed soybean saponins.[13] These effects were demonstrated experimentally in the femoral cells, and the osteoporosis-reducing effect of soybean saponins that were assumed not to be absorbed was confirmed *in vivo* and *in vitro*. Oral administration of soybean saponins provided antilipidemic effects when cholesterol was loaded[14] and showed a synergistic effect, especially when these saponins were fed simultaneously with soybean proteins.[15,16] These effects are derived from increased excretion of acidic or neutral sterols by saponins binding with these sterols.[17–19] Furthermore, various physiological activities of saponins *in vivo* were reported; there are further concerns, including absorption by phytosterol receptors and effects of saponins in the gastrointestinal tract related to biotransformation. Table 9.3 shows the previously reported physiological activities of saponins, and Figure 9.2 shows the relationship between the chemical structure and physiological activity of saponins.

### 9.4.2 ANTICANCER EFFECTS

Soybeans are known as a low risk food for cancer, and a correlation between the intake of soybean foods and the morbidity of cancer, especially colon and prostate cancers, has been reported in an epidemiological survey.[20] Chemical carcinogenesis is a multistage process that includes initiation, promotion, and progression, and many food plants show potent inhibitory effects against carcinogenic promotion.[21] Maeda et al. found that the promotion-inhibitory effect of food plants, especially carrot leaf, oilseed rape, and beans (soybeans, black soybeans, azuki [red] beans), correlated closely with the alkyl peroxide radical scavenging effect.[22]

The anticancer effects of the soybean may mutually involve saponins, protease inhibitors, isoflavones, and inositol-6-phosphate, although there are few reports on the individual anticancer effects of these substances. Konoshima et al. investigated the Epstein-Barr viral antigen activity of triterpenoid saponins of the bean family and reported the antigen activity facilitatory effect of soyasaponin Be (ketone function at C-22), one of the soybean saponins, and a protective

**TABLE 9.3**
**Physiological Properties of Soybean Saponin**

| Physiological Properties | Group A | Group B | Group E |
|---|---|---|---|
| Anticancer | | Konoshima et al. (23, 24) Sung et al. (25) Oh and Sung (26) | Konoshima et al. (23) |
| Antivirus | Nakashima et al. (30) | Nakashima et al. (30) Hayashi et al. (31) | Nakashima et al. (30) |
| Hapatoprotective effect | Ohminami et al. (36) Kinjo et al. (38) | Miyao et al. (37) Kinjo et al. (38, 39) | |
| Antioxidative and/or radical scavenging activity | Nishida et al. (43) | Tsujino et al. (42)[a] Nishida et al. (43)[a] Yoshiki et al. (47, 48)[a] | |
| Anabolic effect on bone | | Ono and Yamaguchi (13) | |
| Antilipidemia activity | Ohminami et al. (36) | | Ueda and Matsumoto (16) Pathirana et al. (15)[b] Oakenfull et al. (18)[b] Topping et al. (19)[b] |
| Prevention of $H_2O_2$ damage | Yoshikoshi et al. (40) | Yoshikoshi et al. (40)[a] | |

[a] Physiological properties obtained from DDMP saponins.
[b] Properties from crude saponin fraction.

effect on Raji cells.[23] However, soyasaponin Bb (hydroxyl group at C-22) with a different partial structure from Be only showed delayed effects of tumor development by treating with 12-$o$-tetradecanoyl phorbol 13-acetate (TPA) and did not have any inhibitory effect as observed in the case of Be, suggesting the importance of the chemical structure of saponins. In addition, Konoshima et al. observed that a combination of soyasaponin Bb with isoflavone (afromosin) provided a dramatic increase in inhibitory effect against tumor development, decreased rate of development, and reduced the number of tumors.[24] Natural substances that inhibit multistage carcinogenesis are now being widely researched.

Soybean saponins may inhibit promotion in a series of multistage carcinogeneses and are expected to show a synergistic effect with coexisting substances, including isoflavones and protein fractions. Long-term administration (48 h) of a soybean saponin fraction (2% saponin) resulted in significant inhibition of the growth and survival of colon tumor cells (HCT-15) and reduction in their overall survival.[25] As described in "biotransformation" of saponins, oral saponins are detected intact in the intestine and colon at high concentrations. This indicates a

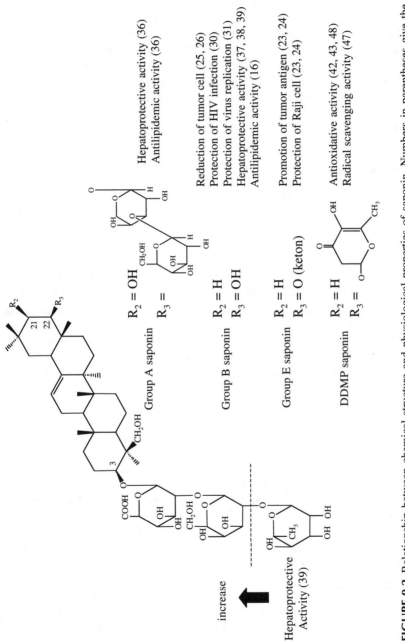

Hepatoprotective activity (36)
Antilipidemic activity (36)

R₂ = OH
R₃ =

Group A saponin

Reduction of tumor cell (25, 26)
Protection of HIV infection (30)
Protection of virus replication (31)
Hepatoprotective activity (37, 38, 39)
Antilipidemic activity (16)

R₂ = H
R₃ = OH

Group B saponin

Promotion of tumor antigen (23, 24)
Protection of Raji cell (23, 24)

R₂ = H
R₃ = O (keton)

Group E saponin

Antioxidative activity (42, 43, 48)
Radical scavenging activity (47)

R₂ = H
R₃ =

DDMP saponin

increase

Hepatoprotective
Activity (39)

**FIGURE 9.2** Relationship between chemical structure and physiological properties of saponin. Numbers in parentheses give the reference number.

prolonged presence of saponins in the intestine, suggesting that the carcinogenesis-inhibitory effect of soybean saponins on colon cancer cells is very strong. It has also been reported, in an experiment using human colon cancer cells (HT-29), that soybean saponins inhibit the growth of cancer cells through the inhibition of TPA-stimulated protein kinase C activity and an increase in carcinoembryonic antigens.[26] The incidence of colon and rectal cancers and other gastrointestinal cancers increases with age and sharply increases after the age of 50. Sung et al. and Oh et al. report that saponins at 600 ppm completely inhibited the growth of cancer cells in cellular experiments.[25,26] Since 100 g of soybeans contains about 0.6 to 6.0 g of saponins,[27] it is likely that saponins have a major inhibitory effect on gastrointestinal tract cancer.

### 9.4.3 ANTIVIRAL EFFECTS

Viruses are infectious particles in which DNA or RNA (the viral genome) is wrapped in a protein capsid. Once DNA viruses invade nonpermissive cells, they are incorporated into the genome of the host cells and replicated or become a plasmid that is replicated. This often causes genetic changes in nonpermissive cells.[28] RNA viruses infect permissive cells, causing genetic changes in the cells.[29] It has recently been revealed that the continuous synthesis of viral protein after these genetic changes causes cell transformation (neoplastic transformation) leading to cancerization, so the antiviral effects of food are now attracting research interest.

The human immunodeficiency virus (HIV), a retrovirus, invades helper T-cells (Th cells) by binding to their membrane protein (CD4). This means there may be two ways to protect against HIV infection: inhibition of reverse transcriptase or binding to Th cells. When the inhibitory effects of Group A (bis-desmoside saponins), Group B (monodesmoside saponins, hydroxyl group at C-22), and Group E (monodesmoside saponins, ketone function at C-22) saponins on HIV infection are compared, Group B saponins show an inhibitory effect that is severalfold greater than that of other saponins.[30] In particular, soyasaponin Bb shows the highest effect, providing almost complete inhibition of cell degeneration and of viral antigen expression caused by HIV. Since soybean saponins themselves do not act directly on HIV, the inhibitory effect of soyasaponin Bb on HIV infection does not provide direct inhibition of the reverse-transcriptional activity of HIV but may protect T4 cells from contact with HIV. The general characteristics of soybean saponins include bubble formability, or the surfactant effect. Group B saponins have greater inhibitory effect on HIV infection than Group A saponins (which have higher bubble formability), suggesting that this inhibitory effect is not derived from the physical characteristics of saponins.

Group B saponins also have an inhibitory effect on the transcription of herpes simplex virus type 1 (HSV-1). This effect was higher in saponins with GlcUA-Ara-Rham (soyasaponin Bc) than those with GlcUA-Gal-Rham (soysaponin Bb).[31] Soyasaponin Bc with arabinose as the second sugar also has an inhibitory effect on human cytomegalovirus (HCMV), influenza A virus, and human immuno-deficiency virus type 1 (HIV-1) and shows a strong antivirus effect, especially on HSV-1 (IC50; 54 $\mu M \pm 5.4 \mu M$). The antivirus effect of soybean saponins not only is a secondary one in which cell permeability and protein synthesis are inhibited but also is a direct one in which viruses (virus particles) are inactivated.

### 9.4.4 HEMOLYTIC EFFECTS

Saponins have long been known to have a hemolytic effect. This has been utilized to quantify the saponin content of plants. The effect comes from the high affinity of saponins to blood cell membrane sterols, which causes the blood cell to burst by changing its membrane permeability. We investigated the hemolytic activity of soybean saponins (0.1 m$M$ soyasaponin Bb and soyasaponin βg) but could not detect it from either saponin. However, high hemolytic activity was observed in soybean extract in 80% methanol. After an attempt to isolate hemolytic compo-nents from soybeans, unsaturated fatty acids such as linoleic acid and linolenic acid were suggested to be involved in the effect. Notably, a high hemolytic activity was observed in 13-hydroxy-9,11-octadecadienoic acid, a possible reac-tion product between lipoxygenase, an oxygenase, and linoleic acid (Y. Yoshiki, unpublished observations). Ginseng saponins also have hemolytic activity that depends greatly on their chemical structure. Hayashi et al. reported that 20-S-protopanaxtriol was highly hemolytic but that 20-S-protopanaxdiol was not hemolytic at all.[32] These results suggest that the polarity of the aglycon is involved in the hemolytic effect. Therefore, soybean neutral saponins are likely to show no hemolytic effect.

In the cancer cell membrane, the lipid and cholesterol content increases mark-edly.[33] Acidic saponins, including gypsophillsaponins, bind to cancer cell mem-brane sterols to increase the transformation of cancer cell surfaces and membrane permeability. By comparing colon cancer cells treated with soybean saponins (neutral saponins) and those treated with gypsophilla saponins (acidic saponins), Sung et al. found that soybean saponins caused neither transformation nor mem-brane permeability of the membrane surface.[25] This result supports reports that soybean saponins have no hemolytic effect mediated by membrane permeability.

Since Birk et al. reported on the hemolytic activity of soybean saponin frac-tions, this activity has attracted attention as a minor characteristic.[34] However, soybean saponin fractions extracted in ethanol or methanol were used in many studies that failed to relate hemolysis to saponins. Recently, it has been reported that soybean saponins were often isolated in the form of artifacts where these saponins bind to unsaturated fatty acids such as linoleic acid.[35] What has been regarded as the hemolytic effect of soybean saponins may be caused by additions to which soybean saponins bind. In addition, no growth inhibition caused by hemolytic activity has been observed in animals fed with soybean saponin fractions showing this activity,[11] indicating that there may be no risk from the hemolytic effect of the soybeans.

### 9.4.5 INHIBITORY EFFECTS ON LIVER DISORDERS

The liver is an important organ that has roles in storing nutrients, producing bile, regulating blood flow, and breaking down alcohol and pharmaceuticals. Excessive intake of alcohol and drugs and viral infections may cause liver disorder (hepatitis), leading to serious liver diseases such as cirrhosis and liver cancer. Soybean saponin fractions have an inhibitory effect on these disorders. Ohminami et al. reported that Group A saponins, or bis-desmoside saponins, have this effect,[36] and Miyao et al. reported the liver-damaging effect of Group B saponins, or monodesmoside saponins.[37] Five Group B saponins have been isolated from soybeans. Soyasaponin Bb, the predominant saponin, effectively inhibits liver disorders induced by carbon tetrachloride, suggesting the usefulness of soybean intake.[37]

Glucoside fractions of other edible beans (azuki beans, kidney beans, and scarlet runner beans) also have inhibitory effects on liver disorders.[38] In experimental systems with immunological liver injury, comparison of the liver disorder prevention rates of bean glycoside fractions revealed that the effectiveness became larger in the order of scarlet runner beans, soybeans, kidney beans, and azuki beans. When the inhibitory effects of the isolated predominant saponins of the beans were compared, the effectiveness of soyasaponin Bb was the highest, followed in descending order by soyasaponin Ba, azukisaponin I, and phaseoside I. These results suggest that the inhibitory effect on liver disorders is higher in saponins with soysapogenol in their aglycon. Kinjo et al. investigated in detail the relationship between C-3 and C-22 chains and the inhibitory effect on liver disorders of saponins isolated from beans.[38,39] An investigation of the C-3 chain revealed that disaccharide had a higher effect than trisaccharide (soyasaponin Bb', Bc' > soyasaponin Bb, Bc) and that, as for the terminal sugar, rhamnose (soyasaponin Bb) showed a higher effect than glucose (soyasaponin Ba, phaseoside I). For the C-22 chain of Group A saponins, glucosyl-arbinose as the terminal sugar was the most effective. The inhibitory effect on cytotoxicity that has often been observed was previously thought to derive from the physical characteristics rather than the chemical properties of soybean saponins.[40] However, a series of studies reported by Kinjo et al. suggests that the inhibitory effect on liver disorders is linked to the chemical properties of saponins, in which the carbohydrate has an important role in the reaction.

### 9.4.6 ANTIOXIDATIVE EFFECTS

Biological oxidation caused by reactive oxygen species (ROS) and free radicals is involved in diseases such as cancer and arteriosclerosis and in biological aging. ROS and radicals are generated by extrinsic factors including exhaust gas, ultraviolet rays, tobacco, and food carcinogens, as well as intrinsic factors including microsomal, peroxisomal, and flavin enzymes. Unsaturated fatty acids or the DNA essential to the living body are often targeted by these radicals; therefore, our body consistently exerts defensive mechanisms against them. Antioxidative mechanisms are divided into four types, depending on the method of defense: (a) preventive antioxidation that inhibits the generation of ROS and radicals; (b) radical-scavenging antioxidation, which eliminates, scavenges, and stabilizes generated ROS and radicals; (c) *de novo* antioxidation, which repairs and reproduces injured sites; and (d) adaptational antioxidation, which induces a defensive function or an antioxidative enzyme at a certain site.[41]

There have been several reports on the antioxidative properties of soybean saponins. These properties are markedly increased when lipid oxidation is induced with radical generators including 2,2′-azobis(2-amidino-propane) (AAPH) and 2,2′-azobis (2,4-dimethylvaleronitrile) (AMVN).[42,43] Nishida et al. reported that the antioxidative effects of Group A saponins were higher than those of Group B saponins in the mouse liver microsome.[43] Radical generators provide a time difference in this antioxidative property, suggesting that the stages at which soybean saponins inhibit the initiation and propagation of lipid oxidation depend on the radical species. The series of soybean saponins newly reported in 1992 (DDMP saponin) show the 2,3-dihydro-2,5-dihydroxy-6-methyl-4$H$-pyran-4-one (DDMP moiety) binding to C-22 of soyasapogenol B.[44-46] Reports on DDMP saponins that are widely distributed among bean species have been inconsistent; some reported antioxidative effects in experimental systems in which oxidation was induced using radical generators, and others reported pro-oxidation effects in lipid autoxidation systems.

Yoshiki et al., who investigated the spin density at the DDMP moiety, demonstrated a high probability of the presence of unpaired electrons at C-6, suggesting that the antioxidative properties of DDMP saponins produce radical scavenging and eliminating, rather than lipid protective effects.[47] One eliminating effect on DPPH radicals, or $O_2^-$, of DDMP saponins, has been reported.[47,48] Pro-oxidating effects in a lipid autoxidation system of DDMP saponins demonstrated a synergistic antioxidative effect in the presence of hydrogen donors such as phenol compounds. This suggests that DDMP saponins have ambivalent effects that include the "negative effect" where hydrogens of unsaturated fatty acids are abstracted due to their radical-scavenging ability and the "positive effect" where interaction with a hydrogen donor (facilitation of radical scavenging ability) prolongs the antioxidative effect. This unique activity is not observed in Group B and E saponins that lack the DDMP moiety, indicating that this behavior is derived from the DDMP moiety. A composite effect with phenol compounds of soybean saponins was reported in the anticancer effect, suggesting the likelihood of a new function.[24] In addition, DDMP saponins have an iron- and copper-chelating effect that is attributable to the DDMP moiety.[49] Iron and copper ions generate hydroxyl radicals through the Fenton reaction to facilitate biological oxidation. DDMP saponins not only have the above-mentioned radical-scavenging antioxidative effect but also have a preventive antioxidant effect that prevents active oxygen from being generated during the chelation of metal ions such as free iron and copper ions. The antioxidative properties of DDMP saponins are shown in Figure 9.3.

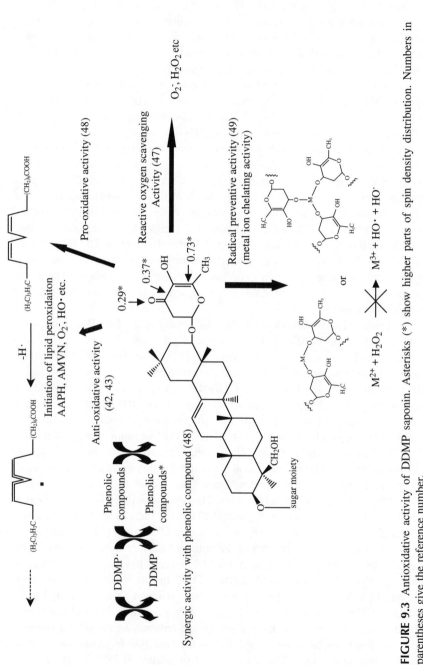

**FIGURE 9.3** Antioxidative activity of DDMP saponin. Asterisks (*) show higher parts of spin density distribution. Numbers in parentheses give the reference number.

## 9.5 CONCLUSIONS

There have been reports on the various effects of soybeans, of which saponins are one of the primary factors showing physiological activity. Kitagawa et al. elucidated the basic structure of soybean saponins in the 1980s.[50] However, saponins, which have amphipathic properties and bubble formability, are difficult to isolate and purify; therefore, many early studies of the physiological activity of saponins used only crude saponin fractions. In this chapter, the characteristics of the structure and physiological activity of saponins were summarized by listing only those studies in which isolated saponins were used or saponin composition was clearly demonstrated. Recently, the synergistic effect obtained by combining saponins with certain compounds (proteins, isoflavones, and phenol compounds) has been reported. The elucidation of complex effects based on the structural characteristics of saponins is currently the focus of much research.

## ACKNOWLEDGMENTS

We are deeply indebted to Ms. Mizuho Okamatsu, Ms. Minobu Managi, Mr. Eric Sheldon, and Ms. Rumi Nogami of World Translation Service, Tsukuba, Japan, for their willingness to assist in translating this chapter into English.

## REFERENCES

1. Fenwick, G.R., Price, K.R., Tsukamoto, C., and Okubo, K., Saponins, in *Toxic Substances in Crop Plants,* D'Mollo, J.P.F., Duffus, C.M., and Duffus, J.H., Eds., Royal Society of Chemistry, Cambridge, UK, 1991, pp. 285–327, 1991.
2. Tsukamoto, C., Kikuchi, A., Harada, K., Kitamura, K., and Okubo, K., Genetic and chemical polymorphisms of saponins in soybean seed, *Phytochemistry,* 34, 1351–1356, 1993.
3. Kudou, S., Tonomura, M., Tsukamoto, C., Uchida, T., Sakabe, T., Tamura, N., and Okubo, K., Isolation and structural elucidation of DDMP-conjugated soyasaponins as genuine saponins from soybean seeds, *Biosci. Biotechnol. Biochem.,* 57, 546–550, 1993.
4. Shimoyamada, M., Kudo, S., Okubo, K., Yamauchi, F., and Harada, K., Distribution of saponins constituents in some varieties of soybean plant, *Agric. Biol. Chem.,* 54, 77–81, 1990.
5. Tsukamoto, C., Kikuchi, A., Kudou, S., Harada, K., Kitamura, K., and Okubo, K., Group A acetyl saponin-deficient mutant from the wild soybean, *Phytochemistry,* 31, 4139–4142, 1992.
6. Tsukamoto, C., Kikuchi, A., Takada, Y., Kono, Y., Harada, K., Kitamura, K., and Okubo, K., Genetic improvement of soybean saponins, in *Proceedings of IV International Soybean Processing and Utilization Conference, PR, Brazil,* 822–829, 2004.
7. Shiraiwa, M., Yamauchi, F., Harada, K., and Okubo, K., Inheritance of "Group A saponin" in soybean seed, *Agric. Biol. Chem.,* 54, 1347–1352, 1990.

8. Kikuchi, A., Tsukamoto, C., Tabuchi, K., Adachi, T., and Okubo, K., Inheritance and characterization of a null allele for Group A acetyl saponins found in a mutant soybean (*Glycine max* (L.) Merrill), *Breed. Sci.,* 49, 167–171, 1999.

9. Shiraiwa, M., Kudo, S., Shimoyamada, M., Harada, K., and Okubo, K., Composition and structure of "Group A saponin" in soybean seed, *Agric. Biol. Chem.,* 55, 315–322, 1991.

10. Tsukamoto, C., Kikuchi, A., Kudou, S., Harada, K., Iwasaki T., and Okubo, K., Genetic improvement of saponin components in soybean, in *ACS Symposium Series 546, Food Phytochemicals for Cancer Prevention I,* Huang, M.T., Osawa, T., Ho, C.T., and Rosen, R.T., Eds., American Chemical Society, Washington, DC, 1994, pp. 372–379.

11. Gestetner, B., Birk, Y., and Tencer, Y., Soybean saponins: fate of ingested soybean saponins and the physiological aspect of their hemolytic activity, *J. Agric. Food Chem.,* 16, 1031–1035, 1968.

12. Yoshikoshi, M., Kahara, T., Yoshiki, Y., Ito, M., Furukawa, Y., Okubo, K., and Amarowicz, R., Metabolism and nonabsorption of soybean hypocotyls saponins in the rat model, *Acta Aliment.,* 24, 355–364, 1995.

13. Ono, R. and Yamaguchi, M., Anabolic effect of soybean saponin on bone components in the femoral tissues of rats, *J. Health Sci.,* 45, 251–255, 1999.

14. Oakenfull, D.G. and Topping, L.D., Saponins and plasma cholesterol, *Atherosclerosis,* 48, 301–303, 1983.

15. Pathirana, C., Gibney, M.J., and Taylar, T.G., The effect of dietary protein source and saponins on serum lipids and the excretion of bile acids and neutral sterols in rabbits, *Br. J. Nutr.,* 46, 421–430, 1981.

16. Ueda, H. and Matsumoto, A., Effects of soybean saponin and soybean protein on serum cholesterol concentration in cholesterol-fed chicks, *Anim. Sci. Technol. Jpn.,* 67, 415–422, 1996.

17. Oakenfull, D.G. and Fenwick, D.E., Adsorption of bile salts from aqueous solution by plant fibre and cholestyramine, *Br. J. Nutr.,* 10, 299–309, 1978.

18. Oakenfull, D.G., Fenwick, D.E., Hood, R.L., Topping, D.L., Illman, R.L., and Storer, G.B., Effects of saponins on bile acids and plasma lipids in the rat, *Br. J. Nutr.,* 42, 209–216, 1979.

19. Topping, D.L., Storer, G.B., Calvert, G.D., Illman, R.J., Oakenfull, D.G., and Weller, R.A., Effects of dietary saponins on fecal bile acids and neutral sterols, plasma lipids, and lipoprotein turnover in the pig, *Am. J. Clin. Nutr.,* 33, 783–786, 1980.

20. Messina, M.J., Persky, V., Setchell, K.D.R., and Barnes, S., Soy intake and cancer risk: a review of the in vitro and in vivo data, *Nutr. Cancer,* 21, 113–131, 1994.

21. Koshimizu, K., Ohigashi, H., Tokuda, H., Kondo, A., and Yamaguchi, K., Screening of edible plants against possible anti-tumor promoting activity, *Cancer Lett.,* 39, 247–257, 1988.

22. Maeda, H., Katsuki, T., Akaike, T., and Yasutake, R., High correlation between lipid peroxide radical and tumor-promoter effect: suppression of tumor promotion in the Epstein-Barr virus/B-lymphocyte system and scavenging of alkyl peroxide radicals by various vegetable extracts, *Jpn. J. Cancer Res.,* 83, 923–928, 1992.

23. Konoshima, T., Kozuka, M., Haruna, M., and Ito, K., Constituents of leguminous plants. XIII. New triterpenoid saponins from *Wistaria brachybotry, J. Nat. Prod.,* 54, 830–836, 1991.

24. Konoshima, T., Antitumor-promoting activities of triterpenoid glycosides: cancer chemoprevention by saponins, in *Saponins Used in Traditional and Modern Medicine: Advances in Experimental Medicine and Biology*, Waller, G.R. and Yamasaki, K., Eds., Plenum Press, New York, 1996, pp. 87–100.

25. Sung, M., Kendall, C.W.C., Koo, M.M., and Rao, A.V., Effect of soybean saponins and gypsophilla saponin on growth and viability of colon carcinoma cells in culture, *Nutr. Cancer,* 23, 259–270, 1995.

26. Oh, Y. and Sung, M., Soybean saponins inhibit cell proliferation by suppressing PKC activation and induce differentiation of HT-29 human colon adenocarcinoma cells, *Nutr. Cancer,* 39, 132–138, 2001.

27. Shiraiwa, M., Harada, K., and Okubo, K., Composition and content of saponins in soybean seed according to variety, cultivation year and maturity, *Agric. Biol. Chem.,* 55, 323–331, 1991.

28. Hausen, H., Viruses in human cancers, *Science,* 254, 1167–1173, 1991.

29. Varmus, H., Retroviruses, *Science,* 240, 1427–1435, 1988.

30. Nakashima, K., Okubo, K., Honda, Y., Tamura, T., Matsuda, S., and Yamamoto, N., Inhibitory effect of glycosides like saponin from soybean on the infectivity of HIV *in vitro, AIDS,* 3, 655–658, 1989.

31. Hayashi, K., Hayashi, H., Hiraoka, N., and Ikeshiro, Y., Inhibitory activity of soyasaponin II on virus replication *in vitro, Planta Med.,* 63, 102–105, 1997.

32. Namba, T., Yoshizaki, M., Tomimori, T., Kobashi, K., Mitsui, K., and Hase, J., Hemolytic and its protective activity of ginseng saponins, *Chem. Pharm. Bull.,* 21, 459–461, 1973.

33. Hilf, R., Goldenberg, H., Michel, I., Orlando, R.A., and Archer, F.L., Enzymes, nucleic acids, and lipids in human breast cancer and normal breast tissue, *Cancer Res.,* 30, 1874–1882, 1970.

34. Birk, Y., Bondi, A., Gestetner, B., and Ishaaya, I., A thermostable maemolytic factor in soybeans, *Nature,* 197, 1089–1090, 1963.

35. Massiot, G., Dijoux, M., and Lavaud, C., Saponins and artifacts, in *Saponins Used in Food and Agriculture: Advances in Experimental Medicine and Biolgy*, Waller, G.R. and Yamasaki, K., Eds., Plenum Press, New York, 1996, pp. 183–192.

36. Ohminami, H., Kimura, Y., Okuda, H., Arichi, S., Yoshikawa, M., and Kitagawa, I., Effects of soyasaponins on liver injury induced by highly peroxidized fat in rats, *Planta Med.,* 50, 440–441, 1984.

37. Miyao, H., Arao, T., Udayama, M., Kinjo, J., and Nohara, T., Kaikasaponin III and soyasaponin I, major triterpene saponins of *Abrus cantoniensis,* act on GOT and GPT: influence on transaminase elevation of rat liver cells concomitantly exposed to $CCl_4$ for one hour, *Planta Med.,* 64, 5–7, 1998.

38. Kinjo, J., Udayama, M., Hatakeyama, M., Ikeda, T., Sohno, Y., Yoshiki, Y., Okubo, K., and Nohara, T., Hepatoprotective effects of oleanene glucuronides in several edible beans, *Nat. Med.,* 53, 141–144, 1999.

39. Kinjo, J., Imagire, M., Udayama, M., Arao, T., and Nohara, T., Structure-hepatoprotective relationships study of soyasaponins I-IV having soyasapogenol B as aglycone, *Planta Med.,* 64, 233–236, 1998.

40. Yoshikoshi, M., Yoshiki, Y., Okubo, K., Seto, J., and Sasaki, Y., Prevention hydrogen peroxide damage by soybean saponins to mouse fibroblasts, *Planta Med.,* 62, 252–255, 1996.

41. Halliwell, B. and Gutteridge, J.M.C., The antioxidants of human extracellular fluids, *Arch. Biochem. Biophys.,* 280, 1–8, 1990.

42. Tsujino, Y., Tsurumi, S., Yoshida, Y., and Niki, E., Antioxidative effects of dihydro-γ-pyronyl-triterpenoid saponin (chromosaponin I), *Biosci. Biotechnol. Biochem.,* 58, 1731–1732, 1994.
43. Nishida, K., Ohta, Y., Araki, Y., Ito, M., Nagamura, Y., and Ishiguro, I., Inhibitory effects of "group A saponin" and "group B saponin" fractions from soybean seed hypocotyls on radical-initiated lipid peroxidation in mouse liver microsomes, *J. Clin. Biochem. Nutr.,* 15, 175–184, 1993.
44. Kudou, S., Tonomura, M., Tsukamoto, C., Shimoyamada, M., and Okubo, K., Isolation and structural elucidation of the major genuine soybean saponin, *Biosci. Biotechnol. Biochem.,* 56, 142–143, 1992.
45. Massiot, J., Lavaud, C., Venkhaled, M., and LeMen-Olivier, L., Saponin VI, a new maltol conjugate from alfalfa and soybean, *J. Nat. Prod.,* 55, 1339–1342, 1992.
46. Tsurumi, S., Takagi, T., and Hashimoto, T., A γ-pyronyl-triterpennoid saponin from *Pisum sativum, Phytochemistry,* 31, 2435–2438, 1992.
47. Yoshiki, Y. and Okubo, K., Active oxygen scavenging activity of DDMP (2,3-dihydro-2,5-dihydroxy-6-methyl-4*H*-pyran-4-one) saponin in soybean seed, *Biosci. Biotechnol. Biochem.,* 59, 1556–1557, 1995.
48. Yoshiki, Y., Kahara, T., Okubo, K., Sakabe, T., and Yamasaki, T., Superoxide- and 1,1-diphenyl-2-picrylhydrazyl radical-scavenging activities of soyasaponin βg related to gallic acid. *Biosci. Biotechnol. Biochem.,* 65, 2162–2165, 2001.
49. Yoshiki, Y., Kudou, S., and Okubo, K., Relationship between chemical structures and biological activities of triterpenoid saponins from soybean, *Biosci. Biotechnol. Biochem.,* 62, 2291–2299, 1998.
50. Kitagawa, I., Saito, M., Taniyama, T., and Yoshikawa, M., Saponin and sapogenol. XXXVIII. Structure of soyasaponin A2, a bisdesmoside of soysapogenol A, from soybean, the seeds of *Glycine max* MERRILL, *Chem. Pharm. Bull.,* 33, 598–608, 1985.

# 10 Role of Soy Lecithin in Lipid Metabolism

*Katsumi Imaizumi*

## CONTENTS

## 10.1   INTRODUCTION

Soy lecithin has been widely used in the food and cosmetic industries because it can emulsify lipid-soluble materials.[1,2] Soy lecithin has also been implicated in absorption, transport, and metabolism of lipids in the intestine, circulation, and liver, thereby contributing to health promotion.[3] However, the precise role of soy lecithin in health and disease related to lipid metabolism has remained elusive. Soy lecithin–derived choline is considered a source of neurotransmitter acetylcholine, and the role of dietary lecithin in neurological disorders has been extensively reviewed by Canty and Zeisel.[4]

Soy lecithin is often used instead of phosphatidylcholine (PC), although commercially available soy lecithin contains triacylglycerols (TGs) and phospholipids other than PC. Phospholipid involvement in various physiological functions has been studied in the field of cell and molecular biology. Although the findings are relevant to the functions of soy lecithin in nutrition, health, and diseases, we must primarily consider how diet-derived soy lecithin influences the concentrations and composition of cellular and extracellular phospholipids and their physiological functions. This chapter reviews as systematically as possible absorption and transport of soy lecithin and the roles in lipid metabolism, based on a series of our studies.[5–16]

## 10.2   HYPOCHOLESTEROLEMIC ACTION OF SOY LECITHIN

### 10.2.1   CHEMICAL COMPOSITION OF SOY LECITHIN

Commercially available crude soy lecithin contains various proportions of neutral and polar lipids.[17] Neutral lipids are mainly TGs, whereas polar lipids consist of phospholipids and glycolipids. Our lecithin preparation contained, by weight, 66% phospholipids, 33% neutral lipids, and less than 0.5% plant sterols.[5–8,11] The major phospholipids were, by weight, 28.1% PC, 28.0% phosphatidylethanolamine (PE), 19.8% phosphatidylinositol (PI), 18.6% phoshatidic acid, and 5.5% lysophosphatidylcholine (lysoPC). Soy lecithin and soybean oil contain similar amounts of linoleic acid: 60.5% in soy lecithin and 58.7% in soybean oil.

## 10.2.2 CHEMICAL COMPOSITION OF MESENTERIC LYMPH LIPOPROTEINS

Dietary lipids are transported in the intestine as chylomicrons (CMs). The particle size of the CM is distributed over a wide range (400 to 6000 Å) and depends on the amount of dietary TG absorbed in the intestine.[18] Large particles (large CMs) are secreted into lymph under active absorption, smaller particles (small CMs) being secreted in the fasting state.[19]

In order to examine how dietary soy lecithin affects the synthesis and secretion of CMs in the intestine of rats during the absorption or postabsorption of dietary lipids, mesenteric lymph was collected from meal-fed (9 A.M. to 10 A.M.) and *ad libitum*–fed rats on purified diets containing 10 g/kg dietary soy lecithin or soy oil for 2 weeks.[5] We did not use duodenum perfusion with a physiological solution to maintain preferable lymph flow, since we wanted to determine the composition of mesenteric lymph in the intact intestine in regularly fed rats. One of the disadvantages of this operation was a low lymph flow (0.3 to 0.8 ml/h) compared to the condition where the duodenum was perfused with physiological saline (1 to 1.5 ml/h). Since the lymph flow rate was comparable between the lecithin- and oil-fed rats, we believed that comparing both dietary treatments is rational.

The concentrations of mesenteric lymph CM obtained from the meal-fed rats given soy lecithin and soy oil were 7- and 11-fold higher, respectively, than those of the *ad libitum*–fed rats, indicating that the CMs and TGs in the meal-fed rats are mainly derived from dietary lipids. In meal-fed rats, the concentration of TGs in the CMs obtained from soy lecithin–fed rats was about 80% of that from the soy oil–fed rats. This means that much of the fatty acids in the phospholipids is utilized for CM–TG because the dietary soy lecithin used in the experiment contained approximately 35% neutral lipids. The utilization of the fatty acids in PC for the formation of the CM–TG was shown by radiolabeling the fatty acids in the PC.[20] The contribution of the glycerophospholipids other than PC to the formation of the CM–TG remains to be established. Since PC accounted for only 30% of the phospholipids of soy lecithin, it is assumed that the fatty acids in glycerophopsholipids other than PC were also utilized for CM–TG.

The lymphatic CMs prepared from rats fed soy lecithin contained more TGs (88.3 vs. 76.8%), and less cholesterol (0.4 vs. 1.0%) and phospholipids (9.1 vs. 15.7%) than those from rats fed soy oil.[11] The average molecular parameters of large and small CMs were estimated from the chemical composition of CMs.[5] The dietary soy lecithin increased the average particle size of the large and small CMs obtained from the meal-fed rats and decreased the average number of particles secreted into the lymph.[5] This means dietary soy lecithin expands the core of the CM particle composed of TG in contrast to the surrounding surface composed of phospholipids, cholesterol, and proteins. This increase in particle size due to soy lecithin feeding was not so prominent in the postabsorptive state (*ad libitum* feeding). The human experiment performed by Beil and Grundy[21] showed the increase in small CMs in plasma due to the feeding of soybean lecithin.

The reason for the alteration of the physicochemical nature of the lymph CMs was not clear, but the following possible mechanisms were proposed. First, dietary soy lecithin might increase the distal absorption of fatty acids from the dietary soy lecithin unabsorbed in the upper part of the intestine. Several workers have shown that large amounts of lecithin perfused into the lumen of the duodenum inhibit the absorption of long chain fatty acids and cholesterol in the proximal intestine[22,23] and that the unhydrolyzed lecithin is absorbed in the distal intestine.[24] CMs produced in the distal intestine are relatively rich in TGs and poor in surface components compared to those in the proximal intestine.[25,26] A second possible reason is that dietary soy lecithin might increase the supply of TG and decrease the supply of surface components for CM synthesis. Competition for the common substrate diacylglycerols between phosphocholinetransferase and diacylglycerol acyltransferase determines *de novo* synthesis of PC and TG.[27] In addition, dietary soy lecithin appeared to decrease the supply of apo A-I, one of the major protein components of CM.[19]

The fatty acid composition of the CM phospholipids was measured to determine whether the 1-acyl lysoPC in the intestinal lumen could be incorporated intact into the CM phospholipids (Table 10.1). The dietary lecithin given to meal-fed rats increased in linoleic acid at the expense of arachidonic acid in the phospholipids.[5] The PC used in the soy lecithin diet contained 53% linoleic acid at the 1-position.[6] Lekim showed that linoleic at the 1-position, but not the 2-position of the oral PC was incorporated intact into the CM–PC when doubly labeled dilinoleoyl PC with [H³] and [C¹⁴] was used.[20] The relative proportion of linoleic acid in the CM–PC increased at the expense of arachidonic acid, and there was no reduction of the saturated fatty acids. Therefore, any direct incorporation of the dietary 1-linoleoyl PC into the counterpart of the CM will be quite small. Our study suggested that the increased proportion of linoleic acid and the decreased proportion of arachidonic acid in rats fed lecithin compared to those fed oil is responsible for the altered activity of Δ6-desaturase.[15] These findings partly explained why the TG form of the arachidonic and docosahexaenoic acid may be more efficacious than the phospholipid source based on increases in both polyunsaturated fatty acids compared with control piglets.[28]

**TABLE 10.1**
**Fatty Acid Composition of Phospholipids in Lymph CM in Rats Fed Soy Lecithin and Soy Oil**

| Fatty Acids | Soy Oil ($n = 5$) | Soy Lecithin ($n = 5$) | $P$ |
|---|---|---|---|
| | (wt%) | | |
| 16:0 | 17.7 | 18.9 | ns |
| 18:0 | 16.4 | 15.2 | ns |
| 18:1 | 9.0 | 8.0 | ns |
| 18:2 | 38.9 | 46.7 | 0.01 |
| 20:4 | 15.4 | 7.8 | 0.01 |

### 10.2.3 Chemical Composition of Bile and Fecal Lipids

Dietary soy lecithin increased the excretion of neutral sterols, but not bile acid, into the feces.[5] In humans, similar results have been reported by Greten et al.[29] A portion of the fecal-neutral sterols could be attributed to the unabsorbed bile cholesterol, since the previous *in vivo* and *in vitro* studies have shown that dietary phospholipids inhibit the intestinal absorption of cholesterol.[21–23,30] In intestinal cell line Caco-2 cells, incubation with PC-containing micelles resulted in reductions in the absorption, esterification, and secretion of cholesterol, whereas pancreatic phospholipase A2 enhanced cholesterol absorption from PC-containing micelles.[31,32]

However, most of the neutral sterols in the feces probably have a source other than bile, because daily excretion of bile cholesterol is about 3 mg, while that into the feces was 10 mg in soy oil–fed rats and 63 mg in soy lecithin–fed rats.[5] The most probable source of fecal sterols appears to be intestinal desquamated cells.[33] Plant sterols contained in the dietary soy lecithin also contributed to the unidentified fecal sterols in rats given soy lecithin, since the highest estimation of the daily intake of plant sterols in the soy lecithin diet was about 10 mg. However, it is not clear whether the desquamation of the intestinal cells due to soy lecithin feeding accompanies increased cell renewal.

### 10.2.4 Serum Lipids and Lipoprotein Profiles

Polyunsaturated phospholipids taken orally decrease serum cholesterol concentrations in rats,[6,34,35] pigs,[36] and monkeys,[37–39] but the mechanism is not known. Some investigators have reported that in humans, polyunsaturated phospholipids prepared from soybean decrease serum cholesterol,[40] and others have not found any significant reduction of cholesterol.[29,41] These discrepancies in humans may be due to the amount of phospholipids ingested or differences in dietary ingredients other than phospholipids. The hypocholesterolemic effect of soy lecithin may be due to the high content of linoleic acid, because linoleic acid lowers serum cholesterol, compared to the saturated fatty acids, in humans[42,43] and experimental animals.[44] In carefully controlled experiments where the amount of linoleic acid in phospholipids and TGs was almost the same, the cholesterol-lowering action of the soybean phospholipids was due to the phospholipid molecule.[38,40]

We compared the chemical composition of the serum lipoproteins in rats fed soy lecithin with those fed neutral lipid containing comparable amounts of linoleic acid (Table 10.2).[6] There was a tendency for linoleic acid to increase at the expense of arachidonic and docosahexaenoic acids in the phospholipids in rats fed soy lecithin (29.4 wt.% vs. 24.6 wt.% for linoleic acid; 13.6 wt.% vs. 19.3 wt.% for arachidonic acid; 2.5 wt.% vs. 4.0 wt.% for docosahexaenoic acid). These results confirmed those of previous experiments in rats,[34] pigs,[36] monkeys,[37,38] and humans[40] that soy lecithin decreases the concentration of serum cholesterol. In addition to the reduction of cholesterol, apo A-I also decreased. The reduction of serum apo A-I due to dietary soy lecithin might be brought about by several possible mechanisms, including a decreased supply of apo A-I from the intestine

TABLE 10.2
Concentration of Serum Lipids and Apolipoproteins
in Rats Fed Soy Lecithin and Soy Oil

| Lipids, Apoproteins | Soy Oil ($n = 10$) | Soy Lecithin ($n = 10$) | P |
|---|---|---|---|
| | (mg/dl) | | |
| Cholesterylesters | 129 | 80.6 | 0.05 |
| Free cholesterol | 19.9 | 19.8 | ns |
| TG | 280 | 296 | ns |
| Phospholipids | 123 | 121 | ns |
| Apo A-I | 84.5 | 54.5 | 0.001 |
| Apo B | 22.4 | 31.1 | 0.01 |
| Apo E | 29.5 | 28.7 | ns |

and liver[45,46] or increased turnover of serum apo A-I. Dietary soy lecithin significantly decreased the secretion of apo A-I from the intestine, as described above.[5]

In contrast to the reduction of serum apo A-I, dietary soy lecithin increased serum
apo B, especially the one with high molecular weight, which is secreted solely
from the liver as very low density lipoproteins (VLDLs).[6] The increased concentration of apo B might be attributable to the lipotropic action of the choline,
inositol, and ethanolamine in the soy lecithin diet,[47] because hepatic TG decreased
remarkably in rats fed soy lecithin (13.9 vs. 22.3 mg/g liver for the soy lecithin
and soy oil groups, respectively; $P < 0.05$). Since an increase in cholesterol ester
was not observed in the $d < 1.063$ g/ml lipoprotein fractions containing VLDLs
and low-density lipoproteins (LDLs), it is not likely that the lipoproteins consisted
of abnormally metabolized TG-rich particles as in the case of type III hyperlipo-
proteinemia in humans.[48]

Epidemiological studies have shown that the reduction of serum apo B and
the enhancement of serum apo A-I are beneficial for the prevention of ischemic
heart diseases.[49] The administration of fat rich in linoleic acid to humans decreases
not only serum cholesterol but also high-density lipoprotein (HDL) cholesterol and
-apo A-I.[43] This effect may be strengthened when linoleic acid is given as phospholipids. Since polyunsaturated phospholipids are used widely as a drug and health
food, further evaluation of the class and amount of polyunsaturated phospholipids
appropriate for human use is necessary.

## 10.2.5 HEPATIC SECRETION OF LIPIDS AND LIPOPROTEINS

To clarify the underlying mechanisms of the alteration of serum lipids and apolipoproteins, secretion of lipids and apolipoproteins from isolated perfused livers of
rats fed soy lecithin and soy oil were compared.[8] The hepatic VLDL prepared
from rats fed soy lecithin contained more TG (81.0 vs. 76.8%) and less cholesterol
(3.8 vs. 5.9%) and phospholipids (11.8 vs. 13.5%) than those from rats fed soy
oil.[11] Soy lecithin significantly decreased the rates of accumulation of apo A-I

(39.4 vs. 108 ng/min/g liver for the soy lecithin and soy oil groups, respectively; $P < 0.05$) and cholesterol (19.0 vs. 34.1 ng/min $\times$ g liver for the soy lecithin and soy oil groups, respectively; $P < 0.05$) in the liver perfusate. The secretion of newly synthesized apo A-I labeled with [$^3$H]lysine into the perfusate also decreased in rats fed soy lecithin (7.1 vs. 12.5 dpm $\times$ $10^{-3}$/g liver for the soy lecithin and soy groups, respectively; $P < 0.05$). The amino acid incorporation studies using the liver perfusion experiment suggest that the altered secretion of labeled apolipoproteins reflects changes in the synthetic rates as well as changes in intracellular or entrapped pool sizes of the surface of the liver.[50,51] The secretion patterns of TGs and apolipoproteins other than apo A-I were similar for rats fed both diets. These *in vitro* studies suggest that decreased secretion of apo A-I and cholesterol from the liver and intestine is responsible for the plasmic reduction of apo A-I and cholesterol in soy lecithin–fed rats.

In contrast to the *in vitro* study, in rats injected with Triton WR-1339, concentrations of serum TG and high-molecular-weight apo B at 20 h after injection were increased by soy lecithin feeding, whereas until 2 h postinjection the accumulation of serum TG was similar for rats fed both diets. These soy lecithin–dependent effects can be attributed to the decreased clearance of TG-rich lipoproteins derived from the liver, since the concentration of TG and apo Bh in serum $d < 1.063$ g/ml lipoproteins at 20 h after Triton injection was higher in the soy lecithin group than in the soy oil group (Table 10.3). Thus, soy lecithin affects not only secretion of hepatic lipoproteins but also metabolism of TG-rich lipoproteins derived from the liver.

## 10.2.6 CATABOLISM OF SERUM LIPOPROTEINS

Feeding soy lecithin to rats caused a lower concentration of serum apo A-I and cholesterol and a higher concentration of serum apo B, especially apo Bh, than feeding soy oil.[6] Secretion of cholesterol and apo A-I, but not apo B, from the liver and intestine was lower in rats fed soy lecithin.[5,8] To investigate the underlying mechanism, catabolism of newly formed TG-rich lipoproteins from the liver

---

**TABLE 10.3**
**Concentration of Lipids and apo B in Serum $d < 1.063$ g/ml Lipoproteins at 20 h after Triton Injection in Rats Fed Soy Lecithin and Soy Oil**

| Lipids, Apoproteins | Soy Oil ($n = 6$) | Soy Lecithin ($n = 6$) | $P$ |
|---|---|---|---|
| | (mg/dl) | | |
| TG | 814 | 1095 | 0.05 |
| Cholesterylesters | 107 | 114 | ns |
| Apo Bh | 26 | 43 | 0.05 |
| Apo Bl | 50 | 51 | ns |

**TABLE 10.4**
**Chemical Composition of Lymph CM in Rats
Fed Soy Lecithin and Soy Oil**

| Lipids, Protein | Soy Oil ($n = 2$) | Soy Lecithin ($n = 2$) |
|---|---|---|
| | (wt%) | |
| TG | 76.8 | 88.3 |
| Cholesterylesters | 4.2 | 1.0 |
| Free cholesterol | 1.0 | 0.4 |
| Phospholipids | 15.7 | 9.1 |
| Protein | 2.4 | 1.1 |

and intestine and of serum HDL were compared in rats fed soy lecithin and rats fed soy oil.[11]

### 10.2.6.1 Catabolism of CM

[³H]oleate-labeled CMs were prepared in rats fed a soy lecithin– or soy oil–containing diet. Recipient rats were fed the diets and injected with the CMs. The CMs prepared from rats fed soy lecithin contained more TGs and less cholesterol and phospholipids than those from rats fed soy oil, indicating bigger CMs (Table 10.4). The labeled CMs disappeared in a biphasic manner within 45 min after dosing. When given their own CMs, less CM radioactivity was recovered at 3, 5, and 10 min after the dose from rats fed soy lecithin than from rats fed soy oil. The disappearance curves were analyzed by computer-assisted curve fitting, with the assumption that clearance was at least biexponential. The general form was disappearance $(t) = A(^{-\alpha t}) + B(^{-\beta t})$.[52] The initial phase of clearance $(t_{1/2}\alpha)$ was faster in rats fed soy lecithin than in rats fed soy oil when their own CMs were infused (2.7 vs. 4.4 min; $P < 0.05$). The second phase of clearance $(t_{1/2}\beta)$ was considerably slower than the first but was not significantly different between groups.

In an attempt to examine whether the difference in clearance could be attributed to the infused CMs or to the recipient rats, the $t_{1/2}$ was also examined in rats given CMs prepared from rats fed different diets. The $t_{1/2}$ was not significantly different for rats fed the two diets when rats were infused with CMs prepared under the other dietary regimen. Nevertheless, rats fed soy lecithin had shorter $t_{1/2}\alpha$ for the CMs prepared from rats fed soy oil than did rats fed soy oil and infused with their own CMs (2.4 vs. 4.4 min; $P < 0.05$). The data, therefore, indicate that faster clearance in rats fed soy lecithin may be partially accounted for by a CM factor: namely, large CMs infused in rats are cleared faster from the circulation than smaller ones,[53] due to the different affinity of CMs and their remnants to peripheral lipoprotein lipase[54] and hepatic receptors.[55]

To estimate the role of adipose tissue in CM catabolism *in vivo*, the radioactivity of [³H]oleate-labeled CMs remaining in the adipose tissue was examined when rats were killed 45 min after the injection of CMs. The recovery of the radioactivity tended to be greater in rats fed soy oil than in rats fed soy lecithin when their own CMs were infused (0.88 vs. 0.42%/g; $P = 0.057$). Rats fed soy oil contained greater radioactivity of [³H]oleate-labeled CMs in the adipose tissue than rats fed soy lecithin when rats were infused with CMs prepared under the other dietary regimen (1.54 vs. 0.32%/g; $P < 0.05$). These results indicate that an intrinsic factor such as uptake or lipoprotein lipase may be a major determinant in the less efficient peripheral uptake of the labeled CM–TG in rats fed soy lecithin. However, among rats fed soy oil, the recovery of the radioactivity appeared to be greater in those infused with larger particles (CMs prepared from rats fed soy lecithin) than in the rats infused with small particles (CMs prepared from rats fed soy oil) (1.54 vs. 0.88; $P = 0.063$). Therefore, this observation could be in part explained by a structural difference or a substrate factor.

## 10.2.6.2   Catabolism of VLDL

Radioactive hepatic VLDLs containing [³H]lysine and [³H]oleate were prepared from the perfusate of isolated livers of rats fed soy lecithin– and soy oil–containing diets.[11] The VLDLs were injected into the recipient rats via a femoral vein; blood was taken by abdominal aorta at 5, 10, and 20 min after the injection; and the radioactivity of apolipoproteins and lipids of a density less than 1.063 g/ml was measured. Higher retention of [³H]oleate and [³H]apo B at 5 and 10 min after the injection was observed in rats fed soy lecithin than in rats fed soy oil. At 10 min after the injection, the recovery of [³H]oleate was greater in liver (30.3 vs. 20.0%/whole; $P < 0.05$) and muscle (0.13 vs. 0.06%/g; $P < 0.05$), but not adipose tissue, from rats fed soy oil than from rats fed soy lecithin. At 20 min after the injection, however, the recovery of [³H]oleate was not affected by diet.

In contrast to the peripheral uptake of TG-rich lipoproteins, the effect of feeding soy lecithin on the disappearance patterns of the [³H]oleate from plasma differed between hepatic and lymphatic TG-rich lipoproteins. Although the metabolic fate of CM and hepatic VLDL in the circulation is assumed to be similar in rats, several differences have been observed in catabolism in the liver after partial removal of TG in the peripheral tissues[55,56] as follows. (a) The half-life in the circulation is definitely shorter for CM than for hepatic VLDL due to the higher affinity of CM–TG to the peripheral lipoprotein lipase. (b) Efficiency (*Km*) in the hepatic uptake of the remnants of CM and VLDL is higher in CM, which depends on the apo E receptor, than in hepatic VLDL, which depends on the apo B,E receptor, while the maximum uptake rate (*Vmax*) in the liver appears to be similar. Dietary soy lecithin suppressed peripheral removal of TG of both TG-rich lipoproteins. Therefore, both substrate factor and intrinsic factor, especially hepatic uptake of their remnants, might be involved in the differences seen after dietary manipulation.

**TABLE 10.5**
**Metabolic Parameters of [$^{125}$I]HDL in Serum from Rats**
**Fed Soy Lecithin and Soy Oil**

| Parameters | Soy Oil ($n = 6$) | Soy Lecithin ($n = 6$) | P |
|---|---|---|---|
| T1/2 (h) | 22.8 | 23.9 | ns |
| FCR (%/h) | 15.4 | 14.3 | ns |
| Catabolic rate (mg/h) | 3.03 | 2.38 | 0.05 |

### 10.2.6.3 Catabolism of HDL

Serum HDL was isolated from rats fed a commercial nonpurified diet and labeled with [$^{125}$I]. The HDL was injected into the recipient rats via a femoral vein. The disappearance of the radioactivity from blood serum was determined from blood taken from the tail vein.[11] An excellent fit was obtained to the equation, disappearance $(t) = A^{(-\alpha t)} + B^{(-\beta t)}$. The [$^{125}$I]HDL disappeared similarly, in rats fed soy lecithin and soy oil, in a biphasic manner over a 50-h period after the dose. The fractional catabolic rate (FCR) was not affected by the dietary manipulation (Table 10.5). However, the catabolic rate calculated by multiplying the FCR by the intravascular pool of apo HDL was greater in rats fed soy oil than in rats fed soy lecithin. Accordingly, the reduction of HDL components from the serum appeared to be attributable to their decreased secretion from the liver and intestine. Alternatively, the catabolic alteration of TG-rich lipoproteins might have some relevance to the reduction of serum HDL, because dietary soy lecithin suppressed peripheral removal of CM– and VLDL–TG.

The recovery of [$^{125}$I]HDL in liver was greater in rats fed soy lecithin than in those fed soy oil (0.42 vs. 0.27% of dose/liver for soy lecithin and soy oil, respectively; $P < 0.05$). Accordingly, livers isolated from rats fed soy lecithin and soy oil diets were perfused with the medium containing [$^{125}$I]HDL, and the rate of catabolism of [$^{125}$I]HDL in the perfused liver was subsequently measured by the production of trichloroacetic acid-soluble [$^{125}$I]HDL in the perfusate plasma and by the radioactivity recovered in the bile.[11] The rate of HDL degradation, expressed by the linear increment of total non-protein-bound [$^{125}$I] in the liver perfusate, was greater in rats fed soy lecithin than in rats fed soy oil ($Y = 7.0 \times 10^{-3}X + 0.39$ and $Y = 4.2 \times 10^{-3}X + 0.50$ for soy lecithin and soy oil, respectively). The FCR of HDL in the perfused liver was 1.6-fold higher after feeding soy lecithin than after feeding soy oil (0.83 vs. 0.53%/h for soy lecithin and soy oil, respectively; $P < 0.05$). Such a limited increase of the FCR catabolic rate by the liver appeared not to be great enough to alter the serum FCR *in vivo* since the liver contributed only 10 to 20% to the catabolism of circulating HDL.[11] Furthermore, total recovery of [$^{125}$I]HDL in the bile for 240 min was greater in rats fed soy lecithin than in rats fed soy oil (1.72 vs. 1.12% of dose for soy lecithin and soy oil, respectively; $P < 0.05$). These results suggest that greater hepatic uptake of serum HDL may accelerate the reversed cholesterol transport from the peripheral tissues to the liver.[57]

## 10.3  AN ACTIVE COMPONENT OF SOY LECITHIN THAT LOWERS SERUM CHOLESTEROL CONCENTRATIONS

### 10.3.1  Effect of Dietary Phospholipids and Their Constituent Bases on Serum Lipids and Apolipoproteins

The effects of purified phospholipids and phospholipid bases were studied in rats[7] to evaluate alterations of serum lipoproteins, liver lipids, and fecal sterol excretion caused by feeding a soy lecithin that contained phospholipids as well as neutral lipids, as described in the previous sections. To discover which phospholipid is responsible for the observed effect, we fed rats purified phospholipids and their constituent bases. Since in our previous experiment,[6] the addition of 4% crude soy lecithin to a basal diet caused a reduction of serum cholesterol, we supplemented the diet with this amount of either purified soy lecithin (96.9% PC and 3.4% lysoPC), hydrogenated purified soy lecithin (92.4% PC and 7.6% lysoPC), purified egg yolk lecithin (70.6% PC, 23.4% PE, 3.1% PI, 1.2% lysoPC, and 1.6% sphingomyelin), or a PI-rich preparation (93% as phospholipids, of which 75% was PI, 6% was phosphatidic acid, and 12% was unidentified components) from safflower oil. Supplementation of a soybean PC preparation, hydrogenated purified soybean PC, and PI rich–phospholipid preparations, compared with no supplementation, resulted in no effect on serum lipoproteins and liver lipids. However, supplementation of egg yolk lecithin, which contains PE as well as PC, caused a decrease in serum cholesterol (54.3 vs. 91.8 mg/dl $P < 0.05$) and apo A-I (48.1 vs. 64.3 mg/dl; $P < 0.05$) and an increase in serum apo B (5.86 vs. 3.93 mg/dl; $P < 0.05$) and liver cholesterol (2.4 vs. 1.1 mg/g; $P < 0.05$) compared with no supplementation.

The reduction of serum cholesterol and apo A-I caused by egg yolk lecithin was most prominent in HDL. These alterations in rats fed egg yolk lecithin were comparable to those observed in rats fed crude soy lecithin.[6] All phospholipids tested increased fecal excretion of neutral sterols to a similar extent (Table 10.6). The increase caused by purified soybean PC feeding in fecal excretion of neutral sterol had been reported in humans by Greten et al.,[29] but they showed no reduction of serum cholesterol. Conflicting results on the cholesterol-lowering action of oral phospholipids in humans,[29,40] therefore, could be attributed to PE in diets.

The effect of a phospholipid base on the concentration of serum lipids was examined.[7] It had been reported that choline in the form of PC is absorbed more than as a free form.[58] To increase the availability of bases, each base (in grams/kilogram of diet, 0.083 choline, 0.043 ethanolamine, and 0.073 inositol) was added in a molar ratio of twice as much as that from a diet containing 10% crude soy lecithin.

**TABLE 10.6**
**Excretion of Sterols into Feces in Rats Fed Different Types of Purified Phospholipids**

| Feces, Sterols | None (n = 5) | Purified Soy Lecithin (n = 5) | Hydrogenated Soy Lecithin (n = 5) | Egg Lecithin (n = 5) |
|---|---|---|---|---|
| Feces wt (g/d) | 1.53 | 1.27 | 1.24 | 1.26 |
| Cholesterol (mg/d) | 1.36 | 2.64[a] | 3.40[a] | 2.82[a] |
| Coprostanol (mg/d) | 2.67 | 3.96[a] | 6.34[a] | 7.23[a] |

[a] Significantly different from the no supplement group at $P < 0.05$.

The addition of these bases did not affect food intake and body weight gain. Supplementation of ethanolamine, compared with no supplementation, decreased the level of serum cholesterol (69.2 vs. 125 mg/dl; $P < 0.05$) and apo A-I (51.3 vs. 83.2 mg/dl; $P < 0.05$) and increased apo B (6.61 vs. 4.99 mg/dl; $P < 0.05$). Choline and inositol showed no effect on these lipoprotein components. The results suggest that PE-derived ethanolamine is responsible for altering the serum lipoprotein profiles. Namely, the difference in the component bases but not the fatty acids in the dietary phospholipids showed remarkable influence on serum lipoprotein levels.

## 10.3.2 CONTRASTING EFFECT OF DIETARY PE AND PC ON SERUM AND LIVER LIPIDS

The effect of dietary PE and PC added to cholesterol-free semipurified diet on serum lipoproteins was compared to the effect on rats fed soy oil.[9] PE was prepared via transphosphatidylation of soy PC by cabbage phospholipase D.[59] Thus, the fatty acid composition of the PE and PC was similar. The fatty acid composition of PC in the serum HDL and the liver was markedly altered by dietary PE, but not by PC (Table 10.7); there was an increase in the percentage of linoleate and a decrease in arachidonate.

Dietary PE, compared with PC, caused a decrease in serum cholesterol esters (91.6 vs. 118 mg/dl; $P < 0.05$), phospholipids (123 vs. 185 mg/dl; $P < 0.05$), and apo A-I (56.9 vs. 98.0 mg/dl; $P < 0.05$) and an increase in high-molecular-weight apo B (5.32 vs. 4.59 mg/dl; $P < 0.05$). The simultaneous addition of PC and ethanolamine, compared with PC alone, also decreased serum apo A-I (56.2 vs. 82.2 mg/dl; $P < 0.05$) and cholesterol (120 vs. 158 mg/dl; $P < 0.05$). PE and PC increased to a similar extent the excretion of fecal neutral sterols (11.2, 10.3, and 6.3 mg/day for the PE, PC, and soy oil groups, respectively; $P < 0.05$) and hepatic 3-hydroxy-3-methylglutaryl-coenzyme A reductase activity (585, 431, and 247 pmol/min · mg protein for the PE, PC, and soy oil groups, respectively; $P < 0.05$) compared to soy oil. These results suggest that not only PC but also

**TABLE 10.7**
**Fatty Acid Composition of PC in Serum HDL and Liver**
**in Rats Fed PC- or PE-Containing Diets**

| | Serum HDL | | | Liver | | |
|---|---|---|---|---|---|---|
| Fatty Acids | PE | PC | *P* | PE | PC | *P* |
| | | | (wt %) | | | |
| 16:0 | 21.5 | 22.0 | ns | 20.4 | 18.3 | ns |
| 18:0 | 22.5 | 24.8 | ns | 17.7 | 19.2 | ns |
| 18:1 | 12.0 | 11.5 | ns | 9.0 | 8.6 | ns |
| 18:2 | 31.8 | 22.5 | 0.05 | 19.6 | 12.7 | 0.05 |
| 20:4 | 13.0 | 8.2 | 0.05 | 24.6 | 31.3 | 0.05 |
| 22:6 | 2.5 | 4.0 | 0.05 | 5.2 | 7.6 | 0.05 |

PE in the diet interrupts the reabsorption of biliary cholesterol in the intestine and probably the subsequent transport of cholesterol as CM. These intestinal events, however, appeared to have no direct relevance to the serum cholesterol and apolipoprotein levels in rats fed a cholesterol-free diet. Namely, the constituent base of PC and PE, after being absorbed, might affect the metabolism of serum lipoproteins and hepatic lipids differently.

The supplementary PE, compared with the PC, increased the relative proportion of PE (29.4 vs. 24.6%; $P < 0.05$) and decreased PC (45.4 vs. 57.2%; $P < 0.05$) in the liver phospholipids. The distribution of phospholipid subclasses in the hepatic microsomes was also similarly altered in the group fed PE or PC plus ethanolamine. It had been reported that ethanolamine added to the medium of freshly isolated hepatocytes increases the synthesis of PE via the CDP-ester pathway and does not affect PC synthesis via the methylation pathway.[60] Since the PC, but not PE, is the major phospholipid in the serum phospholipids secreted from the liver and intestine, the decreased ratio caused by the addition of dietary PE or PC to PE in the hepatic microsomes, where lipoproteins are synthesized, might have some relevance to the reduction of serum phospholipids. However, the amount of VLDL secreted from the isolated perfused liver was almost identical between the rats fed soybean lecithin and those fed soy oil.[8] Therefore, the consequence of the altered distribution of hepatic phospholipids caused by the supplementary PE must be examined in terms of the secretion of nascent HDL or hepatic uptake of serum lipoproteins.

We examined the phospholipid composition of intestine, liver, adrenal gland, kidney, heart, lung, testis, adipose tissue, and brain. A significant increase of PE was observed only in the liver. This transient increase of PE in the liver might cause an alteration of membrane composition and electron transport gradient related to the methyl donor system. These alterations might modify serum lipoprotein metabolism.

## 10.4   ABSORPTION AND TRANSPORT OF PE AND PC

### 10.4.1   INTESTINAL ABSORPTION OF PHOSPHOLIPID BASES

PE played the major role in altering serum lipoproteins.[9] These effects of dietary
PE appeard to be due to the constituent base ethanolamine, since ethanolamine, but
not choline and inositol, causes a similar alteration of serum lipoprotein patterns
in rat.[7] Therefore, it was important to understand the absorption and transport of
dietary PE as well as PC.

Earlier studies suggested that the fatty acid at the second position of PC is
hydrolyzed by pancreatic phospholipase A2 in the intestinal lumen.[61] This lysoPC
is incorporated into intestinal mucosa cells and then either reesterified to PC or
degraded further in the cells, the proportion going to each pathway varying with
the amount of fat given.[61,62] Intestinal mucosal lysophospholipase and glycerophosphorylcholine diesterase participate in the formation of water-soluble metabolites of lysoPC.[63] Although little is known about the further metabolism of
lysoPC in the intestinal lumen, several studies have pointed out that extensive
hydrolysis of lysoPC may occur. Parthasarathy et al. showed that at 90 min after
injection of [$^{32}$P]PC, considerable amounts of [$^{32}$P]glycerophosphorylcholine and
glycerophosphate were found in both lumen and mucosal cells.[64]

On the basis of the previous reports, we compared the absorption and transport
of the base moieties of [ethanolamine-$^3$H]PE and [choline-$^{14}$C]PC that were fed
to rats.[12] Rats were killed 2 h after feeding. The same amount of each label was
recovered in the intestinal mucosa. The jejunal mucosa contained more than 90%
of both radioactivities in the whole intestinal mucosa. The recovery of the labeled
PE and PC in the jejunal and ileum contents was considerably lower than that in
the mucosa (Table 10.8). In contrast to the earlier studies, we observed that large
amounts of the radioactivities from both choline-labeled PC and ethanolamine-
labeled PE were found in the water-soluble fraction in the intestinal content
(relative percentage in water-soluble fraction: 68.4 for $^3$H-labeled PE and 41.0
for $^{14}$C-labeled PC) as well as in the mucosal cells (relative percentage in water-
soluble fraction: 35.6 $^3$H-labeled PE and 37.8 $^{14}$C-labeled PC).

Detailed analyses with thin-layer chromatography revealed that the major part
of the water-soluble fraction in the intestinal contents were glycerophosphorylethanolamine (49.9% for $^3$H-labeled PE), glycerophosphorylcholine (30.8% for
$^{14}$C-labeled PC), ethanolamine (15.8% for $^3$H-labeled PE), and choline (7.6% for
$^{14}$C-labeled PC). As expected, the major radioactivities in the lipid-soluble fractions
in the intestinal contents were lysoPC (58.6% for $^{14}$C-labeled PC) and lysoPE
(33.6% for $^3$H-labeled PE). It was highly likely, therefore, that these water-soluble
metabolites in the lumen were formed by lysophospholipase and phosphodiesterase
contained in the intestinal desquamated cells or secreted directly from the mucosal
cells into the lumen.[65] The possibility remained, however, that lysophospholipase
derived from bile and pancreatic juice might be responsible for the formation of
glycerophosphorylcholine and glycerophosphorylethanolamine, since our preliminary study, in which phospholipids were incubated with a bile and pancreatic juice

**TABLE 10.8[a]**

**Distribution of Ethanolamine-Labeled PE and Choline-Labeled PC in the Lipids and Water Soluble Fractions of Jejunal Mucosa and Jejunal Contents**

| Fractions | Jejunal Mucosa | | Jejunal Content | |
|---|---|---|---|---|
| | PE | PC | PE | PC |
| % of dose | 27.2 | 27.0 | 1.43 | 3.41 |
| | Relative % | | | |
| LPE or LPC | 9.7 | 7.1 | 16.0 | 13.3 |
| PE or PC | 46.9 | 48.9 | 10.1 | 41.3 |
| Ethanolamine or choline | 24.9 | 21.1 | 15.8 | 7.6 |
| GPE or GPC | 9.6 | 16.7 | 49.9 | 30.8 |

[a] Radiolabeled PE and PC were administered into the stomach. The intestine was isolated 2 h after their administration.

GPC, glycerophosphorylcholine; GPE, glycerophosphorylethanolamine.

mixture, also showed the formation of glycerophosphoryl compounds (K. Ikeda, K. Imaizumi, M. Sugano, unpublished observation).

## 10.4.2 TRANSPORT OF PC AND PE IN BLOOD SERUM AND THORACIC DUCT LYMPH

Several studies have reported on the absorption of choline-labeled PC in the intestine, while only we have reported on ethanolamine-labeled PE.[12] Nilsson showed that when [³H]choline-labeled PC and [¹⁴C]oleic acid were fed to rats, the recovery of [³H] was lower than that of [¹⁴C] in lymph collected for 48 h.[62] Le Kim and Betzing also showed that about 50% of [¹⁴C]choline radioactivity of the glycerophosphorylcholine backbone was found in lymph CM and the other half in the liver in rats with lymph fistulae,[66] suggesting that half of the choline was transported to the liver via the portal vein as water-soluble components. Our results demonstrated that less than 10% of the administered [¹⁴C]ethanolamine-labeled PE is transported into the lymphatic systems in rats by 8 h after administration, and the lymphatic transport of choline-labeled PC is more than twofold that of ethanolamine-labeled PE (17.0 vs. 7.8% for base-labeled PC and PE, respectively). The radioactivity of choline-labeled PC in lymph was detected mainly as PC (77.5%), while the radioactivity of ethanolamine-labeled PE was detected not only in PE, but also in PC (55.3% for PE and 14.5% for PC).

Our study showed that transport of ethanolamine-labeled PE and choline-labeled PC via a nonlymphatic route was at least sixfold (7.8 vs. 48%) and 1.3-fold

**TABLE 10.9[a]**
**Distribution of Ethanolamine-Labeled
PE and Choline-Labeled PC in the Lipids
and Water-Soluble Fractions of Liver**

| Fractions | PE | PC |
|---|---|---|
| % of dose | 48.1 | 22.7 |
| **Relative %** | | |
| LPC | 2.7 | 3.2 |
| LPE | 2.6 | 2.3 |
| PC | 22.2 | 33.9 |
| PE | 34.1 | 1.1 |
| Water soluble | 30.0 | 53.5 |

[a] Base-labeled PE and PC were administered into the stomach in lymph diverted rats.

(17 vs. 23%) higher than that via a lymphatic route, respectively (Table 10.9).[12] Major radioactivity from choline-labeled PC and ethanolamine-labeled PE was detected in the PC fraction and in the PE and PC fractions, respectively. These data suggest that the major route of transport of the base part of PE is the portal vein, while both lymphatic and portal vein routes are important for the transport of the choline moiety of PC. In the liver, approximately twice the amount of [14C]ethanolamine as compared with [14C]choline remained as lipid fractions (mainly PE and PC). Smaller amounts of choline-derived lipids remaining in the liver were considered to be due to active excretion of labeled PC as lipoproteins.[67] Since intestinal mucosal cells can methylate PE to PC,[68] it was thought that a considerable amount of labeled ethanolamine transported in the liver as water-soluble components is resynthesized to PE and then is methylated to PC. Therefore, the concentration of PE in the liver might temporarily increase. This eventual difference in the liver in terms of the handling of both bases might explain why exogenous feeding of ethanolamine or PE, but not choline or PC, caused an increased mass of PE in the liver.[9]

### 10.4.3 EFFECT OF DIETARY PE ON TISSUE ETHANOLAMINE AND PHOSPHOETHANOLAMINE CONCENTRATIONS

Rats were fed a purified diet containing either PC or PE prepared by trans-phosphatidylation of PC, after which the amounts of some of the metabolites of the ethanolamine portion of the dietary PE in the liver and blood plasma were determined.[16] The level of serum ethanolamine and liver phosphoethanolamine was 1.5- and 5.8-fold higher, respectively, in rats fed PE than in those fed PC (53.2 vs. 36.4 $\mu M$/l for serum ethanolamine and 7.38 vs. 1.28 $\mu M$/g for phosphoethanolamine). The concentration of serum PC was lower and that of the PE was higher in rats fed PE (83.5 vs. 116 mg/dl for PC and 2.50 vs. 0.93 mg/dl for PE). The concentration of liver phosphoethanolamine in rats fed PE was highly inversely correlated to the level of serum cholesterylester ($r$ = 0.98). Ethanolamine acts as a precursor of PE in cells. The first step of this pathway involves phosphorylation by a kinase that has a broad specificity (i.e., it phosphorylates ethanolamine as well as choline).[69] Porter and Kent showed that ethanolamine/choline kinase is the same enzyme, and choline and ethanolamine are mutually competitive inhibitors.[69] Thus, in the presence of a high ethanolamine concentration, phosphorylation of choline might be diminished and less phosphorylcholine produced, leading to a relatively high synthesis of PE vs. PC. It is therefore possible that lower availability of newly synthesized PC would lead to slower synthesis of VLDL.[70]

Phosphoethanolamine exists in most animal tissues,[71] but its biological importance is unknown, apart from its role as a possible intermediate in the metabolism of phospholipids.[72] However, the role of phosphoethanolamine as a cholinergic-enhancing factor in rat brain[73] and as a growth promoting factor for carcinoma cells[74] deserves attention. Our study showed a five- to sixfold greater accumulation of phosphoethanolamine in the liver in rats fed PE than in those fed PC. Therefore, further possible physiological functions of the metabolites of exogenous PE, other than lipid metabolism, remain to be determined.

From these results, it was suggested that inadequate utilization of PC for a component of secretory lipoproteins in the liver and for a substrate donor for cholesterylester formation in the blood serum might be relevant to the cholesterol-lowering action of dietary PE.

## 10.5 HYPOCHOLESTEROLEMIC ACTION OF ETHANOLAMINE-CONTAINING PHOSPHOLIPIDS

### 10.5.1 HYPOCHOLESTEROLEMIC ACTION IN DIET-INDUCED HYPERCHOLESTEROLEMIA

This study was carried out to determine whether dietary phospholipids containing PE exert hypocholesterolemic action in rats given a high cholesterol diet.[14] Rats were fed a basal diet containing 1% cholesterol and 0.25% Na-cholate. The basal diet was supplemented with egg yolk phospholipids (82.1% PC, 17.1% PE, 0.3% sphingomyelin, and 0.5% LysoPC) or its hydrogenated forms (84.0% PC, 15.5% PE, 0.2% sphingomyelin, and 0.3% LysoPC) and egg yolk PC (98.7% PC, 0.5% sphingomyelin, and 0.8% LysoPC) or its hydrogenated forms (99.1% PC, 0.4% sphingomyelin and 0.5% LysoPC). Egg yolk phospholipids suppressed the elevation of serum cholesterol irrespective of its fatty acid composition, while purified PC and its hydrogenated form had no effect (158, 169, 323, and 251 mg/dl for egg yolk phospholipids, the hydrogenated forms, egg yolk PC, and the hydrogenated

PC, respectively), suggesting that the ethanolamine portion is responsible for this hypocholesterolemic effect.

### 10.5.2 HYPOCHOLESTEROLEMIC ACTION IN EXOGENOUSLY HYPERCHOLESTEROLEMIC RATS

Simultaneous addition of cholesterol and bile acid to a diet results in a profound effect on cholesterol metabolism in rats.[75] ExHC rats are a strain that exhibits hypercholesterolemia when fed a cholesterol-containing diet but does not require simultaneous addition of bile acid for elevating serum cholesterol.[76] Accordingly, ExHC rats were fed the purified diet containing 1% cholesterol and either PE or PC as a control at 2% each for 2 weeks. The elevation of serum cholesterylester level was lower in rats fed PE than in those fed PC (128 vs. 186 mg/dl for the PE and PC groups, respectively; $P < 0.05$).[16] Fecal steroid excretion was not influenced by the type of dietary phospholipid. This study further confirmed a suppressive effect of dietary PE on serum cholesterol level in rats hyperresponsive to dietary cholesterol.

## 10.6  ROLE OF ETHANOLAMINE-CONTAINING PHOSPHOLIPIDS ON FATTY ACID METABOLISM

Dietary soy lecithin resulted in an increase of linoleic acid and a decrease of arachidonic acid in the lymph CM phospholipids[5] and serum phospholipids[6] in rats. These changes were due to the PE in the soy lecithin, since dietary PE prepared from PC by the transphosphatidylation reaction, compared to dietary PC, increased linoleic acid and lowered arachidonic acid in the serum HDL-PC and the liver PC,[9,15] suggesting a role of dietary PE in hepatic metabolism of linoleic acid. Therefore, Δ6-desaturase activity in hepatic microsomes in rats fed PE and the formation of polyunsaturated fatty acids from linoleic acid in cultured hepatocytes supplemented with ethanolamine were measured.[15]

### 10.6.1  IN VIVO EXPERIMENT

Rats were fed a purified diet containing 2% PC or 2% PE at the expense of soy oil for 2 weeks. In a separate experiment, the PC diet was supplemented with ethanolamine equivalent to the amount of the constituent base of PE in the PE diet on a molar basis. PE was synthesized via the transphosphatidylation reaction for soy PC and ethanolamine•HCL.[9] The dietary PE suppressed the formation of arachidonic acid from linoleic acid and possibly the synthesis of docosahexaenoic acid from α-linolenic acid in the liver. Synthesis of arachidonic acid is regulated by several factors such as microsomal Δ6-desaturase,[77] chain-elongation reaction,[78] and oxidation of linoleic acid.[79] Activity of hepatic Δ6-desaturase was markedly suppressed by dietary PE, but not PC when compared to the soy oil diet (0.238, 0.400, and 0.551 nmol/min/mg protein for PE, PC, and control diet, respectively).

Supplementation of ethanolamine to the PC diet also lowered the desaturase activity (0.365 and 0.722 nmol/min/mg protein for ethanolamine and control diet, respectively). These actions of ethanolamine, lowering serum cholesterol and hepatic desaturase activity, were confirmed by Shimada et al.[80]

Flow of acetyl-coenzyme (CoA)-utilization either to $CO_2$ or malonyl CoA is assumed to be the limiting step to the synthesis of longer chain fatty acids, since malonyl-CoA is utilized for the chain-elongation reaction.[81] Thus, $CO_2$ production from [$^{14}$C]acetate was examined in liver slices. Labeled $CO_2$ production increased significantly in rats fed PE and ethanolamine compared to rats fed PC and the control diet (4810, 5910, 2770, and 2280 dpm/g liver for PE, ethanolamine, PC and control, respectively). These results suggest that dietary PE as well as ethanolamine accelerates the flow of acetate into the oxidative pathway and might decrease the formation of malonyl-CoA, which is utilized for chain elongation of linoleic acid.

### 10.6.2 METABOLISM OF LINOLEIC ACID IN CULTURED HEPATOCYTES

Several hormones such as epinephrine,[82] adrenocorticotropin,[83] corticosterone,[84] and glucagon[85] regulate hepatic microsomal Δ6-desaturase activity. Therefore, dietary PE and ethanolamine might indirectly alter the desaturase activity. Conversely, we considered the possibility of the direct effect of ethanolamine on the metabolism of linoleic acid by cultured hepatocytes. For this purpose, monolayered hepatocytes prepared from rats were incubated for 16 h with or without ethanolamine. The addition of 0.1 m$M$, which is slightly higher than the physiological level of free ethanolamine (36.6 μmol/L) in the circulating blood of rats,[15] caused a decreased formation of polyunsaturated fatty acids (mainly γ-18:3 and 20:4) from [$^{14}$C]linoleic acid (Table 10.10). The direct action of ethanolamine to the hepatocytes was also observed in the oxidation of linoleic acid and secretion of VLDL. The addition of ethanolamine to the hepatocytes increased the formation of acid-soluble products that were assumed to be a measure of oxidation rate

### TABLE 10.10
### Desaturation, Esterification, and Oxidation of [$^{14}$C]Linoleic Acid by Cultured Rat Hepatocytes in Medium Containing Ethanolamine

| Parameters | Ethanolamine (m$M$) | | P |
|---|---|---|---|
| | 0 | 0.1 | |
| Desaturation % | 7.00 | 3.84 | 0.05 |
| Oxidation products (dpm $\times$ 10$^{-4}$/mg protein) | 5.38 | 6.10 | 0.05 |
| Medium VLDL (dpm $\times$ 10$^{-4}$/mg protein) | 4.12 | 3.25 | 0.05 |

[a] Hepatocytres were prepared from rats and incubated with serum-free medium containing ethanolamine for 16 h.[15]

and decreased the secretion of [$^{14}$C]linoleic acid as VLDL. These results suggest that ethanolamine directly intervenes in the formation of arachidonic acid, oxidation of fatty acids, and secretion of VLDL in the liver. Furthermore, the incorporation of [$^{14}$C]linoleic acid into the lysoPC fraction in the hepatocytes was decreased by the addition of ethanolamine (2.3 and 1.6% for zero ethanolamine and 0.1 m$M$ ethanolamine, respectively; $P < 0.05$). The latter observation might be related to phospholipase A2(1) activity. In short, these results suggest that ethanolamine derived from the dietary PE plays a regulatory role in linoleate metabolism in the liver.

### 10.6.3 METABOLISM OF GLYCEROL BY CULTURED HEPATOCYTES

To test whether the ethanolamine added to the hepatocyte culture medium influences differently the fate of a lipid precursor, the incorporation of [$^{3}$H]glycerol into the cellular and the medium lipids was investigated. Ethanolamine at the level of 0.1 m$M$ caused an increased incorporation of [$^{3}$H]glycerol into the cellular PE (30,600 and 45,700 dpm/mg protein for zero ethanolamine and 0.1 m$M$ ethanolamine, respectively; $P < 0.05$) and a decreased secretion of medium PC (2,400 and 1,550 dpm/mg protein for zero ethanolamine and 0.1 m$M$ ethanolamine, respectively; $P < 0.05$). These results suggest that mass distribution of hepatic PE is determined by the availability of the phospholipid base. According to Noga et al.,[86,87] PC derived from PE by PE $N$-methyltransferase is required for the secretion of VLDL. However, the increased PE synthesis did not result in an increased pool size of PC via the PE $N$-methylation pathway and therefore lowered VLDL-TG secretion by the liver.

## 10.7 CONSUMPTION OF PHOSPHOLIPIDS

The estimated daily intakes of PC and PE in Sweden are 0.9 to 1.9 and 0.3 to 0.6 mmol, respectively, according to Åkesson.[88] In our preliminary analysis, the daily intakes of PC and PE of students eating in our university refectory were 0.5 to 1.9 and 0.3 to 0.9 mmol, respectively.[10] Since the daily excretion of biliary phospholipids in humans is estimated to be 6 to 23 mmol,[89] which are composed of about of 90% PC and 5% PE,[90] the daily excretion of biliary PC and PE is calculated to be 5.4 to 20 and 0.3 to 1.1 mmol, respectively. Therefore, the daily intake of PE appears to be as much as that secreted as biliary PE, while the daily supply of dietary PC is much less than that of the biliary PC. Hence, the dietary PE may play an important regulatory function in serum lipoprotein metabolism.

## 10.8 APPLICATIONS

We have identified several interesting areas for future lecithin-related research. The exact mechanisms whereby lecithin is involved in hypocholesterolemic action and fatty acid metabolism have not been fully elucidated. However, the active principle appears to be PE and the breakdown product, ethanolamine. The hypocholesterolemic action of dietary PE might be provoked by an enhanced uptake of serum lipoprotein cholesterol and a decreased secretion of VLDL-cholesterol by the liver. Excretion of sterols into feces appears not to be related to the hypocholesterolemic action of dietary PE, because the fecal sterol excretion is enhanced to a similar extent by the dietary PE and PC. It remains to be determined whether the increase in microsomal PE concentration and the suppression of linoleic acid metabolism are associated with the hypocholesterolemic action of ethanolamine. Once the basic mechanisms are elucidated, there will surely be a lot of health-related conditions in which there will be a rationale for the involvement of lecithin as a stimulator for improving lipid metabolism.

# REFERENCES

1. Dashiell, G.L., Lecithin in food processing applications, in *Lecithins: Sources, Manufacture & Uses*, Szuhaj, B.F., Ed., American Oil Chemists' Society, Champaign, IL, 1989, pp. 213–224.

2. Baker, C., Lecithin in cosmetics, in *Lecithins: Sources, Manufacture & Uses*, Szuhaj, B.F., Ed., American Oil Chemists' Society, Champaign, IL, 1989, pp. 253–260.

3. Houtsmuller, U.M.T., Metabolic fate of dietary lecithin, in *Nutrition and the Brain*, Vol. 5, *Choline and Lecithin in Brain Disorders*, Barbeau, A., Growdon, J.H., and Wurtman, R.J., Eds., Raven Press, New York, 1979, pp. 83–94.

4. Canty, D.J. and Zeisel, S.H., Lecithin and choline in human health and disease, *Nutr. Res.*, 52, 327–339, 1994.

5. Imaizumi, K., Murata, M., and Sugano, M., Effect of dietary polyunsaturated phospholipid on the chemical composition of mesenteric lymph chylomicrons and the excretion of steroids into bile and feces in rat, *J. Nutr. Sci. Vitaminol.*, 28, 265–280, 1982.

6. Imaizumi, K., Murata, M., and Sugano, M., Effect of dietary polyunsaturated phospholipids on the chemical composition of serum lipoproteins in rat, *J. Nutr. Sci. Vitaminol.*, 28, 281–294, 1982.

7. Murata, M., Imaizumi, K., and Sugano, M., Effect of dietary phospholipids and their constituent bases on serum lipids and apolipoproteins in rat, *J. Nutr.*, 112, 1805–1808, 1982.

8. Murata, M., Imaizumi, K., and Sugano, M., Hepatic secretion of lipids and apo-lipoproteins in rat fed soybean phospholipids and soybean oil, *J. Nutr.*, 113, 1708–1716, 1983.

9. Imaizumi, K., Mawatari, K., Murata, M., Ikeda, I., and Sugano, M., The contrasting effect of dietary PE and phopshatidylcholine on serum lipoproteins and liver lipids in rat, *J. Nutr.*, 113, 2403–2411, 1983.

10. Imaizumi, K., Murata, M., Ohe, M., and Sugano, M., Phospholipid content of dietary meals in the university refectory, *J. Jpn. Soc. Nutr. Food Sci.*, 37, 185–187, 1984.

11. Murata, M., Imaizumi, K., and Sugano, M., Catabolism of newly formed triglyceride-rich lipoproteins and serum high density lipoproteins in rats fed soybean phospholipid and soybean oil, *J. Nutr.*, 115, 994–1004, 1985.

12. Ikeda, I., Imaizumi, K., and Sugano, M., Absorption and transport of base moieties of PC and phoshatidylethanolamine in rats, *Biochim. Biophys. Acta,* 921, 245–253, 1987.
13. Ishida, T., Koba, K., Sugano, M., Imaizumi, K., Watanabe, S., and Minoshima, R., Cholesterol levels and eicosanoid production in rats fed phosphatidylinositol or soybean lecithin, *J. Nutr. Sci. Vitaminol.,* 34, 237–244, 1988.
14. Imaizumi, K., Sakono, M., Sugano, M., Shigematsu, Y., and Hasegawa, M., Influence of saturated and polyunsaturated egg yolk phospholipids on hyperlipidemia in rats, *Agr. Biol. Chem.,* 53, 2469–2474, 1989.
15. Imaizumi, K., Sakono, M., Mawatari, K., Murata, M., and Sugano, M., Effect of phosphatidylethanolamine and its constituent base on the metabolism of linoleic acid in rat liver, *Biochim. Biophys. Acta,* 1005, 253–259, 1989.
16. Imaizumi, K., Sekihara, K., and Sugano, M., Hypocholesterolemic action of dietary phosphatidylethanolamine in rats sensitive to exogenous cholesterol, *J. Nutr. Biochem.,* 2, 251–254, 1991.
17. Cherry, J.P. and Kramer, W.H., Plant sources of lecithin, in *Lecithins: Sources, Manufacture & Uses,* Szuhaj, B.F., Ed., American Oil Chemists' Society, Champaign, IL, 1989, pp. 16–31.
18. Fraser, R., Size and lipid composition of chylomicrons of different Svedberg units of flotation, *J. Lipid Res.,* 11, 60–65, 1970.
19. Imaizumi, K., Fainaru, M., and Havel, R.J., Composition of proteins of mesenteric lymph CM in the rat and alterations produced upon exposure of chylomicrons to blood serum and serum lipoproteins, *J. Lipid Res.,* 19, 712–722, 1978.
20. Lekim, D., On the pharmacokinetics of orally applied essential phospholipids (EPL), in *Phosphatidylcholine,* Peeters, H., Ed., Springer-Verlag, Heidelberg, 1976, pp. 48–65.
21. Beil, F.U. and Grundy, S.M., Studies on plasma lipoproteins during absorption of exogenous lecithin in man, *J. Lipid Res.,* 21, 525–536, 1980.
22. Rampone, A.J. and Long, L.R., The effect of phosphatidylcholine and lysophosphatidylcholine on the absorption and mucosal metabolism of oleic acid and cholesterol *in vitro, Biochim. Biophys. Acta,* 486, 500–510, 1977.
23. Hollander, D. and Morgan, D., Effect of plant sterols, fatty acids and lecithin on cholesterol absorption *in vivo* in the rat, *Lipids,* 15, 395–400, 1980.
24. Arnesjö, B., Nilson, A., Barrowman, J., and Borgström, B., Intestinal digestion and absorption of cholesterol and lecithin in the human, *Scand. J. Gastroenterol.,* 4, 653–665, 1969.
25. Sabesin, S.M., Holt, P.R., and Clark, S.B., Intestinal lipid absorption: evidence for an intrinsic defect of chylomicron excretion by normal rat distal intestine, *Lipids,* 12, 840–846, 1975.
26. Wu, A.-L., Clark, S.B., and Holt, P.R., Composition of lymph CM from proximal or distal rat small intestine, *Am. J. Clin. Nutr.,* 33, 582–589, 1980.
27. Kennedy, E.P. and Weiss, S.B., The function of cytidine coenzyme in the biosynthesis of phospholipids, *J. Biol. Chem.,* 222, 193–214, 1956.
28. Mathews, S.A., Oliver, W.T., Phillips, O.T., Odle, J., Diersen-Schade, D.A., and Harrell, R.J., Comparison of triglycerides and phospholipids as supplemental sources of dietary long-chain polyunsaturated fatty acids in piglets, *J. Nutr.,* 132, 3081–3089, 2002.
29. Greten, H., Raetzen, H., Stiehl, A., and Schettler, G., The effect of polyunsaturated phosphatidylcholine on plasma lipids and fecal sterol excretion, *Atherosclerosis,* 36, 81–88, 1980.

30. Clark, S.B., Chylomicron composition during duodenal triglyceride and lecithin infusion, *Am. J. Physiol.*, 235, E183–E190, 1978.

31. Mackay, K., Starr, J.R., Lawn, R.M., and Ellsworth, J.L., Phosphatidylcholine hydrolysis is required for pancreatic cholesterol esterase- and phospholipase A2-facilitated cholesterol uptake into intestinal Caco-2 cells, *J. Biol. Chem.*, 272, 13380–13389, 1997.

32. Homan, R. and Hamelehle, K.L., Phospholipase A2 relieves phosphatidylcholine inhibition of micellar cholesterol absorption and transport by human intestinal cell line Caco-2, *J. Lipid Res.*, 39, 1197–1209, 1998.

33. Miettinen, A.P. and McNamara, D.J., Origins of fecal neutral steroids in rats, *J. Lipid Res.*, 22, 485–495, 1981.

34. Samochwiec, L., Kadlubowska, D., and Rozewicka, L., Investigations in experimental atherosclerosis. Part 1. The effect of phosphatidylcholine (EPL) on experimental atherosclerosis in white rats, *Atherosclerosis*, 23, 305–317, 1976.

35. Polichetti, E., Diaconescu, N., De La Porte, P.L., Malli, L., Portugal, H., Pauli, A.-M., Lafont, H., Tuchweber, B., Yousef, I., and Chanussot, F., Cholesterol-lowering effect of soyabean lecithin in normolipidaemic rats by stimulation of biliary lipid secretion, *Br. J. Nutr.*, 75, 471–481, 1996.

36. Samochowiec, L., Kadlubowsky, D., Rozewicka, L., Kuzna, W., and Szyszka, K., Investigations in experimental atherosclerosis. Part 2. The effect of phosphatidylcholine (EPL) on experimental atherosclerotic changes in miniature pigs, *Atherosclerosis*, 23, 319–331, 1976.

37. Rosseneu, M., Declercq, B., Vandamme, D., Vercaemst, R., Soetewey, F., Peeters, H., and Blaton, V., Influence of oral polyunsaturated and saturated phospholipids treatment on the lipid composition and fatty acid profile of chimpanzee lipoproteins, *Atherosclerosis*, 32, 141–153, 1979.

38. Wong, E.K., Nocolosi, R.J., Low, P.A., Herd, J.A., and Hayes, K.C., Lecithin influence on hyperlipemia in rhesus monkeys, *Lipids*, 15, 428–433, 1980.

39. Wilson, T.A., Messervey, C.M., and Nicolosi, R., Soy lecithin reduces plasma lipoprotein cholesterol and early atherogenesis in hypercholesterolemic monkeys and hamsters: beyond linoleate, *Atherosclerosis*, 140, 147–153, 1998.

40. Childs, M.T., Bowlin, J.A., Ogilvie, J.T., Hazzard, W.R., and Albers, J.J., The contrasting effect of a dietary soya lecithin product and corn oil on lipoprotein lipids in normolipidemic and familial hypercholesterolemic subjects, *Atherosclerosis*, 38, 217–228, 1981.

41. Cobb, M., Turkki, P., Linscheer, W., and Raheja, K., Lecithin supplementation in healthy volunteers: effect on cholesterol esterification and plasma, and bile lipids, *Nutr. Metabol.*, 24, 228–237, 1980.

42. Kinsell, L.W., Partridge, J., Boling, L., Margen, S., and Michaels, G., Dietary modification of serum cholesterol and phospholipids levels, *J. Clin. Endocrinol. Metab.*, 12, 909–913, 1952.

43. Shepherd, J., Packard, C.J., Patsch, J.T., Gotto, A.M., Jr., and Jaunton, O.D., Effect of dietary polyunsaturated and saturated fat on the properties of high density lipoproteins and the metabolism of apolipoprotein A-I, *J. Clin. Invest.*, 61, 1582–1592, 1978.

44. Malmros, H. and Wigand, G., The effect of diets containing different fat on serum cholesterol, *Lancet*, II, 1–8, 1957.

45. Imaizumi, K., Havel, R.J., Fainaru, M., and Vigne, J.-L., Origin and transport of the A-I and arginine-rich apolipoproteins in mesenteric lymph of rats, *J. Lipid Res.,* 19, 1038–1046, 1978.

46. Wu, A.-L. and Windmueller, H.G., Relative contributions by liver and intestine to individual plasma apolipoproteins in the rat, *J. Biol. Chem.,* 254, 7316–7322, 1979.

47. Best, C.H., Lucas, C.C., Ridout, J.H., and Patterson, J.M., Dose-response curves in the estimation of potency of lipotropic agents, *J. Boil. Chem.,* 186, 317–329, 1950.

48. Havel, R.J. and Kane, J.P., Primary desbetalipoproteinemia: predominance of a specific apoprotein species in triglyceride-rich lipoproteins, *Proc. Natl. Acad. Sci. USA,* 70, 2015–2019, 1973.

49. Miller, G.J. and Miller, N.E., Plasma high density lipoprotein concentration and development of ischemic heart disease, *Lancet,* I, 16–19, 1975.

50. Marsh, J.B. and Sparks, C.E., Hepatic secretion of lipoproteins in the rat and the effect of experimental nephrosis, *J. Clin. Invest.,* 64, 1229–1237, 1979.

51. Guo, L., Hamilton, R.L., Ostwald, R., and Havel, R.J., Secretion of nascent lipoproteins and apolipoproteins by perfused livers of normal and cholesterol-fed guinea pigs, *J. Lipid Res.,* 23, 543–555, 1982.

52. Gurpide, E., Mann, J., and Sandberg, E., Determination of kinetic parameters in a two-pool system by administration of one or more tracers, *Biochemistry,* 3, 1250–1256, 1964.

53. Quarfordt, S.H. and Goodman, D.S., Metabolism of double-labeled chylomicron cholesteryl esters in the rat, *J. Lipid Res.,* 8, 264–273, 1967.

54. Fielding, C.J. and Higgins, J.M., Lipoprotein lipase: comparative properties of the membrane-supported and solubilized enzyme species, *Biochemistry,* 13, 4324–4330, 1974.

55. Cooper, A.D., Shrewsbury, M.D., and Erickson, S.K., Comparison of binding and removal of remnants of triglyceride-rich lipoproteins of intestinal and hepatic origin by rat liver *in vitro, Am. J. Physiol.,* 243, G389–G395, 1982.

56. Noel, S.P. and Dupras, R., The kinetic parameters of the uptake of very-low-density lipoprotein remnant cholesteryl esters by perfused rat liver, *Biochim. Biophys. Acta,* 754, 117–125, 1983.

57. Schwartz, C.C., Vlahcevic, Z.R., Berman, M., and Meadows, J.G., Central role of high density lipoprotein in plasma free cholesterol metabolism, *J. Clin. Invest.,* 70, 105–116, 1982.

58. De La Huerga, J. and Popper, H., Factors influencing choline absorption in the intestinal tract, *J. Clin. Invest.,* 31, 598–603, 1952.

59. Eibl, H. and Kovatchev, S., Preparation of phospholipids and their analogs by phospholipase D, *Methods Enzymol.,* 72, 632–639, 1981.

60. Sundler, R. and Åkesson, B., Regulation of phospholipids biosynthesis in isolated rat hepatocytes, *J. Biol. Chem.,* 250, 3359–3367, 1975.

61. Scow, R.O., Stein, Y., and Stein O., Incorporation of dietary lecithin and lyso-lecithin into lymph chylomicrons in the rat, *J. Biol. Chem.,* 242, 4919–4924, 1967.

62. Nilsson, A., Intestinal absorption of lecithin and lysolecithin by lymph fistula rats, *Biochim. Biophys. Acta,* 152, 379–390, 1968.

63. Van den Bosch, H., *Phosphoglyceride metabolism, Annu. Rev. Biochem.,* 43, 243–277, 1974.

64. Parthasarathy, S., Subbaiah, P.V., and Ganguly, J., The mechanism of intestinal absorption of phosphatidylcholine in rats, *Biochem. J.,* 140, 503–508, 1974.

65. Mansbach, C.M., Pieoni, G., and Verger, R., Intestinal phospholipase, a novel enzyme, *J. Clin. Invest.,* 69, 368–376, 1982.

66. Le Kim, D. and Betzing, H., Intestinal absorption of polyunsaturated phosphatidylcholine in the rat, *Hoppe Seyler's Physiol. Chem.,* 357, 1321–1331, 1976.

67. Vance, J.E., Nguyen, T.M., and Vance, D.E., The biosynthesis of phosphatidylcholine by methylation of phosphatidylethanolamine derived from ethanolamine is not required for lipoprotein secretion by cultured rat hepatocytes, *Biochim. Biophys. Acta,* 875, 501–509, 1986.

68. Pelech, S.L. and Vance, D.E., Regulation of phosphatidylcholine biosynthesis [Review], *Biochim. Biophys. Acta,* 779, 217–251, 1984.

69. Porter, T.J. and Kent, C., Purification and characterization of choline/ethanolamine kinase from rat liver, *J. Biol. Chem.,* 265, 414–422, 1990.

70. Yao, Z. and Vance, D.E., Head group specificity in the requirement of phosphatidylcholine biosynthesis for very low density lipoprotein secretion from cultured hepatocytes, *J. Biol. Chem.,* 264, 11373–11380, 1989.

71. Kataoka, H., Sakiyama, N., Maeda, M., and Makita, M., Determination of phosphoethanolamine in animal tissues by gas chromatography with flame photometric detection, *J. Chromatogr.,* 494, 283–288, 1989.

72. Sundler, R., Biosynthesis of rat liver phosphatidylethanolamines from intraportally injected ethanolamine, *Biochim. Biophys. Acta,* 306, 218–226, 1973.

73. Bostwick, J.R., Landers, D.W., Crawford, G., Law, K., and Appel, S.H., Purification and characterization of a central cholinergic enhancing factor from rat brain: its identity as phosphoethanolamine, *J. Neurochem.,* 53, 448–458, 1989.

74. Kano-Sueoka, T. and Errick, J., Effects of phosphoethanolamine and ethanolamine on growth of mammary carcinoma cells in culture, *Exp. Cell Res.,* 136, 137–145, 1981.

75. Mahley, R.W. and Holcombe, K.S., Alterations of the plasma lipoproteins and apoproteins following cholesterol feeding in rats, *J. Lipid Res.,* 18, 314–324, 1977.

76. Imai, Y. and Matsumura, H., Genetic studies on induced and spontaneous hypercholesterolemia in rats, *Atherosclerosis,* 18, 59–64, 1973.

77. Brenner, R.R., The oxidative desaturation of unsaturated fatty acids in animals, *Mol. Cell Biochem.,* 3, 41–52, 1974.

78. Christophersen, B.O., Hagve, T.A., and Norseth, J., Studies on the regulation of arachidonic acid synthesis in isolated rat liver cells, *Biochim. Biophys. Acta,* 712, 305–314, 1982.

79. Goodridge, A.G.J., Regulation of the activity of acetyl coenzyme A carboxylase by palmitoyl coenzyme A and citrate, *J. Biol. Chem.,* 247, 6946–6952, 1972.

80. Shimada, Y., Morita, T., and Sugiyama, K., Dietary eritadenine and ethanolamine depress fatty acid desaturase activities by increasing liver microsomal phosphatidylethanolamine in rats, *J. Nutr.,* 133, 758–765, 2003.

81. Goodridge, A.G., Regulation of fatty acid synthesis in isolated hepatocytes: evidence for a physiological role for long chain fatty acyl coenzyme A and citrate, *J. Biol. Chem.,* 248, 4318–4326, 1973.

82. De Gómez Dumm, N.T., De Alaníz, M.J., and Brenner, R.R., Effect of epinephrine on the oxidative desaturation of fatty acids in the rat, *J. Lipid Res.,* 17, 616–621, 1976.

83. Mandon, E.C., De Gómez Dumm, N.T., De Alaníz, M.J., Marra, C.A., and Brenner, R.R., ACTH depresses delta 6 and delta 5 desaturation activity in rat adrenal gland and liver, *J. Lipid Res.,* 28, 1377–1383, 1987.

84. De Gómez Dumm, N.T., De Alaníz, M.J., and Brenner, R.R., Effect of glucocorticoids on the oxidative desaturation of fatty acids by rat liver microsomes, *J. Lipid Res.,* 20, 834–839, 1979.

85. De Gómez Dumm, N.T., De Alaníz, M.J., and Brenner, R.R., Effects of glucagon and dibutyryl adenosine 3', 5'-cyclic monophosphate on oxidative desaturation of fatty acids in the rat, *J. Lipid Res.,* 16, 264–268, 1975.

86. Noga, A.A., Zhao, Y., and Vance, D.E., An unexpected requirement for phosphatidylethanolamine N-methyltransferase in the secretion of very low density lipoproteins, *J. Biol. Chem.,* 277, 42358–42365, 2002.

87. Noga, A.A. and Vance, D.E., A gender-specific role for phosphatidylethanolamine N-methyltransferase-derived phosphatidylcholine in the regulation of plasma high density and very low density lipoproteins in mice, *J. Biol. Chem.,* 278, 21851–21859, 2003.

88. Åkesson, B., Content of phospholipids in human diets studied by the duplicate-portion technique, *Br. J. Nutr.,* 47, 223–229, 1982.

89. Northfield, T.C. and Hofmann, A.F., Biliary output during three meals and an overnight fast, *Gut,* 16, 1–6, 1975.

90. Gottfries, A., Nilsson, S., Samuelsson, B., and Schersten T., Phospholipids in human hepatic bile, gallbladder bile and plasma in cases with acute cholecystitis, *Scand. J. Clin. Lab. Invest.,* 21, 168–176, 1968.

# 11 Soy Sterols

*Ikuo Ikeda*

## CONTENTS

## 11.1 INTRODUCTION

Soybean oil contains about 300 to 400 mg of plant sterols per 100 g (Table 11.1). Major components of soy sterols are sitosterol (53 to 56%), campesterol (20 to 23%), and stigmasterol (17 to 21%). The chemical structures of these sterols are shown in Figure 11.1. The chemical structures of plant sterols resemble those of cholesterol but differ in the side chain. Sitosterol has an ethyl group and campesterol has a methyl group at the 24 position of cholesterol. Stigmasterol has a double bond at the 22-23 position of sitosterol. Plant stanols, in which a double bond at the 5-6 positions in the steroid ring of plant sterols is saturated, are also contained in soybean oil in trace amounts. A typical plant stanol, sitostanol, is shown in Figure 11.1.

Soybean germ makes up 2% of whole soybean. Soybean-germ oil can be extracted from hypocotyl-enriched raw soybean. It comprises 1% of soybean oil. It was reported that soybean-germ oil contains relatively high amounts of plant sterols.[1] The plant sterol content is 1.7 g/100 g oil, about 80% of which is in esterified form. Soybean-germ oil contains specific plant sterols, which are Δ7-stigmastenol, Δ7-avenasterol, and citrostadienol (Figure 11.1). These sterols have a double bond at the 7-8 position in the steroid ring. Δ7-Stigmastenol has an

**TABLE 11.1**
**Examples of Composition of Plant Sterols in Soybean and Soybean-Germ Oils**

| Plant Sterols | Soybean Oil | Soybean-Germ Oil |
|---|---|---|
| | mg/100 g Oil (%) | |
| Campesterol | 80 (20.2) | 137 (8.1) |
| Stigmasterol | 74 (18.6) | 135 (8.0) |
| Sitosterol | 213 (53.7) | 899 (53.3) |
| Δ7-stigmastenol | 22 (5.5) | 240 (14.2) |
| Δ7-avenasterol | 8 (2.0) | 88 (5.2) |
| Citrostadienol | n.d. (0) | 189 (11.2) |
| Total plant sterols | 397 | 1688 |

n.d., not detected

*Source:* Data from Ozawa, Y., Sato, H., Nakatani, A., Mori, O., Hara, Y., Nakada, Y., Akiyama, Y., and Morinaga, Y., *J. Oleo Sci.*, 50, 217–223, 2001.

ethyl group at the 24 position of the side chain. Δ7-Avenasterol and citrostadienol have an ethylidene group at the 24 position of the side chain. Citrostadienol has a methyl group at the 4 position of Δ7-avenasterol. A typical composition of soybean-germ sterols is shown in Table 11.1.

## 11.2 PHYSIOLOGICAL FUNCTIONS OF SOY STEROLS

Extensive studies have shown that dietary plant sterols and stanols lower plasma cholesterol concentration in animals and humans.[2,3] Since soy sterols are major sources of plant sterols, soy sterols have been utilized in many studies. Recently the Stresa Workshop summarized the efficacy of plant sterols and stanols on blood cholesterol levels in humans.[2] They summarized more than 40 randomized placebo-controlled trials. The maximum effect of plant sterols and stanols on the reduction of low-density lipoprotein (LDL) cholesterol was estimated to be 11.3% at doses higher than 2.5 g/d in adults. At doses of 0.7 to 1.1, 1.5 to 1.9, and 2.0 to 2.4 g/d, reductions in LDL cholesterol were estimated to be, respectively, 6.7, 8.5, and 8.9% on average. It seems that at least 0.7 to 1 g/d of plant sterols and stanols are necessary to obtain a significant reduction of LDL cholesterol. The researchers also concluded that no additional effect was obtained at doses higher than 2.5 g/d. Because plant sterols and stanols do not reduce very low density lipoprotein (VLDL) and high-density lipoprotein(HDL)-cholesterol concentrations, the reduction of total cholesterol in plasma reflects that of LDL cholesterol.

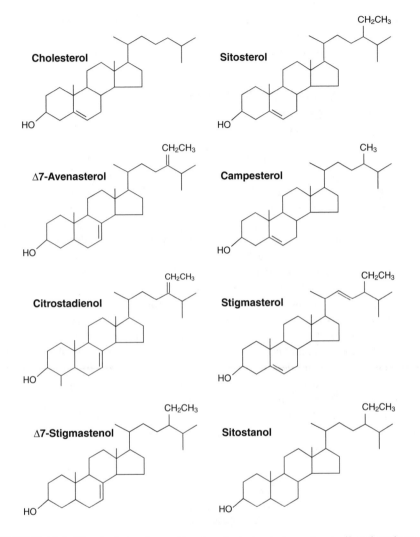

**FIGURE 11.1** Chemical structures of major plant sterols in soybean oil and soybean-germ oil.

## 11.3 MECHANISMS OF THE CHOLESTEROL-LOWERING ACTIVITY OF PLANT STEROLS

Because the feeding of plant sterols and stanols increases fecal excretion of cholesterol and the metabolite coprostanol in humans and experimental animals, it was believed that the reduction of plasma cholesterol concentration by the feeding of plant sterols and stanols is caused by the inhibition of cholesterol absorption in the intestine.[2,3] Our previous study showed that lymphatic transport of cholesterol in rats cannulated in the thoracic duct was lowered when sitosterol was given to the stomach together with cholesterol as an emulsion.[4] The results again support that plant sterols interfere with cholesterol absorption in the intestine.

## 11.4 MECHANISMS OF INHIBITION OF CHOLESTEROL ABSORPTION BY PLANT STEROLS

Dietary cholesterol is emulsified with hydrolysis products by lipases of triacylglycerols, phospholipids, and bile salts in the intestinal lumen. Part of the cholesterol is solubilized in bile salt micelles. After bile salt micelles enter the unstirred water layer, which covers the surface of the intestinal epithelial cells, cholesterol is released from the micelles as a monomer and enters the intestinal epithelial cells through intestinal brush border membranes. After the incorporation of cholesterol into the cells, a large part of the cholesterol is esterified by the action of acyl-CoA cholesterol acyltransferase and incorporated into chylomicrons that are secreted to the lymph.

We previously showed that dietary plant sterols rich in sitosterol limit the micellar solubility of cholesterol *in vitro* and *in vivo*.[5] Plant sterols are solubilized in bile salt micelles to the same or a slightly lower extent than cholesterol. Although almost all cholesterol and plant sterols are emulsified in the intestinal lumen, the solubility of sterols in bile salt micelles is quite limited.[5] Therefore, the solubilization of plant sterols in the micelles limits the solubility of cholesterol. When equal amounts of cholesterol and plant sterols existed in the intestinal contents of rats, the micellar solubility of cholesterol was almost half that of sterol because the other half of the micelles was occupied by plant sterols (Figure 11.2).

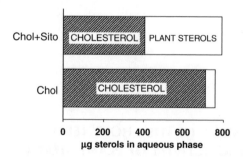

**FIGURE 11.2** Effect of dietary sitosterol and cholesterol on the micellar solubility of sterols in rats. Rats were meal-fed for 1 h with a diet containing 0.5% cholesterol (Chol) or 0.5% cholesterol + 0.5% sitosterol (Chol+Sito) for 1 week. On the last day, 2 h after withdrawal of the diet, the rats were sacrificed and intestinal content was taken. The micellar phase was obtained by untracentrifugation. (Data from Ikeda, I. and Sugano, M., *Biochim. Biophys. Acta*, 732, 651–658, 1983.)

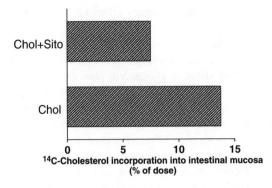

FIGURE 11.3 Effect of sitosterol on incorporation of [14]C-cholesterol into rat intestinal mucosa. Rats were meal-fed a diet containing 0.5% cholesterol (Chol) or 0.5% cholesterol + 0.5% sitosterol (Chol+Sito) as described in Figure 11.2. On the last day, [14]C-cholesterol was mixed in the diets. Two hours after withdrawal of the diet, the rats were sacrificed and intestinal mucosa was scraped. (Data from Ikeda, I. and Sugano, M., *Biochim. Biophys. Acta*, 732, 651–658, 1983.)

The limited solubility of cholesterol in the micelles is reflected by the incorporation of cholesterol into rat intestinal epithelial cells (Figure 11.3) and by lymphatic transport of cholesterol in rats (Figure 11.4). These observations strongly suggest that the limitation of micellar solubility of cholesterol

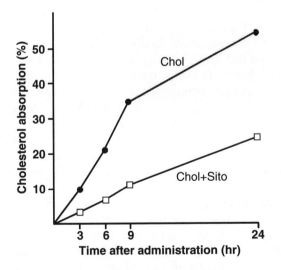

FIGURE 11.4 Effect of sitosterol on lymphatic recovery of [14]C-cholesterol in rats cannulated in the thoracic duct. Rats cannulated in the thoracic duct were given an emulsion containing 25 mg cholesterol (Chol) or 25 mg cholesterol + 25 mg sitosterol (Chol+Sito) via a stomach tube. Lymph fluid was collected for 24 h. (Data from Ikeda, I., Tanaka, K., Sugano, M., Vahouny, G.V., and Gallo, L.L., *J. Lipid Res.*, 29, 1573–1582, 1988.)

by plant sterols determines the inhibitory effect of plant sterols on cholesterol absorption.

The possibility of the direct inhibition of cholesterol absorption by plant sterols was examined in several experimental conditions.[4,5] We prepared bile salt micelles containing cholesterol or cholesterol plus sitosterol. The concentration of cholesterol in the micelles was almost the same in the cholesterol micelles and the cholesterol plus sitosterol micelles. Thus, sitosterol did not interfere with the solubility of cholesterol in these bile salt micelles. When these micelles were used to examine the incorporation of micellar cholesterol into rat intestinal brush border membranes and into rat intestinal epithelium *in situ*, sitosterol did not inhibit cholesterol incorporation.[4,5] Micellar sitosterol also did not inhibit lymphatic transport of cholesterol in rats cannulated in the thoracic duct when cholesterol or cholesterol plus sitosterol completely solubilized in bile salt micelles were continuously infused into the intestinal lumen.[4] Again these observations strongly suggest that the disturbance of the solubilization of cholesterol in bile salt micelles by solubilizing plant sterols may be the major cause of inhibition of cholesterol absorption by plant sterols.

## 11.5 HYPOCHOLESTEROLEMIC EFFECT OF SOYBEAN-GERM OIL

Ozawa et al. reported that serum cholesterol concentration in rats fed soybean-germ oil was significantly lower than in those fed soybean oil when the diets contained cholesterol.[1] Sato et al. observed in a double-blind, controlled study that the intake of 11 g/d of soybean-germ oil for 3 weeks significantly reduced serum cholesterol concentrations in subjects administered two eggs per day during the test period.[6] These subjects had been previously confirmed to have increased serum cholesterol concentrations by the feeding of two eggs per day for 3 weeks. Their average serum cholesterol concentrations were 210 to 230 mg/dl before the test meal. The hypocholesterolemic effect of soybean-germ oil was also examined in normal and mildly hypercholesterolemic volunteers whose cholesterol concentrations were 190 to 260 mg/dl.[7] When 11 g/d of soybean-germ oil was administered for 12 weeks, serum cholesterol concentration was reduced in subjects whose cholesterol concentrations were 220 mg/dl at the beginning of the test meal.

The fatty acid composition of soybean-germ oil is similar to that of soybean oil. Therefore, the effective reduction of serum cholesterol concentration in soybean-germ oil may be ascribed to plant sterols in the oil. Because soybean-germ oil contains 1.7 g/100 g oil of plant sterols, subjects in the studies reported by Sato et al.[6,7] consumed 190 mg of plant sterols per day. As discussed above, many studies have suggested that 0.7 to 1.0 g/d of plant sterols may be the minimum amounts needed to cause a significant hypocholesterolemic effect. The results suggest a possibility that specific plant sterols, Δ7-stigmastenol, Δ7-avenasterol, and citrostadienol, contained in soybean-germ oil have effective cholesterol-lowering activities. More detailed studies using these specific sterols will be necessary to reveal the precise mechanisms of the hypocholesterolemic effects of soybean-germ oil.

## 11.6 CONCLUSIONS

Although it has been well established that plant sterols and stanols lower plasma cholesterol concentration in humans, no evidence is available on the improvement and prevention of atherosclerosis and the reduction of mortality from coronary heart disease in humans.[2,3] In animal studies, Moghadasian et al. have reported that the development of atheroma was reduced by the feeding of plant sterols in apo E–deficient mice.[8] An epidemiological study showed that a 10% reduction of serum cholesterol concentration decreases the incidence of coronary heart disease by 20 to 50% depending on age.[9] These observations strongly suggest that dietary plant sterols and stanols prevent atherosclerosis and contribute to reduced mortality from coronary heart disease. Since plant sterols and stanols are considered to be safe food components, they are useful as materials of functional foods to prevent coronary heart disease.

## REFERENCES

1. Ozawa, Y., Sato, H., Nakatani, A., Mori, O., Hara, Y., Nakada, Y., Akiyama, Y., and Morinaga, Y., Chemical composition of soybean oil extracted from hypocotyl-enriched soybean raw material and its cholesterol lowering effects in rats, *J. Oleo Sci.,* 50, 217–223, 2001.
2. Katan, M.B., Grundy, S.M., Jones, P., Law, M., Miettinen, T., and Paoletti, R., Efficacy and safety of plant stanols and sterols in the management of blood cholesterol levels, *Mayo Clin. Proc.,* 78, 965–978, 2003.
3. Ikeda, I. and Sugano, M., Inhibition of cholesterol absorption by plant sterols for mass intervention, *Curr. Opin. Lipidol.,* 9, 527–531, 1998.
4. Ikeda, I., Tanaka, K., Sugano, M., Vahouny, G.V., and Gallo, L.L., Inhibition of cholesterol absorption in rats by plant sterols, *J. Lipid Res.,* 29, 1573–1582, 1988.
5. Ikeda, I. and Sugano, M., Some aspects of mechanism of inhibition of cholesterol absorption by β-sitosterol, *Biochim. Biophys. Acta,* 732, 651–658, 1983.
6. Sato, H., Ito, K., Sakai, K., Morinaga, Y., Sukegawa, E., Kitamura, T., Shimasaki, H., and Itakura, H., Effects of soybean-germ oil on reducing serum cholesterol level, *J. Oleo Sci.,* 50, 649–655, 2001 (in Japanese).
7. Sato, H., Ito, K., Sakai, K., Morinaga, Y., Tashima, I., Sukegawa, E., Shimasaki, H., and Itakura, H., Effects of soybean-germ oil on reducing serum cholesterol levels in a double-blind controlled trail in healthy humans, *J. Oleo Sci.,* 53, 9–16, 2004.
8. Moghadasian, M.H., Mcmanus, B.M., Pritchard, P.H., and Frohlich, J.J., Tall oil-derived phytosterols reduce atherosclerosis in apoE-deficient mice, *Arterioscler. Thromb. Vasc. Biol.,* 17, 119–126, 1997.
9. Law, M.R. and Weld, N.J., By how much and how quickly does reduction in serum cholesterol concentration lower risk of ischaemic heart disease?, *Br. Med. J.,* 308, 367–372, 1994.

# 12 The Status of Human Trials Utilizing Bowman–Birk Inhibitor Concentrate from Soybeans

*Ann R. Kennedy*

## CONTENTS

## ABSTRACT

The soybean-derived protease inhibitor known as the Bowman–Birk inhibitor (BBI) has many preventive and therapeutic effects for various diseases and adverse conditions that have led to its use in several human trials. This chapter reviews the status of BBI use in human trials. BBI, in the form of a soybean extract enriched in BBI and known as BBI concentrate (BBIC), achieved investigational new drug (IND) status with the Food and Drug Administration (FDA) in 1992, and human trials began at that time. There are currently six INDs involving BBIC trials in patients with oral leukoplakia, benign prostatic hyperplasia, prostate cancer, esophagitis/lung cancer, ulcerative colitis (UC), and gingivitis. A new prostate cancer prevention program utilizing BBIC has recently begun, and new trial areas utilizing BBIC in patients with multiple sclerosis, muscular dystrophy, and muscle atrophy from bed rest resulting from spinal cord injuries are expected to begin in the near future.

## 12.1 INTRODUCTION

The Bowman–Birk inhibitor (BBI) is a soybean-derived protease inhibitor that was discovered approximately six decades ago by Dr. Donald Bowman;[1] it has been characterized by Dr. Yehudith Birk over the past several decades (e.g., Reference 2) and studied in the Kennedy laboratory for nearly three decades. From the many studies performed in the Kennedy laboratory, it has become clear that BBI has numerous biological effects; some of these effects are listed in Table 12.1.[3–18] Most of the published studies relate to the anticarcinogenic and antiinflammatory activities of BBI.

The early *in vitro* studies of BBI suggested that the compound could be useful in human trials. As the performance of large-scale human trials with pure BBI would be prohibitive in cost, an extract of soybeans enriched in BBI, known as BBI concentrate (BBIC), was developed as a less costly substitute for BBI in human trial work. BBIC has the same cancer preventive properties as BBI in numerous models of carcinogenesis, as has been reviewed elsewhere.[3–7] Both BBI and BBIC have the ability to prevent cancer in many *in vitro* and *in vivo* animal carcinogenesis assay systems (reviewed in References 3–7). These animal carcinogenesis studies have indicated that BBI and BBIC prevent or suppress carcinogenesis in many organs and tissue types (including cells of epithelial origin in the colon, lung, liver, esophagus, and oral epitheliam and cells of connective tissue origin [which give rise to fibrosarcomas, lymphosarcomas, angiosarcomas, etc.]). These studies have indicated that the suppression of carcinogenesis by BBI and BBIC is not dependent on (a) inducing carcinogen, (b) species, (c) organ or tissue, (d) cell type, (e) method of administration, (f) type of cancer, or (g) whether

---

**TABLE 12.1**
**Known Biological Effects of BBI**

Prevents cancer (reviewed in References 3–7)

Antiinflammatory agent (reviewed in References 3, 8, 9)

Prevention of hair and weight loss in animals with cancer[10,11]

Prevention of radiation-induced exencephaly[12]

Increases life span[5]

Enhances cytotoxicity of *cis*-platinum as a chemotherapeutic agent[13–15]

Serves as a radioprotector for normal cells *in vitro*[15]

Has effects on the contractile and relaxant responses of smooth muscle
to various forms of stimulation[16]

Prevents muscle atrophy in artificial microgravity[47] and in animals with
muscular dystrophy[17]

Has beneficial effects in animals with experimental autoimmune encephalomyelitis
(EAE), an animal model system for multiple sclerosis,[18] and in animals with
experimental neuritis, an animal model system for Guillain-Barré syndrome
(Abdolmohamad Rostami, personal communication)

---

**TABLE 12.2**
**History of BBI and BBIC from the Bench to the Clinic**

1975: Original observation that protease inhibitors prevent malignant transformation *in vitro*

1978: First publication reporting that protease inhibitors prevent malignant transformation *in vitro*

1985: First publication reporting that BBI and BBIC prevent cancer in animals

1988: Submission of IND to the FDA for BBIC clinical trial in patients with oral leukoplakia

1992: Approval from FDA to perform BBIC single dosing studies in people

1995: Approval from FDA to perform BBIC multiple dosing studies in people for up to 6 months of treatment

1998: Approval from FDA to perform BBIC multiple dosing studies in people for up to 1.5 years of treatment

or not the animals are genetically susceptible to cancer development.[19] BBI and BBIC also have antiinflammatory activity in animal assay systems (reviewed in References 3, 8, and 9). BBI appears to have particularly strong activity in neuro-inflammatory diseases such as multiple sclerosis[18] and Guillain-Barré syndrome (Dr. A. Rostami, personal communication). It is believed that BBIC will be an effective anticarcinogenic and antiinflammatory agent for many organ systems; it is expected that BBI is responsible for both the anticarcinogenic and anti-inflammatory activities of BBIC.

The development of BBI into a drug useful for human trials has taken many years. The history of BBIC development is shown in Table 12.2. The patient populations in which BBIC human trials have been performed thus far, and the respective FDA investigational new drugs (INDs) covering these trials, are shown in Table 12.3. The status of BBI and BBIC use as a human drug product (toxicity testing) is shown in Table 12.4;[20-29] from the studies that have been performed, there is no evidence that BBI and BBIC are genotoxic, teratogenic or oncogenic,

**TABLE 12.3**
**BBIC Clinical Trials**

| IND Number | FDA Drug Product Division | Patient Population |
|---|---|---|
| 34671 | Oncology and pulmonary | Oral leukoplakia |
| 52642 | Reproductive and urologic | Benign prostatic hyperplasia |
| 51216 | Reproductive and urologic | Prostate cancer |
| 55198 | Gastrointestinal and coagulation | Esophagitis and lung cancer |
| 55798 | Gastrointestinal and coagulation | Ulcerative colitis |
| 60447 | Dermatologic and dental | Gingivitis |

## TABLE 12.4
## Status of BBI and BBIC for Use as Human Drug Product

### Toxicity Testing

Studies of subchronic (3 months)[20,21] and chronic (6 months to 1 year)[22–24] toxicity
testing in dogs and rodents; completed

Genotoxicity: a standard battery for genotoxicity testing of pharmaceuticals[25–27]; completed

Teratology: studies in rabbits[29]; completed

Oncogenicity: studies in heterozygous (±) p53 deficient mice[30]; completed

### Human Trials

A pilot study, a Phase I and a Phase IIa trial in patients with oral leukoplakia have been
completed[30–36]; a Phase IIb extended trial is ongoing (this is thought to be a Phase III
trial for the treatment of oral leukoplakia and a Phase II trial for oral cancer prevention)

Two Phase I/II trials have been completed in patients with benign prostatic hyperplasia
(BPH)[37–39] and ulcerative colitis (UC)[40]; a Phase II trial of BBIC in UC patients is ongoing

Six BBIC INDs exist for patients with oral leukoplakia, BPH, prostate cancer, UC,
esophagitis, and gingivitis

and drug-induced toxicity has not been observed in the animal studies. The
specific human trials that have been or are being performed are shown in
Table 12.4, with publications from these studies indicated.[30–40] BBI and BBIC
dosing information is given in Table 12.5, and information from animal and human
BBI pharmacokinetic studies is given in Table 12.6 (these data are reviewed in
References 3, 41–44).

## TABLE 12.5
## BBI and BBIC Dosing Information

Doses in animals have been given as a percentage of the diet or in chymotrypsin
inhibitor (C.I.) units

Doses of BBI and BBIC in people are measured in C.I. units

   1 C.I. unit = the amount of any substance that will inhibit 1 mg of chymotrypsin

   Example: If 0.5 g of the substance inhibits 3 mg of chymotrypsin, then there are
   3 C.I. units of the substance and the substance is 6 C.I. units per gram

Formulations of BBIC for human use: liquid, tablet, and lozenge

Doses of BBIC used in human trials:

   Oral leukplakia: 25, 200, 400, 600, 800, and 1066 C.I. units per day (the current
   Phase IIB/III trial utilizes a dose of 600 C.I. units per day)

   Benign prostatic hyperplasia: 100, 200, 400, and 800 C.I. units per day

   Ulcerative colitis, prostate cancer, and esophagitis and lung cancer: 800 C.I. units
   per day

   Gingivitis: 400 C.I. units per day

**TABLE 12.6**
**BBI Pharmacokinetic Studies**

In animals and people, BBI in blood and urine is detected with antibodies that react with
reduced BBI; thus, it is assumed that BBI is reduced *in vivo* (reviewed in Reference 3)

Ingested BBI peaks in the urine of people within 9 h (mean time: 2 to 3 h) after ingestion[42]

Ingested BBI excreted via the urine is still capable of inhibiting proteases[43]

In animals, the half-life of BBI in the serum or rats or hamsters is 10 h[3]

Approximately 40 to 50% of ingested BBI is taken up into the bloodstream[43] or into
epithelial cells of the gastrointestinal tract[44]; 50 to 60% is excreted via the feces[43]

At 3 h after ingestion, BBI is widely distributed throughout the body[43]

## 12.2 DETAILS OF THE FOUR COMPLETED HUMAN BBIC TRIALS

Four human trials utilizing BBIC have recently been completed and several
publications exist for these studies.[30–40] The completed trials utilized patients with oral
leukplakia, benign prostatic hyperplasia (BPH), and ulcerative colitis. In addition,
results are available from a single patient with metastatic prostate cancer who
was treated with BBIC for a 6-month period. Summaries of the results of these
trials are given below.

### 12.2.1 ORAL LEUKOPLAKIA

A Phase I and a Phase IIa study of BBIC in patients with oral leukoplakia was
performed in collaboration with investigators at the University of California,
Irvine.[30–37] The Phase I trial indicated no toxicity from BBIC at any dose studied.[30]
In the Phase IIA trial, the following types of information were gathered: oral
leukoplakia lesion size, levels of proteolytic activities in buccal mucosa cells,
levels of proto-oncogene expression in buccal mucosal cells and serum, histopathology of the lesions, and clinical laboratory assays (as part of the safety and
toxicity assessment). Figure 12.1 shows an example of a region exhibiting oral
leukoplakia in one of the patients in the Phase IIa trial before and after BBIC
treatment. Following the BBIC therapy period, the oral leukoplakia lesion in this
patient resolved. Conclusions of the Phase IIa study were as follows. Over the
dose range of 200 to 1066 chymotrypsin inhibitor (C.I.) units per day, BBIC
caused a statistically significant reduction of total oral leukoplakia lesion size
that was linearly correlated with increase in dose; these results are illustrated in
Figure 12.2. The compound was well-tolerated with no evidence of laboratory,
symptom, or clinical side effects. The surrogate end point biomarkers (SEB)
utilized in the study were buccal cell proteolytic activity and erbB-2/neu protein
levels in buccal mucosal cells and in serum. The results of the SEB indicated
that changes in the protease activity in oral mucosal cells after BBIC treatment
correlated with the changes in the erbB-2/neu protein levels in oral mucosal cells,

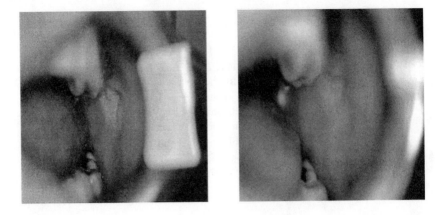

**FIGURE 12.1** Example of the response of a patient with oral leukoplakia to BBIC treatment. Photograph of mouth of patient with oral leukoplakia in the BBIC Phase IIa trial before (left) and after (right) BBIC treatment period. The details of this trial have been described.[33] The oral leukoplakia lesion (left, center) was considered to be resolved following the BBIC treatment period. (Photographs courtesy of Frank L. Meyskens, M.D., University of California, Irvine.)

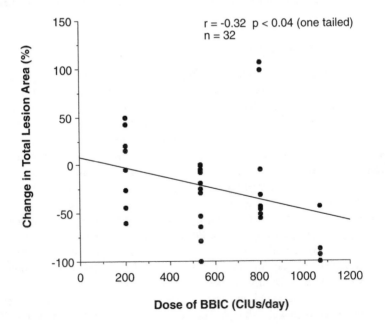

**FIGURE 12.2** Clinical response of oral leukoplakia in relation to the dose of BBIC administered. The size of oral leukoplakia lesions before and after BBIC dosing is shown. BBIC treatment led to a decrease in area of total leukoplakia lesions following the 4-week treatment period. (Data from Armstrong, W.B. et al., *Clin. Cancer Res.*, 6, 4684–4691, 2000.)

suggesting that protease activity can be as useful as erbB-2/neu oncogene expression as SEB in oral carcinogenesis human trials.[34]

## 12.2.2 Benign Prostatic Hyperplasia

A randomized, double-blind trial of BBIC in patients with BPH has also been performed.[37–39] This trial involved 6 months of BBIC treatment involving dosage levels of 100 to 800 C.I. units per day in oral tablet form. The following end points were monitored in this trial: serum prostate-specific antigen (PSA) levels, urinary functions (American Urological Association score), sexual functions (International Index of Erectile Function [IIEF] score), quality of life score (urinary activities), size (ultrasound measurement) and histopathological analysis of prostate (optional), toxicity and adverse side effects (scored by the National Cancer Institute [NCI] common toxicity criteria, BBI pharmacokinetic studies, and clinical laboratory assays (performed as part of the safety and toxicity assessment). The results from this trial are discussed in detail elsewhere.[37–39] Briefly, the results of this BBIC trial were as follows:

- There was no dose-limiting toxicity for BBIC.
- There was a statistically significant decrease in serum levels of PSA in BBIC-treated patients compared to the placebo-treated controls ($P = 0.04$). The decrease in PSA levels was particularly marked in patients from the highest dose groups ($P = 0.023$ for the 400 and 800 C.I. unit dose groups combined).
- There was a statistically significant decrease in serum triglyceride levels in BBIC-treated patients (the mean serum triglyceride level decreased by 24.1% [$P < 0.05$]), representing improved status.
- There was a decrease in prostate volume in BBIC-treated patients; mean pretherapy: 65.3 ± 4.8 cc; mean posttherapy: 46.6 ± 6.9; mean decrease: 28.7%.
- For patients who attempted to achieve erection, BBIC treatment resulted in a statistically significant increase in IIEF scores, representing improved sexual activities (mean IIEF score increased by 31% [$P < 0.05$]). For control subjects, there was a decrease in IIEF scores that was not statistically significant.
- The scores recorded in response to a urinary symptom questionnaire indicated improved urinary activities in the BBIC-treated patients; however, the control subjects exhibited similar improvements in urinary activities during the course of the trial.
- For patients ($n = 6$) who had initial serum levels of cholesterol that were abnormally high (>200 mg/dl), BBIC treatment resulted in a reduction in serum cholesterol levels ($P < 0.05$).
- Prostate biopsy tissues taken pre- and posttreatment were only available for two patients in the trial; both of them were in the lowest dosage group (100 C.I. units per day). The prostate tissue from one of these patients

indicated BPH that was essentially unchanged by BBIC treatment. Histopathological analysis of the prostate tissue from the other patient also indicated BPH and prostatitis, with approximately the same amount of prostatic intraepithelial neoplasia (PIN) pre- and posttreatment. However, his benign prostatic tissue indicated areas of atrophy and focal atrophy, and a decreased amount of prostatitis, upon completion of the BBIC treatment.

The published results from the trial were limited to group mean values utilizing patient results from the beginning and end of the trial.[38,39] Data for the end points evaluated were collected at several points within the BBIC trial period for each patient as well, and analysis of these data can give further information about the effects of BBIC in the patients in the trial. Data from several different time points taken from some of the patients in the trial have been published[37] and are shown in Figure 12.3 to Figure 12.5. Data on the PSA measurements made for all patients in the 400 C.I. unit per day dose cohort are shown in Figure 12.3. In Figure 12.3 there is a downward trend for the PSA measurements over time in the BBIC-treated patients; such a downward trend was not observed for the patient taking placebo in the 400 C.I. unit per day dose cohort.

Figures 12.4 and 12.5 represent the data from a single patient in the trial for all types of data collected; this patient received BBIC therapy as part of the 100 C.I. unit per day dose cohort. This patient agreed to have ultrasound measurements made and have prostate biopsies taken pre- and posttherapy. Several trends are indicated in Figure 12.4a. There was a downward trend for the serum PSA levels, starting from a level that was higher than normal (>4 ng/ml) and progressing toward levels within the normal range for serum PSA concentrations. Values for urinary activities (I-PSS/AUA and Quality of Life scores) showed downward trends over time, suggesting improved status, and his IIEF scores indicated an upward trend, also suggesting improved status. His prostate volume decreased by 23% over the BBIC trial period (pretherapy: 70 cc, posttherapy: 54 cc), indicating improved status, as indicated in Figure 12.4b. Histopathological analysis revealed that pretherapy, there was BPH and prostatitis, and posttherapy, there was BPH with focal atrophy and reduced inflammation. For this patient, the BBIC treatment appeared to have several beneficial effects.

## 12.2.3 ULCERATIVE COLITIS

A human trial of patients with UC has recently been completed.[40] As part of this trial, patients with UC (left-sided disease or pancolitis) received BBIC or placebo tablets over a 3-month treatment period. The following end points were monitored: serum levels of inflammation markers α-1-antichymotrypsin, C-reactive protein and serum amyloid A protein, extent of disease (sigmoidoscopy), histopathology (biopsy), symptoms (bleeding, urgency, frequency, etc.), BBI pharmacokinetic studies, levels of proteolytic activity in biopsy samples, erythrocyte sedimentation rate analysis, and clinical laboratory assays (as part of the toxicity

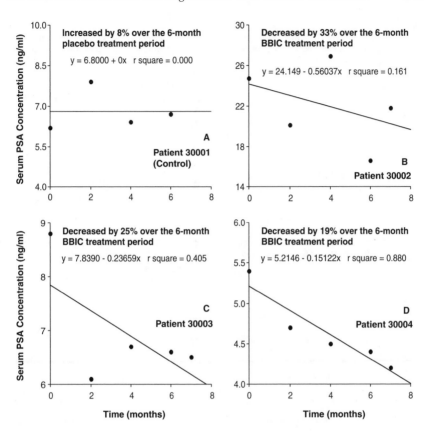

**FIGURE 12.3** Effects of BBIC (400 C.I. units per day) and placebo medication on the serum PSA concentration in patients with BPH. BBIC treatment led to a reduction in serum PSA levels in the BBIC treated patients (panels B, C, and D), while the placebo medication led to a slight, but not statistically significant, increase in the serum PSA levels in this trial. (From Kennedy, A.R. and Wan, X.S., in *Soy & Health 2002: Clinical Evidence, Dietetic Applications*, Descheemaeker, K. and Debruyne, I., Eds., Garant Publishers, Antwerp-Apeldoorn, 2002, pp. 129–136. With permission.)

and adverse side effects assessment). This was a randomized, double-blind, placebo-controlled trial: 50% of the patients received placebo tablets and 50% received BBIC tablets at a dosage of 800 C.I. units per day. A total of 28 patients were enrolled in the trial: 23 patients completed the trial and 5 patients withdrew or were dismissed. Fourteen patients were treated with BBIC in this trial. The primary goals of the trial were to assess the safety of the drug, BBIC, in patients with UC and to assess the effect of BBIC on serum inflammation markers and tissue protease levels, which would serve as disease markers for future trials.

No serious adverse events occurred during the trial. Some nausea and disease symptom exacerbation was observed, but these occurred in equal frequency in

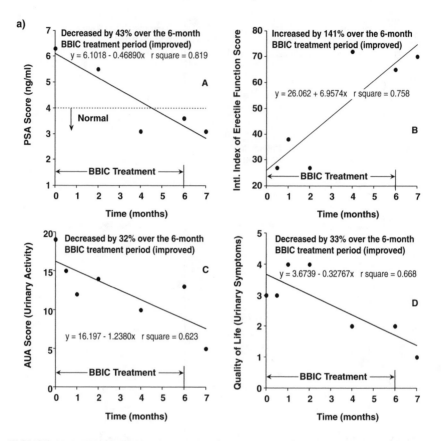

**FIGURE 12.4** Effects of 100 C.I. units of BBIC per day in a patient with BPH. (a) Results of sequential measurements assessing the serum PSA concentration, urinary activities, and sexual functions during the BBIC treatment period. See text for details. (b) Effects of BBIC on prostate volume. See text for details. These data are presented in References 37 and 38. (Part a from Kennedy, A.R. and Wan, X.S., in *Soy & Health 2002: Clinical Evidence, Dietetic Applications,* Descheemaeker, K. and Debruyne, I., Eds., Garant Publishers, Antwerp-Apeldoorn, 2002, pp. 129–136. With permission.)

the active drug group and the placebo group (Lichtenstein, et al., unpublished data). While isolated blood test results received Eastern Cooperative Oncology Group (ECOG) toxicity scores other than 0, these were, if anything, more common in the placebo group than in the active drug group. No significant differences were observed between treatment groups in serum inflammation markers or tissue protease levels. Secondary goals of the trial included clinical assessments of the patients. A BBIC dose of 800 C.I. units per day for a 3-month period resulted in regression of disease in patients with UC.[40] The data indicated several trends, including a trend in the primary clinical end point, the Sutherland Disease Activity Index (an index that consists of four criteria as follows: stool frequency, rectal

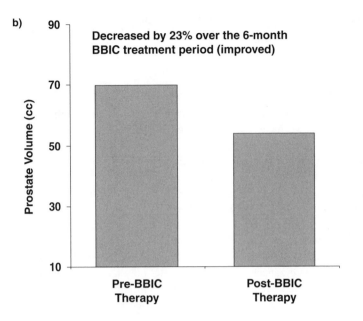

FIGURE 12.4 (Continued).

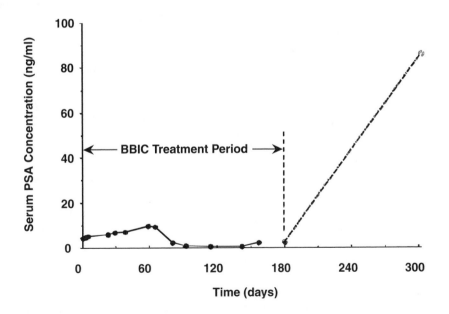

**FIGURE 12.5** Effects of 6 months of BBIC (800 C.I. units per day) treatment on serum PSA levels in a patient with metastatic prostate cancer. The serum PSA levels remained at an approximately constant level over the 6-month BBIC treatment period but rose to a high level after the BBIC therapy period ended.

bleeding, mucosal appearance, and physician rating of disease activity). Because of the encouraging results from this pilot trial, a Phase II trial for this indication has begun.

## 12.2.4 PROSTATE CANCER

A single patient with metastatic prostate cancer was treated with BBIC for 6 months. Data for serum PSA measurements during BBIC treatment are shown in Figure 12.5. Serum PSA levels were maintained at approximately a constant level during the BBIC therapy period but rose to a much higher level following BBIC treatment. In preparation for this study, a number of studies in cells and animals were performed to assess the effects of BBIC on prostate cancer. BBI and BBIC treatment was shown to inhibit the growth of human prostate cells *in vitro*[45] and in nude mice.[46] BBI and BBIC were directly cytotoxic to abnormal prostate cells (including prostate cancer cells[45]), without having cytotoxic effects on normal prostate epithelial cells. The results of PSA measurements for the patient with metastatic prostate cancer suggest that BBIC may have had a growth inhibitory effect on the prostate cancer cells during the treatment period; these results are promising and suggest the possible use of BBIC in prostate cancer patients.

## 12.2.5 SUMMARY OF HUMAN BBIC TRIALS PERFORMED TO DATE

The BBIC studies performed in patients with oral leukoplakia, BPH, prostate cancer, ulcerative colitis, gingivitis, and esophagitis and lung cancer involve the treatment of patients with BBIC doses up to 1066 C.I. units per day for as long as 6 months (and up to 1.5 years in the case of some patients with oral leukoplakia who are participating in the extended Phase IIb trial). Thus far, 86 patients are known to have been treated with BBIC for up to 6 months. This includes patients from the Phase I (24 patients) and Phase IIa (32 patients) trials of patients with oral leukoplakia, the Phase I trial of patients with benign prostatic hyperplasia (15 patients), the Phase I trial of patients with ulcerative colitis (14 patients), and the single patient with metastatic prostate cancer.

In addition, it is expected that many other patients have been treated with BBIC. There are two patients with lung cancer and esophagitis and nine patients with gingivitis who are expected to have received daily BBIC treatments (lozenge formulation) for 3 months. In the Phase IIb trial of patients with oral leukoplakia, 44 patients have completed the trial and been treated with BBIC or placebo for at least 6 months (as of February 5, 2004); it is expected that approximately 22 of these patients have been or are being treated with BBIC. Thus, the total number of patients treated with BBIC up until the present time is approximately 119. There have been two serious adverse events reported to the FDA as part of the BBIC trials; these adverse events are in each case considered to be unrelated to drug treatment, as described below. While some side effects have been reported by patients in the trials, it is not clear whether the observed adverse events are drug related in most cases. In the completed trials, the adverse event rates in patients receiving BBIC therapy have been comparable to those observed for patients taking the placebo medication.

Thus far, there have been two serious adverse events reported for patients in the BBIC human trials. Details of these adverse events follow:

- Adverse event in the extended Phase IIb trial of patients with oral leukoplakia, which is currently ongoing. This Phase IIb trial is a randomized, double-blind, placebo-controlled trial involving patient treatment for 6 months. Patients in remission at 6 months are expected to continue the drug therapy up to a maximum of 1.5 years on BBIC (at 600 C.I. units per day) or placebo tablets. One adverse event has been reported from this trial. This adverse event occurred in an elderly man (over 81 years old) who experienced chest pain while at work and was hospitalized for 5 d. The patient had "a history of hypothyroidism, HTN, coronary artery disease with CABG in 1981 and angioplasty with stent placement in 1999." This adverse event was considered to be unrelated to drug treatment by Frank L. Meyskens, Jr., M.D., principal investigator for the trial. This patient has continued in the protocol; it is not known whether the patient is or was taking BBIC or placebo medication at the time of the adverse event, as the code for the trial has not yet been broken.
- Serious adverse event in the BBIC gingivitis trial. This serious adverse event occurred in an elderly man (over 88 years old) who stopped taking the medication within 5 d after he became enrolled in the trial. He stopped taking the medication at some point before having a quintuple bypass procedure. As he had chest pains, he drove himself to the hospital, where it was determined that he needed bypass surgery. At the time of entry into the trial, it was noted that he had preexisting heart disease and was taking one aspirin per day, blood pressure medication (Atenolol), and nitroglycerin as needed for chest pain. Dr. Roy Feldman, the dentist following the patient in the trial and serving as the principal investigator on the protocol, believed the adverse event was not related to his participation in the research protocol.

At this point in the human drug experience with BBIC, some gas or bloating can be considered an expected side effect. This is a common side effect associated with consumption of soybeans and other types of beans. This side effect is expected to last only for approximately 1 week after the beginning of high levels of soybean or bean consumption. This side effect has been relatively rare in the BBIC trials performed thus far. This is presumably because BBIC is essentially a protein extract of soybeans, and flatulence or bloating from bean products is due to difficulties in the digestion of the soybean carbohydrates.

In conclusion, based on the results of the clinical trials that have been performed thus far, BBIC appears to be highly promising as a drug for various human conditions.

## ACKNOWLEDGMENTS

The human trial work described in this report has been supported by several different sources of funding. The trials of patients with oral leukoplakia were supported in part by Grants U01-CA46496 and P30CA 62203 from the National Cancer Institute (principal investigator: Frank L. Meyskens, M.D.); the trial in patients with ulcerative colitis was supported by NIH Grant R43 GM55469 (principal investigator: Dr. Jeffrey H. Ware); the trial of patients with BPH and prostate cancer was supported by ProtoMed, Inc. (Lake Forest, IL). Ann R. Kennedy has a financial interest (equity) in ProtoMed, Inc.

## REFERENCES

1. Bowman, D.E., Differentiation of soybean antitryptic factors, *Proc. Soc. Exp. Biol. Med.*, 63, 547–550, 1946.
2. Birk, Y., Purification and some properties of a highly active inhibitor of trypsin and α-chymotrypsin from soybeans, *Biochim. Biophys, Acta*, 54, 378–381, 1961.
3. Kennedy, A.R., Chemopreventive agents: protease inhibitors, *Pharmacol. Ther.*, 78, 167–209, 1998.
4. Kennedy, A.R., Overview: anticarcinogenic activity of protease inhibitors, in *Protease Inhibitors as Cancer Chemopreventive Agents*, Troll, W. and Kennedy, A.R., Eds., Plenum, New York, 1993, pp. 9–64.
5. Kennedy, A.R., Szuhaj, B.F., Newberne, P.M., and Billings, P.C., Preparation and production of a cancer chemopreventive agent, Bowman–Birk inhibitor concentrate, *Nutr. Cancer*, 19, 281–302, 1993.
6. Kennedy, A.R., Prevention of carcinogenesis by protease inhibitors, *Cancer Res.* (Suppl.), 54, 1999s–2005s, 1994.
7. Kennedy, A.R., *In vitro* studies of anticarcinogenic protease inhibitors, in *Protease Inhibitors as Cancer Chemopreventive Agents*, Troll, W. and Kennedy, A.R., Eds., Plenum, New York, 1993, pp. 65–91.
8. Hawkins, J.V., Emmel, E.L., Feuer, J.J., Nedelman, M.A., Harvey, C.J., Klein, H.S., Rozmiarek, H., Kennedy, A.R., Lichtenstein, G.R., and Billings, P.C., Protease activity in a hapten-induced model of ulcerative colitis in rats, *Dig. Dis. Sci.*, 42, 1969–1980, 1997.
9. Ware, J.H., Wan, X.S., Newberne, P., and Kennedy, A.R., Bowman–Birk Inhibitor Concentrate reduces colon inflammation in mice with dextran sulfate sodium-induced ulcerative colitis, *Dig. Dis. Sci.*, 44, 986–990, 1999.
10. Evans, S.M., Szuhaj, B.F., Van Winkle, T., Michel, K., and Kennedy, A.R., Protection against metastasis of radiation induced thymic lymphosarcoma and weight loss in C57Bl/6NCr1BR mice by an autoclave resistant factor present in soybeans, *Radiat. Res.*, 132, 259–262, 1992.
11. Kennedy, A.R., The impact of protease inhibitors from soybeans on the carcinogenic process, In *Adjuvant Nutrition in Cancer Treatment*, Quillin, P. and Williams, R.M., Eds., Cancer Treatment Research Foundation, Arlington Heights, IL, 1993, pp. 129–143.
12. von Hofe, E., Brent, R., and Kennedy, A.R., Inhibition of x-ray induced exencephaly by protease inhibitors, *Radiat. Res.*, 123, 108–111, 1990.

13. Wan, X.S., Hamilton, T.C., Ware, J.H., Donahue, J.J., and Kennedy, A.R., Growth inhibition and cytotoxicity induced by Bowman–Birk Inhibitor Concentrate in cisplatin-resistant human ovarian cancer cells, *Nutr. Cancer,* 31, 8–17, 1998.

14. Zhang, L., Wan, X.S., Donahue, J., Ware, J.H., and Kennedy, A.R., Effects of the Bowman–Birk inhibitor on clonogenic survival and cisplatin or radiation induced cytotoxicity in human breast, cervical and head and neck cancer cells, *Nutr. Cancer,* 33, 165–173, 1999.

15. Kennedy, C.W., Donahue, J.J., and Wan, X.S., Effects of the Bowman–Birk protease inhibitor on survival of fibroblasts and cancer cells exposed to radiation and cis-platinum, *Nutr. Cancer,* 26, 209–217, 1996.

16. Malkowicz, S.B., Liu, S.P., Broderick, G.A., Wein, A.J., Kennedy, A.R., and Levin, R.M., Effect of the Bowman–Birk inhibitor (a soy protein) on *in vitro* bladder neck/urethral and penile corporal smooth muscle activity, *Neurourol. Urodyn.,* 22(1), 54–57, 2003.

17. Morris, C.A., Morris, L.D., Kennedy, A.R., and Sweeney, H., *Functional improvement of mdx mouse muscle following treatment with protease inhibitors,* Presented at the New Directions in Biology and Disease of Skeletal Muscle Meeting, Jan. 25–27th, 2004, San Diego, CA.

18. Rostami, A., Gran, B., Tabibzadeh, N., Ventura, E., Ware, J.H., and Kennedy, A., *Oral administration of Bowman–Birk Inhibitor Concentrate, a soybean-derived protease inhibitor, suppresses EAE in the Lewis rat: a potential oral therapy for multiple sclerosis,* Abstract P02.013, Presented at the 56th Annual Meeting of the American Academy of Neurology, San Francisco, April 27, 2004.

19. Kennedy, A.R., Beazer-Barclay, Y., Kinzler, K.W., and Newberne, P.M., Suppression of carcinogenesis in the intestines of Min mice by the soybean-derived Bowman–Birk inhibitor, *Cancer Res.,* 56, 679–682, 1996.

20. Page, J.G., Heath, J.E., May, R.D., and Martin, J.F., *13-Week Toxicity Study of Bowman–Birk Inhibitor Concentrate (BBIC) in Rats,* Report SRI-CBE-94-060-7482, Southern Research Institute, Birmingham, AL, 1994.

21. Page, J.G., Rodman, L.E., Giles, H.D., Farnell, D.R., and Wood, R.D., *13-Week Toxicity Study of Bowman–Birk Inhibitor Concentrate in Dogs,* Report SRI-CBE-94135-7482, Southern Research Institute, Birmingham, AL, 1994.

22. Serota, D.G., *Six-Month Oral Toxicity Study of Bowman–Birk Inhibitor Concentrate (BBIC) in Mice,* Report 560-057, MPI Research, Mattawan, MI, 2000.

23. Serota, D.G., *One-Year Oral Toxicity Study of Bowman–Birk Inhibitor Concentrate in Dogs,* Report 560-058, MPI Research, Mattawan, MI, 2000.

24. Wan, X.S., Serota, D.G., Ware, J.H., Crowell, J.A., and Kennedy, A.R., Detection of Bowman–Birk inhibitor (BBI) and anti-BBI antibodies in sera of humans and animals treated with Bowman–Birk Inhibitor Concentrate (BBIC), *Nutr. Cancer,* 43(2), 167–173, 2002.

25. Mirsalis, J.C., *Evaluation of Bowman–Birk Inhibitor Concentrate (BBIC) in the Salmonella Escherichia coli/Microsome Preincubation Assay,* Report SRI Study No. G069-99, SRI International, Menlo Park, CA, 2000.

26. Mirsalis, J.C., *Evaluation of Bowman–Birk Inhibitor Concentrate (BBIC) in the L5178Y Mouse Lymphoma Cell tk +/–, tk –/– Gene Mutation Assay,* Report SRI Study No. G071-99, SRI International, Menlo Park, CA, 2000.

27. Mirsalis, J.C., *Evaluation of Bowman–Birk Inhibitor Concentrate (BBIC) in the Mouse Bone Marrow Micronucleus Assay,* Report SRI Study No. G070-99, SRI International, Menlo Park, CA, 2000.

28. Johnson, W.D. and McCormick, D.L., *A Developmental Toxicity Study of Orally Administered Bowman–Birk Inhibitor Concentrate in Rabbits,* Final Report, IITRI Project No. 11659, IIT Research Institute, Chicago, 2004.

29. Johnson, W.D. and McCormick, D.L., *Six-Month Oral (Gavage) Toxicity/Oncogenicity Study of Bowman–Birk Inhibitior Concentrate in Heterozygous (+/−) p53 Deficient Mice,* Final Report, IITRI Project No. 1640, IIT Research Institute, Chicago, 2004.

30. Armstrong, W.B., Kennedy, A.R., Wan, X.S., Atiba, J., McLaren, C.E., and Meyskens, F.L., Jr., Single dose administration of Bowman–Birk Inhibitor Concentrate (BBIC) in patients with oral leukoplakia, *Cancer Epidemiol. Biomarkers Prev.,* 9, 43–47, 2000.

31. Armstrong, W.B., Kennedy, A.R., Wan, X.S., Taylor, T.H., Nguyen, Q.A., Jensen, J., Thompson, W., Lagerberg, W., and Meyskens, F.L., Jr., Clinical modulation of oral leukoplakia and protease activity by Bowman–Birk inhibitor concentrate in a Phase IIa chemoprevention trial, *Clin. Cancer Res.,* 6, 4684–4691, 2000.

32. Armstrong, W.B., Wan, X.S., Kennedy, A.R., Taylor, T.H., and Meyskens, F.L., Development of the Bowman-Birk inhibitor for oral cancer chemoprevention and analysis of Neu immunohistochemical staining intensity with Bowman-Birk Inhibitor Concentrate treatment, *Laryngoscope,* 113(10), 1687–1702, 2003.

33. Meyskens, F.L., Jr., Armstrong, W.B., Wan, X.S., Taylor, T., Jenson, J., Thompson, W., Nguyen, Q.A., and Kennedy, A.R., Bowman–Birk inhibitor concentrate (BBIC) affects oral leukoplakia lesion size and neu protein levels and proteolytic activity in buccal mucosal cells, *Proc. Am. Assoc. Cancer Res.,* 40, 432, 1999 (Abstract #2855).

34. Wan, X.S., Meyskens, F.L., Jr., Armstrong, W.B., and Kennedy, A.R., Relationship between a protease activity and neu oncogene expression in patients with oral leukoplakia treated with the Bowman–Birk inhibitor, *Cancer Epidemiol. Biomarkers Prev.,* 8, 601–608, 1999.

35. Meyskens, F.L., Development of Bowman–Birk inhibitor for chemoprevention of oral head and neck cancer, *Ann. NY Acad. Sci.,* 952, 116–123, 2001.

36. Wan, X.S. and Kennedy, A.R., Cancer prevention by the soybean-derived Bowman–Birk inhibitor, in *Proceedings of the International Symposium on Soybeans & Human Health,* November 16, 2000, Seoul, Korea, pp. 67–84, 2001.

37. Kennedy, A.R. and Wan, X.S., Biological effects of a soybean-derived protease inhibitor, the Bowman–Birk inhibitor, in *Soy & Health 2002: Clinical Evidence, Dietetic Applications,* Descheemaeker, K. and Debruyne, I., Eds., Garant Publishers, Antwerp-Apeldoorn, 2002, pp. 129–136.

38. Malkowicz, S.B., McKenna, W.G., Vaughn, D.J., Wan, X.S., Propert, K.J., Rockwell, K., Marks, S.H.F., Wein, A.J., and Kennedy, A.R., Effects of Bowman–Birk inhibitor concentrate in patients with benign prostatic hyperplasia, *Prostate,* 48, 16–28, 2001.

39. Malkowicz, S.B., Broderick, G.A., Zoltick, B., Marks, H.F., Treat, J., Tomaszewski, J., Propert, K., Wein, A.J., and Kennedy, A.R., Phase I study of oral Bowman–Birk Inhibitor Concentrate (BBIC), a soy protein, on patients with lower urinary tract symptoms, *J. Urol.,* 161, 228, 1999.

40. Lichtenstein, G.R., Deren, J., Katz, S., Kennedy, A.R., and Ware, J.H., The Bowman Birk protease inhibitor: a novel therapy for patients with active ulcerative colitis, *Gastroenterology,* 122, A-60, 2002.

41. Wan, X.S., Koch, C.J., Lord, E.M., Manzone, H., Billings, P.C., Donahue, J.J., Odell, C.S., Miller, J.H., Schmidt, N.A., and Kennedy, A.R., Monoclonal antibodies differentially reactive with native and reductively modified Bowman–Birk protease inhibitor, *J. Immunol. Methods,* 180, 117–130, 1995.
42. Wan, X.S., Lu, L.-J.W., Anderson, K.E., Miller, J.H., Ware, J.H., Donahue, J.J., and Kennedy, A.R., Urinary excretion of Bowman–Birk inhibitor in humans after soy consumption as determined by a monoclonal antibody-based immunoassay, *Cancer Epidemiol. Biomarkers Prev.,* 9, 741–747, 2000.
43. Billings, P.C., St. Clair, W.H., Maki, P.A., and Kennedy, A.R., Distribution of the Bowman–Birk protease inhibitor in mice following oral administration, *Cancer Lett.,* 62, 191–197, 1992.
44. Billings, P.C., Brandon, D.L., and Habres, J.M., Internalization of the Bowman–Birk protease inhibitor by intestinal epithelial cells, *Eur. J. Cancer,* 27, 903–908, 1991.
45. Kennedy, A.R. and Wan, X.S., Effects of the Bowman–Birk inhibitor on growth, invasion and clonogenic survival of human prostate epithelial cells and prostate cancer cells, *Prostate,* 50, 125–133, 2002.
46. Wan, X.S., Ware, J.H., Zhang, L., Newberne, P.M., Evans, S., Clark, L.C., and Kennedy, A.R., Treatment with the soybean-derived Bowman–Birk inhibitor increases the serum prostate specific antigen concentration while suppressing the growth of human prostate cancer xenografts in nude mice, *Prostate,* 41, 243–252, 1999.
47. Morris, C.A., Morris, L.D., Kennedy, A.R., and Sweeney, H.L., Dietary intake of a soy-derived protease inhibitor attenuates the skeletal muscle mass loss associated with disuse atrophy in mice, *FASEB J.,* 17, Abst. 594.11, 2003.

# 13 Bioactive Peptides Derived from Soy Protein

*Masaaki Yoshikawa and Takahiro Tsuruki*

## CONTENTS

## 13.1 INTRODUCTION

It is widely accepted that soy has many beneficial effects in preventing life-style-related diseases. Some of them have been attributed to protein and peptides in soy. However, the preventive effect against breast cancer, which has been attributed to soy protein, is now ascribed to isoflavones.[1] In some cases, the beneficial effects of soy can be ascribed not to protein or peptides per se but to the amino acids constituting them. This chapter describes the physiological effects that are truly attributable to protein and peptides in soy.

## 13.2 HYPOCHOLESTEROLEMIC PEPTIDES

It has been reported that plant proteins are generally more hypocholesterolemic than animal proteins.[2] The hypocholesterolemic nature of soy proteins is the highest among plant proteins. Iwami found that the hydrophobicity of pepsin, and the bile acid–binding ability of pepsin digest of soy protein were the highest among proteins.[3] Sugano et al. found that the hypocholesterolemic activity of soy protein could be mainly ascribed to a high-molecular-weight peptide fraction remaining after gastrointestinal digestion.[4,5] The undigested fraction (UDF) binds bile acids tightly and inhibits their reabsorption because of its hydrophobic nature. This leads to increased fecal excretion of bile acids and reduction of cholesterol in serum and liver. The hypocholesterolemic activity was reserved after phospholipids, saponines, and isoflavones have been washed with organic solvent, suggesting that the UDF itself is the essential component.

Makino et al., suggested that glycinin A1a and A2 are the bile acid–binding proteins.[6,7] They identified a hydrophobic peptide corresponding to residues 114 to 161 of glycinin A1a as the bile acid–binding site. They also suggested that this peptide might be responsible for potentiation of insulin action.[6] Choi et al., identified VAWWMY, which corresponds to residues 129 to 134 of glycinin A1a, as a bile acid–binding site from experiments using a deoxycholic acid column.[8]

Lovati et al. found that the β-conglycinin α' subunit stimulated expression of the LDL-receptor in Hep G2 cells.[9] They suggested that a peptide, LRVPAGT TFYVVNPDNDENLRMIA, corresponding to residues 127 to 150 of the α' subunit is responsible for the activity.[9]

## 13.3  HYPOTRIGLYCERIDEMIC PROTEIN

It has been reported that soy protein or peptides stimulate fat metabolism and have an antiobesity effect. Saito observed stimulation of the sympathetic nervous system after injestion of soy peptides.[10] Aoyama et al. found that the hypotriglyceridemic effect is ascribable to β-conglycinin.[11] Moriyama et al. observed a reduction of serum tryglyceride level and an increase of serum growth hormone level after ingesting ethanol-washed 7S-rich protein.[12] Fecal excretion of triglyceride was also increased. In the liver, β-oxidation was stimulated and fatty acid synthesis was suppressed. Stimulation of β-oxidation and elevation of serum growth hormone level could be ascribed to a specific amino acid composition of soy protein.[13]

## 13.4  PEPTIDES REGULATING FOOD INTAKE

Nishi et al. found that peptides rich in Arg residues stimulate cholecystokinin (CCK) release by binding to intestinal mucosal cells in rats.[14] They found that a synthetic VRIRLLQRFNKRS that corresponds to residues 51 to 63 of the β-conglycinin β subunit suppressed food intake by way of stimulation of CCK release. They also found that some other synthetic Arg-rich peptides found in β-conglycinin suppressed food intake by similar mechanisms. However, it is uncertain whether such trypsin-sensitive peptides could exist in the intestine after soy protein ingestion.

## 13.5  HYPOTENSIVE PEPTIDES

The hypotensive effect of soy protein has been reported.[15] Inhibitors for the angiotensin I–converting enzyme (ACE) have been isolated from natto fermented soy.[16] Nonpeptidic nicotianamin in soy also has inhibitory activity for ACE.[17] However, it is also reported that ACE inhibition does not account for the antihypertensive effect of dietary soy in mature SHR.[18]

## 13.6 ANTICANCER PROTEINS AND PEPTIDES

Proteins and polypeptides in soy might be effective for cancer chemoprevention. It has been suggested that the Bowman–Birk trypsin inhibitor might suppress carcinogenesis induced by chemicals or radiation.[19] The Kunitz trypsin inhibitor might also suppress metastasis of ovarian cancer cells by blocking urokinase up-regulation.[20] Soybean lectin is expected to be effective for cancer prevention and diagnosis.[21] Another candidate for anticarcinogenic peptides in soy is lunacin, a 43–amino acid polypeptide derived from 2S albumin (Gm2S-1).[22] Lunacin has an Arg-Gly-Asp (RGD) cell adhesion motif and a helix with a structural homology to a conserved region of chromatin-binding proteins.[23] Commercial soy products contain amounts of lunacin, ranging from 5.48 mg/g of protein (defatted soy flour) to 16.52 mg/g protein (soy concentrate) (Figure 13.1). Lunacin is heat stable and resistant to gastrointestinal digestion. It is found in the Bowman–Birk trypsin inhibitor preparation and constitutes its major anticancer component.[24] In SENCAR mice, lunacin reduced skin tumor incidence by approximately 70%, decreased tumor yield per mouse, and increased tumor latency period after dermal application.[25] The cancer-preventing property of lunacin might be related to its chromatin-binding affinity.[26]

A hydrophobic peptide, MLPSYSPY, which has cytotoxicity against a mouse monocyte macrophage cell line P388D1, has been isolated from thermoase digest of soy protein by a Korean group.[27]

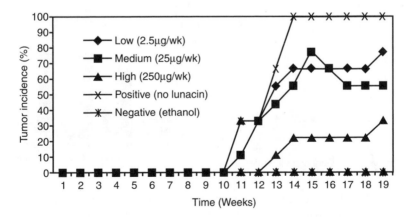

**FIGURE 13.1** Effect of lunacin on DMBA-initiated, TPA-promoted skin tumorigenesis in female SENCAR mice.[24] DMBA = 2,4-dimethylbenzoic acid, TPA = 12-$O$-tetradecanoylphorbol-13-acetate, SENCAR = sensitivity to carcinogenesis.

## 13.7  IMMUNOMODULATING PEPTIDES

Immunomodulating peptides have been found in soy proteins. HCQRPR, derived from glycinin A1aB1b, stimulates phagocytosis in a similar manner to tuftsin (TKPR), which is derived from immunoglobulin G.[28]

Another peptide that stimulates phagocytosis by human polymorphonuclear leukocytes has been isolated from tryptic digest of soy protein. The structure of tridecapeptide obtained was Met-Ile-Thr-Leu-Ala-Ile-Pro-Val-Asn-Lys-Pro-Gly-Arg, derived from residues 173 to 185 of the β-conglycinin α′ subunit.[29] The peptide was named soymetide since the Met residue at the amino terminus is essential for the immunostimulating activity; the des-Met peptide has no activity. Synthetic homologues of soymetide-13 in α and β subunits have no immunostimulating activity since the essential Met residue is replaced by Leu or Ile in these subunits. The immunostimulating activity of soymetides is elevated by deletion of residues from the carboxyl terminus (Figure 13.2).

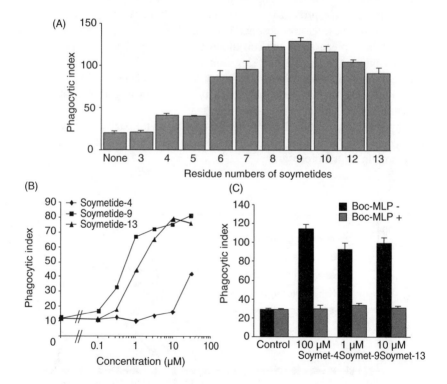

**FIGURE 13.2** (A) Activation of phagocytosis by soymetides with C-terminal deletions. Human neutrophils were incubated with opsonized fluorescent beads and 30 $\mu M$ soymetides ($n = 3$). Values are expressed as the mean ± standard error (SE). (B) Concentration-dependent activation of phagocytosis by soymetide-4, -9, and -13 ($n = 2$). (C) Effect of the fMLP antagonist Boc-MLP (100 $\mu M$) on phagocytosis activated by soymetides ($n = 4$). Values are expressed as the mean ± SE.

Soymetide-9, Met-Ile-Thr-Leu-Ala-Ile-Pro-Val-Asn, exhibits the highest activity, and its activity is reduced by further deletion. The shortest peptide showing immunostimulating activity is soymetide-4, that is, Met-Ile-Thr-Leu. Soymetide was compared with formyl-Met-Leu-Phe (fMLP) since it is as an immunostimulating peptide containing essential Met residue. Soymetides show weak affinity for fMLP receptors (Table 13.1). Furthermore, immunostimulating activities of soymetide-4, -9, and -13 are all blocked by Boc-MLF, an fMLP antagonist. fMLP has been designed to mimick bacterial proteins or peptides carrying formyl Met at their amino terminus and induces chemotaxis and phagocytosis of polymorphonuclear leukocytes. Thus, bacterial infection is detected by a receptor for formyl peptides.

Although not formylated, soymetide has weak affinity for the formyl peptide receptor. This means that the human body stimulates the immune system by recognizing as if bacterial infection has occurred when we take soy. At concentrations higher than $10^{-6}$ $M$, fMLP induces reactive oxygen species to kill phagocytosed bacteria, which also leads to inflammation. Thus, fMLP is regarded as an inflammatory substance. However, soymetide-4 does not stimulate reactive oxygen production because of its weak affinity for the fMLP receptor (Table 13.2). Soymetide-4 is expected to be a safe immunostimulating peptide without risk of inflammation. Immunostimulating activity of soymetide-4 is marginal after intraperitoneal (i.p.) administration. However, in stimulating release of tumor necrosis factor $\alpha$ (TNF-$\alpha$) after oral administration, soymetide-4 was more active than soymetide-9 and -13 (Table 13.2). This is probably because intestinal absorption of soymetide-4 is better than that of soymetide-9 and -13.

Soymetide-4 prevented hair loss (alopecia) induced by cancer chemotherapy. The alopecia induced by etoposide in neonatal rats was suppressed almost completely after oral administration of soymetide-4 at a dose of 300 mg/kg for 8 consecutive days (Figure 13.3).[30] fMLP also inhibited alopecia induced by etoposide after i.p. injection at a dose of 30 mg/kg for 4 d, though it was ineffective after oral administration.[31] This is probably due to the restricted permeability of $N$-formylpeptides through the intestinal mucosa.

**TABLE 13.1**
**Affinities of Soymetide-13 and Its Derivatives for fMLP Receptor**

| Peptides | $IC_{50}$ ($\mu M$) |
|---|---|
| MITLAIPVNKPGR (soymetide-13) | 50 |
| MITLAIPVN (soymetide-9) | 25 |
| MITL (soymetide-4) | 450 |
| fMLF (fMLP) | 0.03 |

Binding assay was performed in the presence of [$^3$H]-fMLP (25 n$M$) using human neutrophils.

**TABLE 13.2**
**Immunostimulating Properties of Soymetide-4, -9, and -13**

| Peptides | Phagocytosis (*in vitro*) | $O_2$ Production (*in vitro*) | TNF-$\alpha$ Secretion (p.o.) |
|---|---|---|---|
| Soymetide-4 | + | ± | ++ |
| Soymetide-9 | +++ | ++ | + |
| Soymetide-13 | ++ | + | − |

Hair loss, thinning of the skin layer, and thickening of the epidermis induced by etoposide were also suppressed by oral administration of soymetide-4 (Figure 13.4). The shape of the hair follicles in rats given both etoposide and soymetide-4 was normal. The etoposide-induced hair loss and skin layer thinning were also suppressed by intraperitonealy injected fMLP. However, etoposide-induced thickening of the epidermis was not inhibited by fMLP. fMLP and soymetide-4 did not cause inflammatory infiltration of macrophages and granulocytes to skin tissues under these conditions.

The antialopecia effect of orally administered soymetide-4 is reversed by indomethacin, a cyclooxigenase (COX) inhibitor, suggesting the involvement of

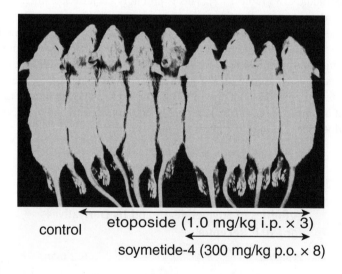

**FIGURE 13.3** Protective effects of soymetide-4 against etoposide-induced alopecia. Etoposide was injected at a dose of 1.0 mg/kg intraperitonealy for 3 consective days to 11-d-old rats. Soymetide-4 was administered orally at a dose of 300 mg/kg for 8 consecutive days beginning 5 d before the first etoposide injection. Pictures were taken 7 d after the last injection.

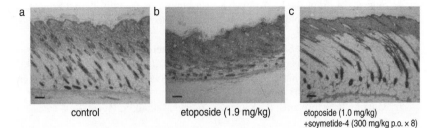

FIGURE 13.4 Light micrographs of hematoxylin-eosin–stained dorsal skin sections from neonatal rats treated with saline (a), etoposide (1.0 mg/kg, i.p. × 3), (b) or etoposide (1.0 mg/kg, i.p. × 3) + soymetide-4 (300 mg/kg, p.o. × 8) (c). Scale bars: 100 μm.

COX metabolites in the antialopecia effect.[32] Prostaglandin $E_2$ ($PGE_2$) is a prostaglandin involved in hair growth. There are four subtypes of $PGE_2$ receptors: $EP_1$, $EP_2$, $EP_3$, and $EP_4$. AH-23848B, an antagonist of the $EP_4$ receptor subtype, blocks the anti-alopecia effect of soymetide-4. However, AH-6809, an antagonist of the $EP_1$, $EP_2$, and $EP_3$ receptor subtypes, does not inhibit the antialopecia effect. These results suggest that the antialopecia effects of soymetide-4 are mediated via $EP_4$.

Etoposide-induced alopecia is caused by apoptosis of hair follicle cells. NF-κB is a nuclear factor that prevents apoptosis and is activated by various factors including $PGE_2$. PDTC, an inhibitor of NF-κB activation, abolishes the antialopecia effect of soymetide-4, suggesting that activation of NF-κB is involved in the antialopecia effect of orally administered soymetide-4.

## 13.8 ANTIOXIDATIVE PEPTIDES

Proteins, peptides, and amino acids have antioxidative activity. Six antioxidative peptides have been isolated from soy protein digest by Muramoto's group.[33] Muramoto also isolated peptides inhibiting crystallization of calcium phosphate from soy protein digest.[34]

## REFERENCES

1. Fritz, W., Coward, L., Wang, J., and Lamartiniere, C.A., Dietary genistein: perinatal mammary cancer prevention, bioavailability and toxicity testing in the rat, *Carcinigenesis,* 19, 2151–2158, 1998.
2. Hamilton, R.M. and Carroll, K.K., Plasma cholesterol levels in rabbits fed low fat, low cholesterol diets: effects of dietary proteins, carbohydrates and fibre from different souces, *Atherosclerosis,* 24, 47, 1976.
3. Iwami, K., Sakakibara, K., and Ibuki, F., Involvement of post-digestion "hydrophobic peptide" peptides in plasma cholesterol-lowering effect of dietary plant proteins, *Agric. Biol. Chem.,* 50, 1217–1222, 1986.

4. Sugano, M., Yamada, K., Yoshida, K., Hashimoto, Y., Matsuo, T., and Kimoto, M., The hypocholesterolemic action of the undigested fraction of soybean protein in rats, *Atherosclerosis,* 72, 115–122, 1988.
5. Sugano, M., Goto, S., and Yamada, Y., Cholesterol-lowering activity of various undigested fractions of soybean proteins in rats, *J. Nutr.,* 120, 977–985, 1990.
6. Makino, S., Nakashima, H., Minami, K., Moriyama, R., and Takao, S., *Agric. Biol. Chem.,* 52, 803–809, 1986.
7. Minami, K., Moriyama, R., Kitagawa, Y., and Makino, S., *Agric. Biol. Chem.,* 54, 511, 1990.
8. Choi, S.K., Adachi, M., and Utsumi, S., Identification of the bile-acid binding region in the soyglycinin A1aB1b subunit, *Biosci. Biotechnol. Biochem.,* 66, 2395–2401, 2002.
9. Lovati, M.R., Manzoni, C., Gianazza, E., Arnoldi, A., Kurowska, E., Carroll, K.K., and Sirtori, C.R., Soy protein peptides regulate cholesterol homeostasis in Hep G2 cells, *J. Nutr.,* 130, 2543–2549, 2000.
10. Saito, T., Effect of soy protein and peptide on sympathetic nerve system, Report of Soy Protein Res. Committee, Japan, 11, 95–97, 1990.
11. Aoyama, T., Kohno, M., Saito, T., Fukui, K., Takamatsu, K., Yamamoto, T., Himoto, Y., Hirotsuka, M., and Kito, M., Reduction of phytate-reduced soybean β-conglycinin of plasma triglyceride level of young and adult rats, *Biosci. Biotechnol.,* 65, 1071–1075, 2001.
12. Moriyama, T., Kishimoto, K., Nagai, K., Urade, R., Ogawa, T., Utsumi, S., Maruyama, N., and Maebuchi, M., Soybean β-conglycinin diet suppresses serum triglyceride levels in normal and genetically obese mice by induction of β-oxidation, downregulation of fatty acid synthase, and inhibition of triglyceride absorption, *Biosci. Biotechnol. Biochem.,* 68, 352–359, 2004.
13. Maebuchi, M., Machidori, M., Urade, R., Ogawa, T., Maruyama, N., and Moriyama, T., Hypolipidemic effect of dietary soybean, *J. Nutr.,* 134, 1274S, 2004.
14. Nishi, T., Hara, H., Asano, K., and Tomita, F., The soybean β-conglycinin β51-63 fragment suppresses appetite by stimulating cholecystokinin release, *J. Nutr.,* 133, 2537–2542, 2003.
15. Kimura, S., Chiang, M.R., and Fujimoto, H., Effect of eicosapentanoic acid and soybean protein on plasma cholesterol, blood pressure, and platelet aggregation in stroke-prone spontaneously hypertensive rats, *Diet. Proteins Cholesterol Metab. Atheroscler.,* 16, 26–35, 1990.
16. Okamoto, A., Hanagata, H., Kawamura, Y., and Yanagida, F., Anti-hypertensive substance in fermented soybean, natto, *Plant Foods Hum. Nutr.,* 47, 39–47, 1995.
17. Kinoshita, E., Yamakoshi, J., and Kikuchi, M., Purification and identification of an angiotensin I-converting enzyme inhibitor from soy sauce, *Biosci. Biotechnol. Biochem.,* 57, 1107–1110, 1993.
18. Martin, D.S., Williams, J.L., Breitkopf, N.P., and Eyster, K.M., Pressor responsiveness to angiotensin in soy-fed spontaneously hypertensive rats, *Can, J. Physiol. Pharmacol.,* 80, 1180–1186, 2002.
19. Kennedy, A.R., Chemopreventive agents: protease inhibitors, *Pharmacol. Ther.,* 78, 167–209, 1998.
20. Kobayashi, H. and Suzuki, M., Soybean Kunitz trypsin inhibitor suppresses ovarian cell invasion by blocking urokinase upregulation, *Soy Protein Res. Jpn.,* 7, 137–144, 2004.

21. Ganguly, C. and Das, S., Plant lectins as inhibitors of tumour growth and modulators of host immune response, *Chemotherapy,* 40, 272–278, 1994.
22. Hellerstein, M., Antimitotic peptide characterized from soybean: role in protection from cancer?, *Nutr. Rev.,* 57, 359–361, 1999.
23. Jeong, H.J., Park, J.H., Lam, Y., and de Lumen, B.O., Characterization of lunasin isolated from soybean, *J. Agric. Food Chem.,* 51, 7901–7906, 2003.
24. de Mejia, E.G., Bradford, T., and Hasler, C., The anticarcinogenic potential of soybean lectin and lunasin, *Nutr. Rev.,* 61, 239–246, 2003.
25. Galvez, A.F., Chen, N., Macasieb, J., and de Lumen, B.O., Chemopreventive property of a soybean peptide (lunasin) that binds to deacetylated histones and inhibits acetylation, *Cancer. Res.,* 61, 7473–7478, 2001.
26. Galvez, A.F. and de Lumen B.O., A soybean cDNA encoding a chromatin-binding peptide inhibits mitosis of mammalian cells, *Nat. Biotechnol.,* 17, 495–500, 1999.
27. Kim, S.E., Kim, H.H., Kim, J.Y.,Kang, Y.I., Woo, H.J., and Lee, J.L., Anticancer activity of hydrophobic peptides from soy proteins, *BioFactors,* 12, 151–155, 2000.
28. Yoshikawa, M., Kishi, K., Takahashi, M., Watanabe, A., Miyamura, T., Yamazaki, M., and Chiba, H., Immumomodulating peptide derived from soybean protein, in *Immunomodulatinh Drugs, Annals of the New York Academy of Sciences,* Vol. 685, St. Georgiev, V. and Yamaguchi, H., Eds., 1993, pp. 375–377.
29. Tsuruki, T., Kishi, K., Takahashi, M., Tanaka, M., Matsukawa, T., and Yoshikawa, M., Soymetide, an immunostimulating peptide derived from soybean β-conglycinin, is an fMLP agonist, *FEBS Lett.,* 540, 206–210, 2003.
30. Tsuruki, T., Takahata, K., and Yoshikawa, M., A soy-derived immunostimulating peptide inhibits etoposide-induced alopecia in neonatal rats, *J. Invest. Dermatol.,* 122, 848–850, 2004.
31. Tsuruki, T., Ito, A., Takahata, K., and Yoshikawa, M., FPRL1 receptor agonist peptides prevent etoposide-induced alopecia in neonatal rats peptide inhibits etoposide-induced alopecia in neonatal rats, *J. Invest. Dermatol.,* 123, 242–243, 2004.
32. Tsuruki, T., Takahata, K., and Yoshikawa, M., Anti-alopecia mechanism of soymetide-4, an immunostimulating peptide derived from soy β-conglycinin, *Peptides,* 26, 707–711, 2005.
33. Chen, H.-M., Muramoto, K., and Yamauchi, F.J., *Agric. Food Chem.,* 43, 574, 1995.
34. Jin, D.H., Zhang, Y., Suzuki, Y., Naganuma, T., Ogawa, T., Hatakeyama, E., and Muramoto, K., Inhibitory effect of protein hydrolysates on calcium carbonate crystallization, *J. Agric. Food. Chem.,* 48, 5450–5454, 2000.

# 14 Soy Peptides as Functional Food Material

*Kiyoharu Takamatsu*

## CONTENTS

## 14.1 INTRODUCTION

Peptides are unique components of living organisms and appear in many biological capacities, nutritional activities, and fermentation processes. Many types of biologically active peptides in the body, such as peptide hormones, participate in inter- and intracellular communication and activities. Proteins in the diet are hydrolyzed to amino acids in the gastrointestinal system, and in the course of this, various peptides with different chain lengths and sequences are generated as intermediates and some of these are composed with several amino acids absorbed directly from the intestine by peptide-specific transport systems (Figure 14.1).

Partially fermented foods contain various peptides and amino acids due to microbial activity and result in specific tastes in traditional foods. Much attention has been paid to food-derived peptides because of their good absorbability compared to amino acids. Early peptide research began in the 1960s.[1-4] Since nutritionists and food manufacturers expect the nutritional advantages of food-derived peptides and use them as food materials, development of peptide foods for clinical nutrition has been under intense study. However, much research on food processing has been performed to determine the physiological function of soybean and

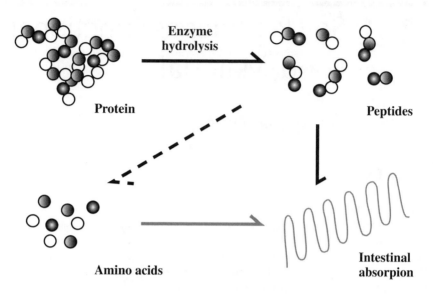

**FIGURE 14.1** Protein peptides and amino acids.

soy products, and thus their nutritional values and health benefits are increasing markedly.[5,6]

Concerning the functionality of dietary soy protein hydrolysates (defined and abbreviated as soy peptides), Hoff et al. suggested that there are some differences in lipid-lowering effects among soy protein, soy peptides, and amino acid mixtures that simulate soy protein amino acid composition.[7] Further studies have been performed to determine what kinds of molecules have dominant roles in lipid lowering. Yashiro et al. found that the high-molecular-weight fraction (HMF) of digested soy protein has a significant role in the cholesterol-lowering effect of soy protein compared with the low molecular weight of digested soy protein.[8] These studies suggest that the digestion of soy protein results in the presence various physiologically active peptides in the gastrointestinal tract. Indeed, subsequent research revealed benefits of soy peptides for life-style-derived diseases, including antiobesity, hypotensive, antifatigue, and other effects.

In this chapter, the story of commercial soy peptides, which result from soy protein digestion using proteolytic enzymes, is summarized, and possibilities for the use of soy peptides are discussed.

## 14.2  SOY PEPTIDE MANUFACTURING

Fermented soybean (natto), soy paste, and soy sauce are traditional foods and seasonings that have a history of over 1000 years in Japan and contain various types of peptides depending on their rate of hydrolysis. However, since both soybean paste and soy sauce contain a lot of salt, some limitations exist in their direct use as health foods. Moreover, almost of all of the protein in soy sauce has been degraded to amino acids, and there are thus few peptides in it. In the case of fermented soybean, the protein degradation rate is variable and not high. Partially hydrolyzed soy protein is thus the most suitable way to make soy peptides into food products, especially for health use.

Many processing methods using enzymes, acids, and heating are used for protein hydrolysis to produce peptides. In particular, enzyme hydrolysis has the advantage of high sequence specificity, low energy cost, and avoidance of side effects. Industrialized soy peptide production by enzyme hydrolysis started in the early 1980s in Japan with the growth of soy protein manufacturing. Agricultural, nutritional, and clinical scientists performed several physiological and nutritional studies of soy peptides in parallel with this development.

Food manufacturers are also interested in the solubility, low viscosity, and good absorbability of peptides, which improve the quality of foods. However, since peptides generally are bitter, before the industrial production of peptides was possible, development of a processing technology to eliminate the bitterness was necessary.[9,10] The typical reaction system used to remove the bitterness from the hydrophobic amino acids of the carboxyl terminal, which is caused by the action of the endo-protease with the exo-protease, was developed to restrain the formation of bitterness that consists mainly of two types of proteases.

Practical commercial soy peptide production consists of the following processes. The soybean protein curd from whole soybean first undergoes delipidation, water extraction, and isoelectric point precipitation. Enzymes are added to the curd, and hydrolysis is maintained in suitable conditions for several hours. Processes such as centrifugation, sedimentation, and filtration follow to separate debris from the reaction mixture. The scheme of production of soybean peptides is shown in Figure 14.2.

A mixture of polypeptides of various lengths and sequences is used for commercial products as shown in Table 14.1. To control the taste and solubility of peptides for various uses, several enzyme mixtures are used for hydrolysis, and various hydrolysis rates have been chosen, so the soy peptide products consist of various types of peptides. The product quality is generally defined by solubility for TCA solution, average amino acid chain lengths, and content of free amino acids. Table 14.2 shows examples of amino acid compositions of type a and b soy peptides compared with those of soy protein isolate. As shown, these peptides differ slightly in amino acid composition from soy protein isolate because they differ in enzyme processing rate and have almost the same purification processes.

There are several definitions of soy peptides. The Foundation of Japan Health Food and Nutritional Food has established a quality standard for healthy peptide foods. In that standard, peptide foods are defined as hydrolyzed protein mixtures in which at least 85% of the protein has a molecular weight below 15 kDa. Almost all of the soy peptides listed in Table 14.2 meet the Japanese standard.

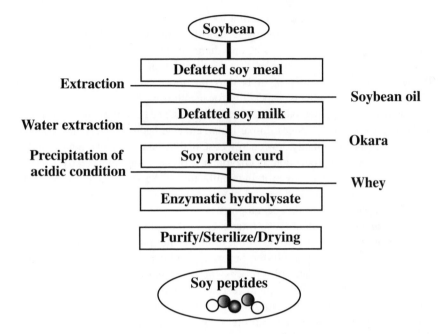

**FIGURE 14.2** Soy peptide manufacturing.

The CODEX description lists partially hydrolyzed protein for peptides and polypeptides used for the food-derived peptides.[11] According to this standard, 3 to 85% of peptide bonds in the proteins must be hydrolyzed. Thus, the quality of the soy peptides in commercial use indicated in Table 14.1 almost meets these two standards.

**TABLE 14.1**
**Characteristics of Commercial Soy Peptides**

| Type | A | B | C | D | E |
|---|---|---|---|---|---|
| Crude protein (%) | 87–92 | 87–91 | 87–91 | 79 | 63–66 |
| 15% TCA solubility (%) | 86–99 | 23–49 | 75–99 | 98–99 | 93–98 |
| Average peptide length (AvPL) | 3–4 | — | 5–6 | 5–6 | 3–4 |
| Free amino acids (%) | 10–14 | < 2 | < 2 | < 2 | 6–8 |
| Additive | — | — | — | Organic acid | — |
| pH (10% solution) | 6.8–6.9 | 6.5–6.8 | 6.3 | 4.5–4.6 | 6.3–6.8 |
| Appearance (solution) | Transparent, ~cloudy | Cloudy | Transparent, ~cloudy | Transparent | Cloudy |

**TABLE 14.2**
**Amino Acid Composition of Soy Peptide**
**Products (g/100 g)**

| Amino Acid | Soy Peptide Products | | SPI |
|---|---|---|---|
| | Type A | Type B | |
| Thr | 3.05 | 3.15 | 3.0 |
| Tyr | 3.11 | 3.21 | 3.2 |
| Phe | 4.15 | 4.23 | 4.5 |
| Cys | 1.04 | 1.03 | 1.1 |
| Met | 1.01 | 1.07 | 1.1 |
| Val | 3.77 | 3.81 | 4.1 |
| Ile | 3.76 | 3.79 | 4.1 |
| Leu | 6.37 | 6.55 | 6.7 |
| Lys | 4.95 | 5.03 | 5.2 |
| Trp | 1.07 | 1.12 | 1.1 |
| His | 2.06 | 2.24 | 2.3 |
| Asx | 9.47 | 9.14 | 9.9 |
| Ser | 4.13 | 4.21 | 4.2 |
| Glx | 16.2 | 16.2 | 17.0 |
| Pro | 4.32 | 4.31 | 4.6 |
| Gly | 3.36 | 3.45 | 3.4 |
| Ala | 3.35 | 3.53 | 3.4 |
| Arg | 6.32 | 6.32 | 6.6 |

Asx, Asp + Asn; Glx, Glu + Gln

## 14.3 HISTORY OF DIETARY PEPTIDES IN NUTRITION

It has been recognized in recent decades that protein is simply absorbed from the small intestine as amino acids as a result of protein hydrolysis by digestive enzymes in the gastrointestinal tract. In the 1960s to 1970s, frontier research revealed the peptide characters in absorption event in the gastrointestinal tract. Craft et al. reported that di- and triglycine peptides are absorbed rapidly compared with the same amount of free glycine in the human intestine.[2] In addition, experiments on absorption of peptide mixtures revealed that blood amino acid patterns reflect well the original composition of peptides. However, in the case of ingested amino acids that have the same composition as the peptide mixture, the blood amino acid pattern does not reflect the original composition of amino acids.[3] Many studies have suggested the existence of a peptide-specific transporter, which was cloned and characterized as an H(+)-coupled transporter of oligopeptides named PepT1. It displays broad substrate specificity, unlike amino acid transporters. These studies clearly show that peptides are absorbed with their primary structures maintained. Thus, it is thought that in the intestine, the peptide transporter constitutes a major mechanism for absorption of the products of protein digestion.[12]

The absorbability of soy peptides has been confirmed by animal experiments. Soy peptides have rapid absorption ratios compared with proteins and amino acid mixtures in normal and several intestinal disorder models.[13–15] Using an intestinal everted sac, Chun et al. studied the influence of the chain length of soy peptides on intestinal absorption.[16] Preliminary clinical trials of soy peptides have also been performed for Crohn's disease[17] and subjects with malnutrition syndromes using oligopeptide rich liquid food,[18] and in many cases soy peptides yielded nutritional improvements.

These results show that the peptide transport system efficiently absorbs peptides in hydrolyzed food protein, and the low osmotic pressure of peptides compared with amino acid mixtures affected subdominantly for good absorbability[19] (Table 14.3 and Table 14.4).

## TABLE 14.3
## Clinical Studies of Soy Peptides[a]

| Experimental Condition | Subjects | Results | References |
|---|---|---|---|
| 10–30 g soy peptides; 20 w, 10 w | 4 malabsorption subjects | Improved nitrogen balance | Komatsu, 1988 |
| 7–10 d 1000-kcal diet treatment with 30-g soy peptides | 11 obese children, age 7–14 | Basal energy expenditure maintained; body weight reduced | Komatsu, 1989 |
| 12-month, 1800-kcal diet with 55-g soy peptides | Crohn's disease patient | Well nourished | Bamba et al., 1989[17] |
| 8-d 1000-kcal diet with 21 g of soy peptides or lactalbumin | 5 obese children, age 5–6 | Basal energy expenditure changed soy peptides; +2.3 kcal, lactalbumin; −4.8 kcal | Komatsu, 1990 |
| 8-d 1000-kcal diet with 21 g of soy peptides or lactalbumin | 23 obese children, age 6–7 | Basal energy expenditure soy peptides > lactalbumin | Komatsu, 1991 |
| 14-d diet with 14 g of soy peptides | 14 healthy subjects | Cholesterol tended to decrease in the higher cholesterol subjects | Chikamochi, 1991 |
| 800-kcal basal diet with 15 g of lactalbumin, soy protein, or soy peptides | 6 males | Diet-induced thermogenesis measured; lactalbumin: 35.9 kcal, soy protein: 34.6 kcal, soy peptide: 44.3 kcal | Komatsu, 1992 |

[a] Type A soy peptides in Table 14.1 used.

**TABLE 14.4**
**Antiobesity Effects Observed in Animals Fed Soy Peptides**

| Subject | Condition Adopted for Feeding | Results Body Fat and Body Weight | Thermogenesis | Brown Adipose Tissue | Others | References |
|---|---|---|---|---|---|---|
| Rats | High-calorie diet used | Decreased | Up-regulated | Increased | Increased UCP | Shimazu, 1992 |
| GTG mice | Peptides force feed | Decreased | — | — | Decreased liver lipids | Niiho, 1993[29] |
| Mice (ddY) | Swimming | Decreased | — | — | Increased muscle | Fushiki, 1996 |
| Rats, mice (diet-induced obese) | Calorie restricted | Decreased | — | — | Maintained body protein | Aoyama, 2000 |
| Rats (diet-induced obese) | Calorie restricted | Decreased | — | — | Maintained body protein | Aoyama, 2001 |
| Mice (diet-induced obese) | Calorie restricted | Decreased | — | — | Increased oxidation of carbohydrates | Ishihara, 2003[38] |

## 14.4 SOY PEPTIDES AS FUNCTIONAL FOODS

The well-known physiological effects of soybean peptides are as follows:

- Relief of muscle fatigue and physical stress
- Antiobesity effect
- Hypoallergenicity
- Hypotensive effect

### 14.4.1 SOY PEPTIDES FOR SPORTS FATIGUE AND STRESS

Degradation of muscle protein following exercise results in muscle protein regeneration. Some evidence suggests that muscle regeneration is a rapid process and that it occurs within about 1 h after exercise.[20–22] However, the blood growth hormone level becomes highest within about 1 h after sleep.[23] Because growth hormone is related to muscle recovery, rapid feeding after exercise and good absorbability of a nitrogen source aid in muscle regeneration, and peptides may be suitable for this. Indeed, many studies have indicated that timing of postexercise nutrient intake is critical for recovery of leg glucose level and protein homeostasis in humans.

Fushiki et al. observed that soy peptides increase muscle mass and suppress body fat accumulation during endurance swimming in mice.[24–26] They suggested that the amino acid composition of soy peptide is a major contributor to those effects. In human experiments, Muramatsu et al. investigated the effect of soy peptide (two times a day, after exercise training and before sleep) intake for 5 months on the performances of judo athletes and observed good effects.[27] Miura et al. examined the effect of soybean peptides and soy protein intake over 6 months on the work capacity of power lifters.[28] The results obtained from both long-term clinical trials were significantly higher in lean body mass (LBM), increasing in several muscle performances and maximal anaerobic power (P max) in soy peptide groups compared with those of control groups. These trails suggested that soy peptides may increase muscle mass and power because of their good amino acid balance and that peptides may be absorbed when growth hormone increases.

Physiological fatigue develops with energy expenditure from muscle, resulting in various biochemical reactions in the body from physical stress, including sports and exercise. Since protein is the dominant constituent of muscle, a nitrogen source is important for maintenance and recovery of muscle.

Niiho et al.[29] examined the pharmacological antifatigue, antiobesity, and hypoglycemia effects of soy peptides (average molecular weight 389) in mice. They found a decrease in movement induced by concussion stress and a larger fatigue recovery rate with soy peptide administration after induced stress than with pretreatment. They also observed that amino acid mixtures with the same peptide amino acid composition did not prevent fatigue. Moreover, they showed the antiobesity effect of soybean peptides in gold thioglucose-induced obese mice.[29]

Nigawa et al. reported that soy protein intake maintained muscle mass and exercise capacity and suppressed the postexercise increase in creatine phospho-kinase activity, a muscle damage marker, compared with casein in rats.[30] In addition, Takenaka et al. reported the effect of soy peptides on paraquat-induced oxidative stress in rats.[31] They demonstrated that intake of either dietary soy protein isolate or soy peptides, but not of an amino acid mixture, reduced paraquat-induced oxidative stress in rats.[31] These findings suggest that the origin and amino acid composition of supplied nitrogen sources play important roles in muscle recovery and stress reduction and that rapid absorbability of peptides may be the hallmark difference between soy protein and soy peptides.

### 14.4.2 OBESITY AND PROTEINS AND PEPTIDES

Obesity is thought to be a basic preclinical status of life-style-related diseases such as hyperlipidemia, diabetes, hypertension, coronary heart disease, and stroke. Various methods are recommended for the treatment of obesity. In general, the first choice for controlling obesity is to reduce energy consumption by reducing food intake and to increase energy expenditure by exercise. Many preliminary studies of dietary treatment for obese subjects have suggested another possibility.[32] Intake of protein produces significantly greater postprandial energy expenditure than intake of the same number of calories from glucose and fat during in humans. Several trials have been performed for obesity treatment with a high-protein diet to determine whether protein consumption will result in higher energy expenditure. Baba et al. found that including soy protein in a high-protein diet affected body fat content, though body protein content was not different.[33]

Saito[34] reported effects of dietary soy peptides (average peptide length: 3 to 4 amino acids) on energy expenditure with special reference to the thermogenic activity of brown adipose tissue (BAT). The energy efficiency of their soy peptide diet group decreased, suggesting an increase in energy expenditure, and GDP binding to BAT mitochondria increased in this group.[34] They also performed a soy peptide diet experiment with gold-thioglucose-induced obese mice and observed that the soy peptide diet group had higher BAT levels.[35]

Komatsu and Yamamoto performed a series of clinical and animal experiments on soybean protein and peptides with obese subjects (Table 14.3). Their experiments revealed that soy peptide intake helps maintain (or increase) body protein and basal energy expenditure and may stimulate lipid metabolism. They also compared the soy peptide with another nitrogen source, lactalbu-min, and observed the advantage of the soy peptides in basal energy expenditure maintenance.[36]

We conducted dietary treatment with genetic and food-induced obese animals to test the soybean-derived protein sources. First, using food-induced obese rats and genetically obese mice, body fat-reducing effects of soy protein and soy peptides groups were observed. The soy peptide group tended to have lower levels than the soy protein group in several parameters, such as body weight, fat percentage, plasma lipids, and plasma glucose.[37] Our subsequent findings showed that regardless of the origin of the protein, peptides show a tendency to increase more than the original protein.

Postprandial thermogenesis is important for energy metabolism and thought to contribute to antiobesity effects. Recently, Ishihara et al.[38] compared the effects of dietary proteins on the oxidation of dietary carbohydrate and lipids in Type II diabetic mice. When diabetic mice were fed a restricted diet, postprandial energy expenditure was higher in the soy peptide group than in the casein group. The researchers suggested that the difference in energy expenditure between the groups was due to an increase in postprandial carbohydrate oxidation in addition to lipid oxidation.[38]

Obesity is thought to be the cause of the "metabolic syndrome," which includes hyperlipidemia, hypertension, diabetes, and so on. The antiobesity effect of soybean peptides is thought to involve the increase of lipid and carbohydrate metabolism. However, because the soybean peptides used by researchers are a mixture of hydrolysates of soybean protein, is possible that a particular peptide or the amino acid composition of the peptides causes the effect. Further examination will be necessary to determine this (Table 14.4).

### 14.4.3 ALLERGENS AND PEPTIDES

Food-derived allergic responses are a serious problem for hypersensitive people and food manufacturers. In the case of soybean, several antigenic substances have been reported, and Gly m Bd30kd is the most severe allergen.[39] Samoto et al. developed an industrial process for removing allergens.[40] This process can remove over 99% of the allergenic protein; however, the clinical validity of a low allergen product has not been proved. Another possibility is removal or degradation of antigenic sites belonging to primary sequences of the proteins. Enzymatic hydrolysis is the predominant method for reducing the allergenicity of a protein. Some peptides have been developed and tested as hypoallergenic foods.[41] Baba et al., reported a long-term clinical trial for allergic patients using a soy peptide beverage.[42] The trial included 11 atopic dermatitis patients, and within 6 months to 1 year, 9 of the 11 subjects had finished the ingestion test with some nutritional improvement and without any avoidance to diet treatment.Though further examination is necessary, this report suggests that soy peptides may be useful as hypoallergenic foods.

### 14.4.4 HYPOTENSIVE EFFECT

Hypertension is a major life-style disease. The renin–angiotensin system plays a dominant role in the regulation of blood pressure, so angiotensin-converting enzyme (ACE) inhibitory activity was chosen for the hypotension factor search study. Since the late 1980s, much attention has been given to the generation of hypotensive active peptides derived from food proteins. ACE inhibitory peptides were discovered and developed from food proteins including casein, sardine muscle, and dried bonito.[44–46] Kawamura indicated that hydrolyzed soy protein has a hypotensive effect *in vitro*.[47] Tadasa et al. also indicated that the appearance of ACE inhibitory activity with soy protein hydrolysis is dependent on the pH specificity of the enzyme used.[48] In animal experiments using the spontaneously hypertensive rat (SHR) model, Kawamura[49] and Wu et al.[50] also showed that soy protein and its hydrolysates, respectively, have antihypertensive activity, though they did not identify the active peptide (average molecular weight, under 1000; average peptide length, 2 to 8).

Recently, oligopeptides from Korean soybean paste and tofuyo, a fermented soybean food, were identified that have ACE inhibitory activity,[51] but their effects on blood pressure have not been confirmed clinically. Sour milk containing ACE-inhibitory active oligopeptides showed a hypotensive effect on patients with high blood pressure and confirmed the existence of the active oligopeptide in the blood vessels of SHRs, which is absorbed intrabody. Thus, sour milk foods contain the active peptides approved as food for specific health use (FOSHU).[52]

## 14.5  RECENT TOPICS IN STRESS AND BRAIN FUNCTION

Some reports have related soy and brain functions such as cognition. Researchers have paid attention to the role endogenous estrogen plays in neuron mainte-nance, especially in postmenopausal women, and soy isoflavone is known to have weak estrogenic activity.[53] However, several amino acids and their metab-olites are the mediators of physiological events such as pain and excitement. Unique and interesting studies have recently been started using soy peptides. Hatakeyama et al. evaluated the modulating effects of soy protein isolate and soy peptides on human brain functions by cerebral blood flow examination and electroencephalography.[54] They found significant increases in the amplitudes of theta, alpha-2, and beta-1 frequency bands after ingestion of soy peptides compared with a placebo group. Further research is needed to confirm these effects physiologically as well as to identify the active components contained in soy products.

## 14.6  CONCLUSIONS

So peptides that are mixture of soy protein hydrolysates contain active compo-nents that in most cases are not defined. However, soy peptides have the ability to prevent some life-style diseases such as obesity, hypertension, and physical stress, in addition to having nutritional advantages. The food market for, and scientific interest in, functionally active food components have grown rapidly in recent years. Soy peptides are a suitable food material for these fields, and may have various functions. It is important to conduct more research on these com-ponents. In particular, the physiological and psychological effects of peptides will become main targets of research.

## REFERENCES

1. Newey, H. and Smyth, D.H., Cellular mechanisms in intestinal transfer of amino acids, *J. Physiol.,* 164, 527–551, 1962.
2. Craft, I.L., Geddes, D., Hyde, C.W., Wise, I.J., and Matthews, D.M., Absorption and malabsorption of glycine and glycine peptides in man, *Gut,* 9, 425–437, 1968.
3. Silk, D.B.A., Marrs, T.C., Addison, J.M., Burston, D., Clark, M.L., and Matthews, D.M., Absorption of amino acids from an amino acid mixture simulating casein and a tryptic hydrolysate of casein in man, *Clin. Sci. Mol. Med.,* 45, 715–719, 1973.
4. Webb, K.E., Jr., Intestinal absorption of protein hydrolysis products: a review, *J. Anim. Sci.,* 68(9), 3011–3022, 1990.
5. Erdman, J.W., Jr., Soy protein and cardiovascular disease: a statement for health-care professionals from the nutrition committee of the AHA, *Circulation,* 102, 2555–2559, 2000.
6. Messina, M., Modern applications for an ancient bean: soybeans and the prevention and treatment of chronic disease, *J. Nutr.,* 125(3S), 567–569, 1995.
7. Huff, M.W., Hamilton, R.M.G., and Carroll, R.R., Plasma cholesterol levels in rabbits fed low fat, cholesterol-free, semipurified diets: effects of dietary proteins, protein hydrolysates and amino acid mixtures, *Atherosclerosis,* 28, 187–195, 1977.
8. Yashiro, A., Oda, S., and Sugano, M., Hypercholesterolemic effect of soybean protein in rats and mice after peptic digestion, *J. Nutr.,* 115(10), 1325–1336, 1985.
9. Matoba, T., Hayashi, R., and Hata, T., Isolation of bitter peptides from tryptic hydrolysate of casein and their chemical structure, *Agric. Biol. Chem.,* 34(8), 1235–1243, 1970.
10. Pedersen, B., Removing bitterness from protein hydrolysates, *Food Technol.,* 48(10), 96–99, 1994.
11. Partially hydrolyzed proteins, in *Food Chemicals Codex,* 4th ed., National Academy Press, Washington, DC, 1996, pp. 282–283.
12. Fei, Y.J., Kanai, Y., Nussberger, S., Ganapathy, V., Leibach, F.H., Romero, M.F., Singh, S.K., Boron, W.F., and Hediger, M.A., Expression cloning of a mammalian proton-coupled oligopeptide transporter, *Nature,* 368(7), 563–566, 1994.
13. Nakabou, Y., Utsunomiya, R., Suzuki, T., Watanabe, M., Hagihira, H., Matsuo, T., Kimoto, M., and Ohshima, Y., Demineralization of enzymic hydrolysate of SPI (Hinute PM) and absorption of desalted preparation in rat small intestine *in vitro, Nutr. Sci. Soy Protein Jpn.,* 10(1), 76–80, 1989.
14. Ihara, M., Miyanomae, T., Kido, Y., and Kishi, K., Effects of soy protein peptide on nutritional state and small intestinal function in short-bowel and methotrexate treated rats, *Nutr. Sci. Soy Protein Jpn.,* 11(1), 87–94, 1990.
15. Nakabou, Y., Suzuki, Y., Okamoto, M., Kuzuhara, Y., and Hagihira, H., Nutritional evaluation of oligopeptide mixture, prepared from soy protein isolate (SPI) in rats resected two-thirds of the small intestine, *Nutr. Sci. Soy Protein Jpn.,* 11(1), 108–112, 1990.
16. Chun, H., Sasaki, M., Fujiyama, Y., and Bamba, T., Effect of peptide chain length on absorption and intact transport of hydrolyzed soybean peptide in rat intestinal everted sac, *J. Clin. Biochem. Nutr.,* 21, 131–140, 1996.
17. Bamba, T., Chikamochi, N., Fuse, K., and Hosoda, T., Usefulness of soy peptide in the patients with Crohn's disease, *Nutr. Sci. Soy Protein Jpn.,* 10(1), 117–121, 1989.

18. Bamba, T., Obata, H., Nishimura, M., Hosoda, T., Chikamochi, N., and Hosono, S., Effect of peptides on brush border transporters in rat intestine and clinical usefulness of soy peptides in the patients with malabsorption syndrome, *Nutr. Sci. Soy Protein Jpn.,* 11(1), 113–119, 1990.

19. Aoyama, T., Fukui, K., and Yamamoto, T., Effect of various forms of force-fed nitrogen sources on gastric transit time in rats, *J. Jpn. Soc. Nutr. Food Sci.,* 49(1), 46–51, 1996.

20. Levenhagen, D.K., Gresham, J.D., Carlson, M.G., Maron, D.J., Borel, M.J., and Flakoll, P.J., Postexercise nutrient intake timing in humans is critical to recovery of leg glucose and protein homeostasis, *Am. J. Physiol. Endocrinol. Metab.,* 280, E982–E993, 2001.

21. Doi, T., Matsuo, T., Sugawara, M., Matsumoto, K., Minehira, K., Hamada, K., Okamura, K., and Suzuki, M., New approach for weight reduction by a combination of diet, light resistance exercise and the timing of ingesting a protein supplement, *Asia Pac. J. Clin. Nutr.,* 10(3), 226–232, 2001.

22. Plotnick, L.P., Thompson, R.G., Kowarski, A., de Lacerda, L., Migeon, C.J., and Blizzard, R.M., Circadian variation of integrated concentration of growth hormone in children and adults, *J. Clin. Endocrinol. Metab.,* 40(2), 240–247, 1975.

23. Wolfe, R.R., Protein supplements and exercise, *Am. J. Clin. Nutr.,* 72, 551S–557S, 2000.

24. Fushiki, T., Matsumoto, K., Uohashi, R., and Inoue, K., Effects of the soybean peptide on an increase in muscle mass during training in mice, *Nutr. Sci. Soy Protein Jpn.,* 15, 51–56, 1994.

25. Fushiki, T., Ishihara, K., Matsumoto, K., Uohashi, R., and Inoue, K., Effects of the soybean peptide on an increase in muscle mass during training in mice, *Nutr. Sci. Soy Protein Jpn.,* 16, 1–3, 1995.

26. Ishihara, K., Matsumoto, K., Uohashi, R., Fushiki, T., Effects of the soybean peptide on suppression of body fat accumulation during endurance swimming in mice, *Nutr. Sci. Soy Protein Jpn.,* 17, 94–97, 1996.

27. Muramatsu, S., Shunsuke Yamazaki, S., Hattori, Y., and Hattori, Y., Effect of soy-peptide intake for long term on exercise performances of judo athletes, *Chiba J. Phys. Edu.,* (18), 41–48, 1994.

28. Miura, K., Takenaka, S., Okuno, M., and Kohara, N., Effect of soy-bean peptide and soy-bean isolated protein intake over 6 months on work capacity of power-lifters, *Bull. Fac. Edu. Okayama Univ.,* 100, 139–150, 1995.

29. Niiho, Y., Yamazaki, T., Hosono, T., Nakajima, Y., Ishizaki, M., and Kurashige, T., Pharmacological studies on small peptide fraction derived from soybean: the effects of small peptide fraction derived from soybean on fatigue, obesity and glycemia in mice, *J. Pharmaceut. Soc. Jpn.,* 113(4), 334–342, 1993.

30. Nigawa, K., Yamamoto, T., Yamaguchi, A., Ohno, T., Nanba, K., Kido, Y., Rokutan, K., and Kishi, K., Effect of soy protein isolate on free radical-induced muscle injury under exercise, *Nutr. Sci. Soy Protein Jpn.,* 15, 45–50, 1994.

31. Takenaka, A., Annaka, H., Kimura, Y., Aoki, H., and Igarashi K., Reduction of paraquat-induced oxidative stress in rats by dietary soy peptide, *Biosci. Biotechnol. Biochem.,* 67(2), 278–283, 2003.

32. Welle, S., Lilavivat, U., and Campbell, R.G., Thermic effect of feeding in man: increased plasma norepinephrine levels following glucose but not protein or fat consumption, *Metabolism,* 30(10), 953–958, 1981.

33. Baba, N., Radwan, H., and Van Itallie, T., Effects of casein versus soyprotein diets on body composition and serum lipid levels in adult rats, *Nutr. Res.*, 12(2), 279–288, 1992.
34. Saito, M., Availability of soy protein peptides for total enteral nutrition, *Nutr. Sci. Soy Protein Jpn.*, 10(1), 81–83, 1989.
35. Saito, M., Effects of soy peptides on energy metabolism in obese animals, *Nutr. Sci. Soy Protein Jpn.*, 12(1), 91–94, 1991.
36. Aoyama, T., Fukui, K., Nakamori, T., Hashimoto, Y., Yamamoto, T., Takamatsu, K., and Sugano, M., Effect of soy and milk whey protein isolates and their hydrolysates on weight reduction in genetically obese mice, *Biosci. Biotechnol. Biochem.*, 64(12), 2594–2600, 2000.
37. Aoyama, T., Fukui, K., Takamatsu, K., Hashimoto, Y., and Yamamoto, T., Soy protein isolate and its hydrolysate reduce body fat of dietary obese rats and genetically obese mice (yellow KK), *Nutrition*, 16, 349–354, 2000.
38. Ishihara, K., Oyaizu, S., Fukuchi, Y., Mizunoya, W., Segawa, K., Takahashi, M., Mita, Y., Fukuya, Y., Fushiki, T., and Yasumoto, K.A., Soybean peptide isolate diet promotes postprandial carbohydrate oxidation and energy expenditure in type II diabetic mice, *J. Nutr.*, 133(3), 752–757, 2003.
39. Ogawa, T., Tsuji, H., Bando, N., Kitamura, K., Zhu, Y.-L., Hirano, H., and Nisikawa, K., Identification of the soybean allergenic protein, Gly m Bd 30K, with the soybean seed 34-kDa oil-body-associated protein, *Biosci. Biotechnol. Biochem.*, 57(6), 1030–1033, 1993.
40. Samoto, M., Fukuda, Y., Takahashi, K., Tabuchi, K., Hiemori, M., Tuji, H., Ogawa, T., and Kawamura, Y., Substantially complete removal of three major allergenic soybean proteins (Gly m Bd 30K, Gly m Bd 28K, and the a-subunits of conglycinin) from soy protein by using a mutant soybean, Tohoku 124, *Biosci. Biotechnol. Biochem.*, 61(12), 2148–2150, 1997.
41. Suzanne, W.J., Terheggen-Lagro, I., Khouw, M.S.L., Schaafsma, A., and Wauters, E.A.K., Safety of a new extensively hydrolysed formula in children with cow's milk protein allergy: a double blind crossover study, *BMC Pediatr.*, 21(5), 929–935, 2000.
42. Iwasaki, E., Maba, M., Kaminogawa, S., Enomoto, J., Totsuka, M., Konishi, N., and Kimoto, M., Allergic and nutritional evaluation of a drink with soy protein hydrolysate in food allergic children, *Jpn. Soc. Ped. Allerg. Clin. Immunol.*, 9(1), 23–31, 1995.
43. Maruyama, S., Mitachi, H., Tanaka, H., Tomizuka, N., and Suzuki, H., Studies on the active site and antihypertensive activity of angiotensin I-converting enzyme inhibitors derived from casein, *Agric. Biol. Chem.*, 56(6), 1581–1586, 1987.
44. Matsui, T., Matsufuji, H., Seki, E., Osajima, K., Nakashima, M., and Osajima, Y., Inhibition of angiotensin I-coverting enzyme by bacillus licheniformis alkaline protease hydrolyzates derived from sardine muscle, *Biosci. Biotechnol. Biochem.*, 57(6), 922–925, 1993.
45. Fujii, M., Matsumura, N., Mito, K., Shimizu, T., Kuwahara, M., Sugano, S., and Karaki, H., Antihypertensive effects of peptides in autolysate of bonito bowels on spontaneously hypertensive rats, *Biosci. Biotechnol. Biochem.*, 57(12), 2186–2188, 1993.
46. Kawamura, Y., Healthy technology for soybeans 10: peptide inhibitor fro angiotensin converting enzyme of soybean protein and its antihypertensive effect, *Food Ind.*, 40(12), 73–82, 1997.

47. Wu, J. and Ding, X., Hypotensive and physiological effect of angiotensin converting enzyme inhibitory peptides derived from soy protein on spontaneously hypertensive rats, *J. Agric. Food Chem.,* 49(1), 501–506, 2001.
48. Tadasa, K., Murakami, Y., and Kayahara, H., Activities of angiotensin-I converting enzyme inhibition in proteolytic hydrolyzate of food proteins: in view of development of physiologically functional peptides, *J. Fac. Agric. Shinshu Univ.,* 26(1–2), 13–18, 1990.
49. Shin, Z.I., Yu, R., Park, S.A., Chung, D.K., Ahn, C.W., Nam, H.S., Kim, K.S., and Lee, H.J., His-His-Leu, an angiotensin I converting enzyme inhibitory peptide derived from Korean soybean paste, exerts antihypertensive activity *in vivo, J. Agric. Food Chem.,* 49(6), 3004–3009, 2001.
50. Kuba, M., Tanaka, K., Tawata, S., Takeda, Y., and Yasuda, M., Angiotensin I-converting enzyme inhibitory peptides isolated from tofuyo fermented soybean food, *Biosci. Biotechnol. Biochem.,* 67(6), 1278–1283, 2003.
51. Masuda, O., Nakamura, Y., and Takano, T., Antihypertensive peptides are present in aorta after oral administration of sour milk containing these peptides to spontaneously hypertensive rats, *J. Nutr.,* 126, 3063–3068, 1996.
52. Kritz-Silverstein, D., Von Muhlen, D., Barrett-Connor E., and Bressel M.A., Isoflavones and cognitive function in older women: the soy and postmenopausal health in aging (SOPHIA) study, *Menopause,* 10(3), 196–202, 2002.
53. Hatakeyama, E., Yamaguchi, F., Muramoto, K., Ito, G., Motohashi, Y., and Higuchi, S., Modulating effects of soy protein isolate and soy protein hydrolysate on human brain function, *Nutr. Sci. Soy Protein Jpn.,* 6, 147–152, 2003.

# 15 Fermented Soybean Components and Disease Prevention

*Hiroyuki Sumi and Chieko Yatagai*

## CONTENTS

## 15.1 INTRODUCTION

Among the traditional Japanese foods with a history of more than 1000 years, miso (soybean paste), shoyu (soy sauce), and natto, which are all produced from soybeans, have come to be mass-produced in modern factories. Based on numerous results of epidemiological research, the effects (functional activity) of these foods made from fermented soybeans have lately been the focus of renewed interest from the viewpoint of preventive medicine. However, not much has been revealed about the substances that make up the functional components of these foods. Soybeans are very rich in nutrition, but the fermented foods mentioned above are created as a result of the changes brought about by the modification process thanks to microorganisms, or of additional substances not contained in the original soybeans. The food that has recently drawn the attention of the public, in particular, is natto, because it contains unique components related to the prevention of many illnesses and disorders that are closely linked with modern life-styles and habits. What follows is a summary of the aspects of these fermented soybean foods that contribute to improving and maintaining our health, chiefly focusing on those aspects for which the functional components have now clearly been identified.

## 15.2  NATTO

Natto, a food with sticky threads, is representative of the so-called salt-free fermented soybean foods produced by the fermentation of boiled or steamed soybeans using *Bacillus subtilis natto*. Natto was introduced overseas as "vegetable cheese natto" by Dr. Yabe in 1894,[1] but its history can be traced back to ancient times, with written records referring to natto remaining from around 600 A.D. in Japan. As described in *Honcho Shokkan*, a food dictionary published during the Edo period (1603 to 1867), natto as "a food with detoxification effects that stimulates one's appetite" is a nutritious fermented food that is highly effective for dealing with intestinal troubles and attenuating viruses and bacteria.[2] It seems that natto played a valuable part in the traditional treatment of patients based on diet and medicine in the days when vitamin pills and cold medicine were not easily accessible. Many of the medicinal benefits of natto were passed down by oral tradition, as follows: is effective for curing colds, prevents getting sick from excessive drinking and a hangover, is effective for stiff shoulders, brings recovery from fatigue or the effects of summer heat, achieves an improvement in liver functions, is effective for angular stomatitis and tuberculosis, is helpful in making the heart and blood vessels stronger, is effective for diarrhea, is helpful in maintaining smooth skin, etc.[2,3] Also, because of its strong antibacterial activity, natto was used by the Japanese army and navy in World War II for the treatment of trichophytosis[4] and the prevention and treatment of cholera, typhoid, and dysentery.[5-7]

### 15.2.1  ANTIBACTERIAL ACTIVITY OF NATTO
####           AND NATTO BACILLUS

One of the antibacterial components of natto that has been identified as a chemical substance is dipicolinic acid (2,6-pyridinedicarboxylic acid), which was discovered by Udo[8] in Japan in 1936. Dipicolinic acid is known not only for its antibacterial effects but also for its effectiveness in the protection from radioactivity. Recently it has also drawn attention for its apoptosis effects against acute leukemia cells.

## TABLE 15.1
## Dipicolic Acid in Natto and *Bacillus subtilis* Natto

| Sample | Sample Weight (g) | Yield (mg) | Content per 100 g (mg) |
|---|---|---|---|
| **Natto Sold on the Market** | | | |
| Kokin (antibacterial) natto | 56.2 | 27.10 | 48.22 |
| Yuki hyakubai (organic) natto | 52.3 | 7.36 | 14.07 |
| Okame natto | 52.1 | 6.08 | 11.67 |
| Maboroshi-no natto | 56.1 | 3.43 | 6.12 |
| Shiso nori natto | 48.1 | 3.80 | 7.91 |
| KSD-1 natto[a] | 20.0 | 17.45 | 87.25 |
| Kokin (antibacterial) natto (not heat-treated) | 62.1 | 4.12 | 6.64 |
| **Prepared Natto** | | | |
| Miyagino-kin bacillus | 37.8 | 6.49 | 17.18 |
| Naruse-kin bacillus | 36.7 | 13.00 | 35.45 |
| Takahashi-kin bacillus | 36.8 | 7.84 | 21.30 |
| Yunnan bacillus SL-001 | 43.4 | 10.02 | 23.07 |
| Product of the fermentation of *Bacillus subtilis* IAM12118 | 34.7 | 0.59 | 1.70 |
| ***B. subtilis* Natto** | | | |
| Nitto-kin bacillus L001 | 1.0 | 12.87 | 1287.00 |
| Nitto-kin bacillus L002 | 1.0 | 17.72 | 1772.00 |
| Meguro-kin bacillus BN-(1)[a] | 1.0 | 5.23 | 523.00 |
| Meguro-kin bacillus BN-(2)[a] | 1.0 | 24.09 | 2409.00 |
| Meguro-kin bacillus BN-(3) (solid state culture)[a] | 1.0 | 36.44 | 3644.00 |
| *Bacillus subtilis* IAM12118 | 1.0 | 1.98 | 198.00 |

[a] Unlike other samples, these are measurement values for a dry product.

*Source:* Sumi, H. and Ohsugi, T., *Nippon Nogei kagaku Kaishi*, 73, 1289–1291, 1999 (in Japanese). With permission.

Table 15.1 shows the results of our tests regarding the concentration of dipicolinic acid in various types of natto sold in Japan and in natto bacillus.[9] The tests revealed that natto contains a substantial amount of dipicolinic acid on average, with $17.60 \pm 17.40$ mg contained per 100 g, and that the content is much higher in natto bacteria, at 1772 to 3644 mg per 100 g, accounting for 2 to 4% of the dry weight of the bacteria. With wide-ranging antibacterial functions, dipicolinic acid is effective against *Aspergillus oryzae, Penicillium* (blue mold), and pathogenic colon bacillus, *Escherichia coli O-157*, as well as against yeasts,[9] which is believed to be related to the traditional prohibition against bringing natto to sake brewing facilities.

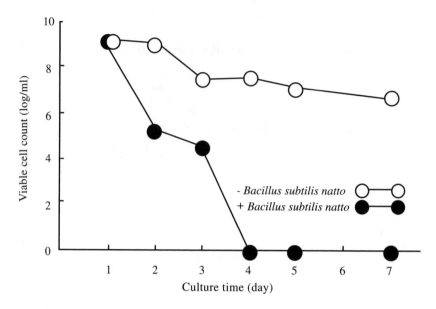

**FIGURE 15.1** The effects on *O-157* as a result of the addition of natto bacillus. This figure shows the growth-inhibiting effects of *O-157* by using $10^6$ cells/ml of *B. subtilis natto*. (From Sumi, H., *Bio Ind.*, 14, 47–50, 1997. With permission.)

Research on natto bacillus has been conducted from a long time ago for the prevention and treatment of infectious diseases such as dysentery and paratyphoid, with the Japanese navy playing a central role. Figure 15.1 shows the results of tests using the mixed culture with *O-157*, from which it is clear that *B. subtilis natto* has strong antibacterial effects.[10] The dipicolinic acid produced by *B. subtilis natto* is soluble in water and thin acetic acid but it is nearly insoluble in alcohol; it has been found, however, that the alcohol-soluble fractions of the fermented products of *B. subtilis natto* contain a strong anti–*Helicobacter pylori* activity[11] (Figure 15.2).

## 15.2.2 FIBRINOLYTIC ENZYME SUBSTANCES CONTAINED IN NATTO

In research conducted on more than 200 types of foods, natto was the only food in which fibrinolytic enzymes were discovered, and this enzyme was named nattokinase.[12] Nattokinase is not contained in the soybean itself; it is produced only as a result of the effects of the *B. subtilis natto* on soybeans. As shown in the photograph in Figure 15.3, natto has very strong fibrinolytic activity (the ability to melt thrombus), which for approximately 100 g of the natto sold (about two packages) is equivalent to about one dose of urokinase (200,000 International Units [IUs]), a therapeutic agent that is clinically administered to patients in critical conditions.

Figure 15.4 shows the amino acid sequence of nattokinase that was determined after the purification process from natto; this is a simple protein without any S-S band, composed of 275 amino acids.[13] As a protease enzyme with a

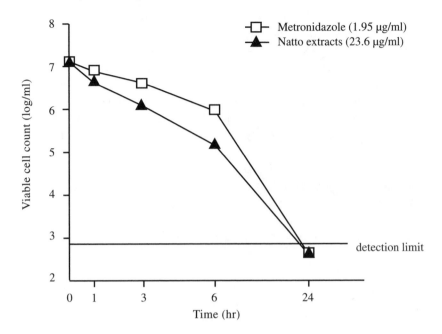

**FIGURE 15.2** The effects on *H. pylori* (Sydney strain) resulting from the addition of natto extracts. (From Sumi, H., *Toyo Sinpo*, 1442, 5, 2002. With permission.)

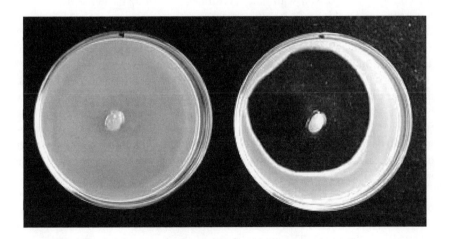

**FIGURE 15.3** Fibrinolytic activity of natto. A piece of natto commonly sold on the market was placed in a petri dish with artificial thrombus. The photographs show the conditions before incubation at 37°C (left) and after 18 h (right). It can be clearly seen that the areas around the natto have dissolved. (From Sumi, H. et al., *Experientia*, 43, 1110–1111, 1987. With permission.)

```
                                       10                                       20
H2N-Ala-Gln-Ser-Val-Pro-Tyr-Gly-Ile-Ser-Gln-Ile-Lys-Ala-Pro-Ala-Leu-His-Ser-Gln-Gly-Tyr-
                                  30    *                               40
Thr-Gly-Ser-Asn-Val-Lys-Val-Ala-Val-Ile-Asp-Ser-Gly-Ile-Asp-Ser-Ser-His-Pro-Asp-Leu-Asn-
                            50                              60               *
Val-Arg-Gly-Gly-Ala-Ser-Phe-Val-Pro-Ser-Glu-Thr-Asn-Pro-Tyr-Gln-Asp-Gly-Ser-Ser-His-Gly-
                    70                                      80
Thr-His-Val-Ala-Gly-Thr-Ile-Ala-Ala-Leu-Asn-Asn-Ser-Ile-Gly-Val-Leu-Gly-Val-Ala-Pro-Ser-
        90                                     100
Ala-Ser-Leu-Tyr-Ala-Val-Lys-Val-Leu-Asp-Ser-Thr-Gly-Ser-Gly-Gln-Tyr-Ser-Trp-Ile-Ile-Asn-
110                                     120                                     130
Gly-Ile-Glu-Trp-Ala-Ile-Ser-Asn-Asn-Met-Asp-Val-Ile-Asn-Met-Ser-Leu-Gly-Gly-Pro-Thr-Gly-
                                    140                                     150
Ser-Thr-Ala-Leu-Lys-Thr-Val-Val-Asp-Lys-Ala-Val-Ser-Ser-Gly-Ile-Val-Val-Ala-Ala-Ala-Ala-
                         160                                   170
Gly-Asn-Glu-Gly-Ser-Ser-Gly-Ser-Thr-Ser-Thr-Val-Gly-Thr-Pro-Ala-Lys-Tyr-Pro-Ser-Thr-Ile-
                    180                                     190
Ala-Val-Gly-Ala-Val-Asn-Ser-Ser-Asn-Gln-Arg-Ala-Ser-Phe-Ser-Ser-Val-Gly-Ser-Glu-Leu-Asp-
        200                                     210
Val-Met-Ala-Pro-Gly-Val-Ser-Ile-Gln-Ser-Thr-Leu-Pro-Gly-Gly-Thr-Tyr-Gly-Ala-Tyr-Asn-Gly-
220     *                                  230                                       240
Thr-Ser-Met-Ala-Thr-Pro-His-Val-Ala-Gly-Ala-Ala-Ala-Leu-Ile-Leu-Ser-Lys-His-Pro-Thr-Trp-
                                    250                                     260
Thr-Asn-Ala-Gln-Val-Arg-Asp-Arg-Leu-Glu-Ser-Thr-Ala-Thr-Tyr-Leu-Gly-Asn-Ser-Phe-Tyr-
                                270
Tyr-Gly-Lys-Gly-Leu-Ile-Asn-Val-Gln-Ala-Ala-Ala-Gln-COOH
```

*active site

**FIGURE 15.4** The molecular structure of nattokinase. 275 residue calculated molecular weight: 27,724. This is a serine enzyme with a single polypeptide structure. (From Sumi, H. et al., *Fibrinolysis*, 6, 86, 1992. With permission.)

molecular weight of 27,724 and an isoelectric point (pI) of 8.7 in isoelectric focusing, the most significant characteristic of nattokinase is its high specificity for fibrins in comparison with other substrates.[14,15] Nattokinase has a far lower Km value and a higher $k_{cat}$ value than any other proteases isolated from *B. subtilis*, or plasmin, which is the only fibrinolytic enzyme found in human blood. The effects of nattokinase have also been confirmed in angiograms after its oral administration in animals in which artificial thrombi were created beforehand[14,16] (Figure 15.5). It has been confirmed that nattokinase can be absorbed from the digestive tract[17] and that its effects after oral administration continue for a few hours. In contrast to this persistence of the effects of nattokinase, the active time (half-time) of the fibrinolytic agents used in hospitals (usually urokinase, streptokinase, or tissue-plasminogen) is very short at 4 to 20 minutes once they enter the blood, and these agents are active only during administration through an intravenous drip[16] (Figure 15.6).

In the body of a healthy person, fibrinolytic activators called tissue type plasminogen activator (t-PA) and urokinase type plasminogen activator (u-PA) are produced from the blood vessel walls (vascular endothelial cells) and gradually released into the blood. The concentration of these activators in the blood of a thrombosis patient is smaller. In addition to the direct fibrinolytic effects, it has been confirmed that nattokinase increases the amount of t-PA produced, activating prourokinase to urokinase[18] and, according to recent research, inactivating PAI-1, which is one of the inhibitors for the fibrinolytic enzymes (plasminogen activators) in the blood.[19]

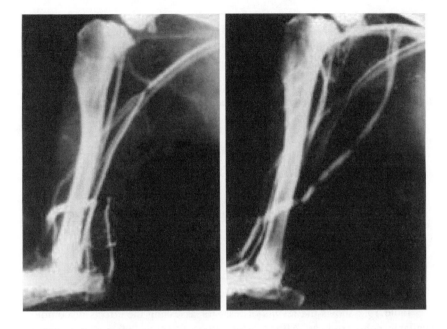

**FIGURE 15.5** Fibrinolytic activity of nattokinase. After the oral administration of four enteric coated capsules (250 mg each) to a 10-kg thrombus model beagle hound, it was confirmed by angiography that a reopening of the blood vessels through thrombolysis occurred within 5 h. (From Sumi, H. et al., *Acta Haematol.*, 84, 139–143, 1990. With permission.)

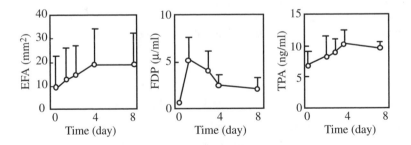

**FIGURE 15.6** Changes in the fibrinolytic parameters in the blood after oral administration of nattokinase to human volunteers. After the oral administration of two enteric coated capsules (650 mg each) to 12 healthy adults (age 21 years to 55 years old), their blood samples were taken at regular intervals. Observations of the samples revealed increases in the euglobulin fibrinolytic activity (EFA), fibrin degradation products (FDPs), and tissue-plasminogen activators (TPAs) in the plasma. (From Sumi, H. et al., *Acta Haematol.*, 84, 139–143, 1990. With permission.)

**TABLE 15.2**
**Fibrinolytic Activity in Human Plasma after Intake of Natto**

| Time after Intake (h) | ELT (h) | | EFA (mm²) | |
|---|---|---|---|---|
| | Intake of Boiled Soybeans | Intake of Natto | Intake of Boiled Soybeans | Intake of Natto |
| 0 | 32.2 ± 6.3 | 31.5 ± 6.2 | 0 | 0 |
| 2 | 33.4 ± 9.0 | 16.4 ± 8.6[a] | 0 | 8.4 ± 5.1[a] |
| 4 | 35.2 ± 4.8 | 16.7 ± 6.6[a] | 0 | 15.2 ± 3.0[a] |
| 8 | 36.1 ± 5.5 | 19.3 ± 12.0[a] | 0 | 5.8 ± 4.1[a] |
| 12 | 34.6 ± 7.3 | 27.4 ± 10.3 | 0 | 1.9 ± 5.2[a] |
| 24 | 34.6 ± 7.7 | 31.9 ± 8.9 | 0.4 ± 0.2 | 0.8 ± 0.6 |

[a] $p < 0.005$

*Source:* Sumi, H., Hamada, H., Nakanishi, H., and Hiratani, H., *Acta Haematol.*, 84, 139–143, 1990. With permission.

Table 15.2 shows the results of tests for assessing the effects of commonly available natto products. After the ingestion of 100 to 200 g of commercially available natto sold by 12 healthy persons, blood samples were taken at regular intervals to measure fibrinolytic activity according to eugloblin lysis time (ELT) and eugloblin fibrinolytic area (EFA). The decrease of ELT and increase of EFA were observed, confirming the increase in fibrinolytic activity during the 2 to 8 h after ingestion. Such phenomena were not observed in the control group, in which the subjects took soybeans that were simply boiled.[16]

Expecting such fibrinolytic activity, the ingestion of natto or the oral administration of nattokinase tablets has recently been used for the treatment of patients suffering from retinal embolism[20] and, lately, the so-called economy-class syndrome[21] and for the prevention of such illnesses and disorders, with good results.

### 15.2.3 DEPRESSOR EFFECTS, CARCINOSTATIC EFFECTS, AND DISSIPATION OF THE EFFECTS OF ALCOHOLIC DRINKS

It is well-known that eating natto results in depressor effects for blood pressure, although the actual substances at work have not yet been identified. Hayashi et al.[22] demonstrated that the intake of alcohol-soluble fractions of natto was effective in bringing down the blood pressures of spontaneously hypertensive rats (SHRs). Figure 15.7 shows the results of the ingestion by adult volunteers of water-soluble fractions of natto commonly sold on the market, with depressor effects observed, particularly in those with the highest blood pressure levels.[23] It was confirmed that the water-soluble fractions of natto also contain nattokinase activity and inhibitor activity against the agglutination of ADP in a human blood platelet[24] (Figure 15.8).

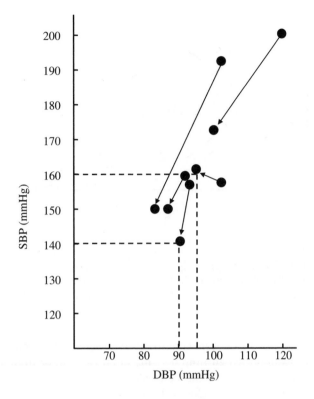

**FIGURE 15.7** The effects of natto extracts on blood pressure. The measurement values after the ingestion of natto extracts equivalent in weight to 200 g are shown. The broken lines show the normal values. (From Maruyama, M. and Sumi, H., in *Basic and Clinical Aspects of Japanese Traditional Food Natto*, Vol. 2, Japan Technology Transfer Association, Tokyo, 1998, pp. 1–3 [in Japanese]. With permission.)

Also well-known are the anticancer effects of *B. subtilis natto*, which were widely reported some time ago in the media. Kameda et al.[25] performed subcutaneous implantation of cancer cells (Ehrlich's carcinoma) in both of the inguinal regions (the base of the feet) of mice, after which natto bacillus was injected into the right inguinal region, and a comparison in the growth of cancer cells was made in the right and left inguinal regions. On day 11 after the implantation of the cancer cells, either no cancer growth was observed in the right inguinal region, or when cancer growth was observed, it was less than half of the growth in the left inguinal region, which was not treated with *B. subtilis natto*. There was also a report of interferons being induced by *B. subtilis natto*.[26]

Natto is also effective in dissipating the effects of alcohol. There were reports that for persons who took a liquid of fermented natto bacillus (100 ml) before drinking 30 to 65 g, in ethanol amount, of whisky, the concentrations of alcohol

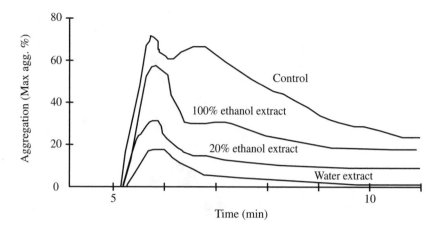

**FIGURE 15.8** The inhibitor activity of platelet aggregation. 5 μl of natto extract was added to 200 μl of human platelet ($220 \times 10^6$/ml), and agglutination was induced using ADP, with the aggregation patterns shown here. The water extract shows the strongest inhibitor activity. (From Sumi, H., Yatagai, C., and Kishimoto, N., *Int. J. Hematol.*, S51, 1996. With permission.)

and aldehyde in their blood were comparatively lowered. The alcohol concentration in their breath decreased from 0.32 mg/l to 0.18 mg/l, or from the level of violation (driving under the influence of alcohol) down to the level of warning according to the Road Traffic Law of Japan.[27]

### 15.2.4 Preventive Effects for Osteoporosis

The rate of occurrence of bone fractures is lower among the Japanese than among Americans or Europeans, in spite of the relatively lower bone-salt density among the Japanese. Some call this phenomenon the "Japanese paradox," and the consumption of natto by the Japanese may be one factor accounting for it. The results of a recent study by Kaneki et al.[28] show that the concentration of vitamin K in the blood is lower among elderly patients who had a bone fracture and that, even though there was virtually no difference in the concentration of vitamin $K_1$ (phylloquinone), which is derived from plants, there were differences in the concentration of vitamin $K_2$ (menaquinone-7), which is derived from microorganisms. The study was based on a group of ten female residents of London who have no habit of eating natto. Another study looked at a group of 49 female residents of Tokyo, of whom more than half eat natto at least twice a week, and another group of 25 female residents of Hiroshima, of whom more than 90% eat natto less than once a week. The $K_2$ concentration of the females in Tokyo was about 15 times higher than the level of the females in London and about five times higher than the level of the females in Hiroshima.

Figure 15.9 shows the results of an analysis of the concentration of menaquinone-7 in the blood of a male student in our laboratory before he ingested

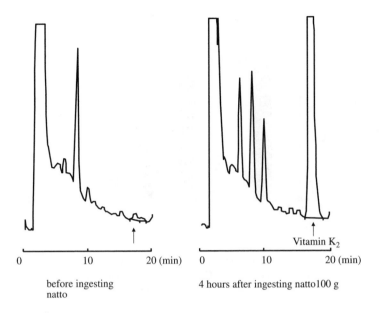

0     10     20 (min)     0     10     20 (min)

before ingesting
natto

Vitamin $K_2$

4 hours after ingesting natto100 g

**FIGURE 15.9** The concentration of vitamin $K_2$ in human blood after the intake of natto. This is the HPLC pattern, with the arrow showing the elution position of MK-7. (From Sumi, H., *J. Home Econ. Jpn.*, 50, 309–312, 1999 [in Japanese]. With permission.)

natto (100 g), and 4 h after ingestion. After ingestion, the peak for menaquinone-7 is substantially higher at approximately 18 min of retention time. The results of another analysis show that, whereas the average value for the concentration of menaquinone-7 in the blood of a healthy person is 1.1 ± 0.5 ng/ml, the amount increases to 11.5 ± 5.0 ng/ml, or about 10 times as much, for those who ate 5 g of natto; to 22.5 ± 5.0 ng/ml, or about 20 times as much, for those who ate 30 g; and to 57.1 ± 7.7 ng/ml, or about 60 times as much, for those who ate 100 g of natto.[29]

The amount of menaquinone-7 produced by *B. subtilis natto* is substantially different according to the bacteria strain used. The characteristics also differ, and most of the menaquinone-7 produced in a culture exists in a water-soluble form that is a complex with a protein, whereas other types of vitamin K are fat soluble; this may account for the characteristic persistence of the effects of menaquinone-7 after ingestion.[30]

Figure 15.10 shows the changes in the concentration of menaquinone-7 in the blood of a healthy person after eating commercially available natto. Figure 15.10 shows that when a person takes 100 g of natto a day for 2 weeks, the concentration of menaquinone-7 in the blood is maintained at significantly high levels, even about 1 week after stopping eating the natto. This is a phenomenon that does not occur as a result of oral administration of purified, free menaquinone-7, so a habit of eating natto, which means an intake of live *B. subtilis natto*, can be described as having "probiotics" effects against osteopathic disorders.[31]

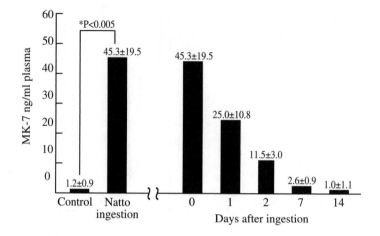

**FIGURE 15.10** Changes in the concentration of menaquinone-7 in plasma after ingestion of natto. (From Sumi, H. and Yatagai, C., *Abstract of XVIIth International Congress on Fibrinolysis and Proteolysis*, 2004, p. 111. With permission.)

The amount of vitamin K deemed necessary for the prevention of osteoporosis according to the U.S. Food and Drug Administration and the Japanese Ministry of Health, Labor, and Welfare is currently about 60 to 80 µg/d for adults;  this is equivalent in content to about 5 to 10 g of natto. Among various types of vitamin $K_2$, menaquinone-7 is found only in natto, with almost no menaquinone-7 contained even in other fermented foods including miso, shoyu (soy sauce), cheese, yogurt, and liquor.

According to the results of the National Survey on Transcervical Fractures recently conducted by the Comprehensive Research Group for the Prevention of Osteoporosis of the Ministry of Health, Labor, and Welfare, the number of transcervical fracture patients was larger in western Japan, where the consumption of natto is generally less. In particular, among females, of which there are more osteoporosis patients than males, a negative correlation was clearly observed between the consumption of natto and the rate of occurrence of transcervical fracture for each prefecture.[32]

Through fermentation with *B. subtilis natto* using such industrial waste as boiled soybean stock, nattokinase and vitamin $K_2$ has been mass-produced. They are also produced through fermentation by *B. subtilis natto* using the residue from the production of tofu (bean curd), called *okara*. In addition to the effects mentioned so far, natto also has fairly strong antioxidant enzymes or active oxygen elimination enzymes (SODs),[33,34] and it has been found through animal tests that, when natto is ingested and the enzymes absorbed by animals, these enzymes lower the lipid peroxide in the animal livers and aortas.[35] The existence of fibrinolysis activators[36] in natto, or the fermented products of *B. subtilis natto*, has also been confirmed, but their bioactive effects and possible applications need to be addressed in the future.

## 15.3 TEMPEH

Tempeh is a salt-free fermented soybean food produced by using the effects on soybeans of microorganisms centering around molds including *Rhizopus*. Tempeh has a history of more than 500 years in Indonesia, originally as a staple food in eastern and central Java.[37] In Indonesia, with its general climate of high temperatures and high humidity, tempeh has drawn attention for its strong antibacterial effects, with its characteristic of not going bad quickly and its effectiveness against dysentery touted through people's experiences over the years.

### 15.3.1 STRONG ANTIBACTERIAL ACTIVITY AND EFFECTIVENESS AGAINST INTESTINAL DISORDERS

Among the Dutch prisoners held in Indonesia during World War II, many of whom were afflicted with dysentery and disorders caused by malnutrition, the digestive organs of those who ate tempeh were relatively healthy, protected by the activity of tempeh. More recently, there have been reports that giving tempeh to patients suffering from chronic diarrhea resulted in improving their digestive and absorbing powers, increasing their weight and the number of hemoglobins in their blood, and enhancing their resistance to infections. Fermentation by the tempeh bacteria results in restraining the generation of gases, so tempeh is acknowledged as being effective for preventing and treating intestinal disorders[38] (Table 15.3). The reason for these effects is believed to be that the antibiotics produced by *Rhizopus* inhibit the propagation of the bacteria that produce intestinal gases. The study conducted by Wang revealed that the tempeh bacteria are particularly effective against Gram-positive bacteria such as *Staphylococcus*.[39]

### 15.3.2 ANTIOXIDANT, ANTIALLERGIC, AND BEAUTY CARE EFFECTS

Although the substances at work have not yet been identified, it is known that eating tempeh leads to lowering cholesterol levels in the blood.[40] Tempeh is also known for its strong antioxidant activity. For example, measurements of the peroxide value (POD) of tempeh powder in storage show a far stronger antioxidation ability than in natto. Recent research has also revealed that a strong SOD activity equivalent to the level in natto is detected in tempeh.[41] The antioxidation activity of tempeh remains effective after eating it. Rilantono et al.[42] gave water extracts of tempeh to rats for 1 week and observed antioxidation, antiinflammatory, and antithrombogenic activities in the rat aortas. Water extracts of tempeh have fibrinolytic enzymes[43,44] different from those in natto, as well as inhibitor activity against the release of histamine from the mast cells of rats.[45] In a study of the antioxidants contained in tempeh, György et al.[46] isolated 6,7,4-trihydroxyisoflavone as a flavonoid, which along with its derivatives were reported

**TABLE 15.3**
**Expired Gas and Intestinal Gas after Intake of Tempeh**

| Sample Food Offered | Amount[b] (g) | Number of Test Subjects | Hydrogen in Expired Gas[a] Peak Emergence Time (Number of Hours after Intake) | Concentration in the Case to the Left (ppm) | Sum Area[c] | Total Passage Amount[d] (ml/6 h) | Intestinal Gas Carbonic Acid Gas (ml/6 h) | Methane (ml/6 h) | Hydrogen (ml/6 h) | Speed of Gas Formation (ml/h) |
|---|---|---|---|---|---|---|---|---|---|---|
| Brand foods (standard foods) | 382 | 28 | 6 ± 2 | 14 ± 9 | 142 ± 61 | 166 ± 79 | 4 ± 3 | 0.4 ± 0.8 | 2 ± 1 | 9 |
| Tempeh | 199 | 6 | 9 ± 1 | 20 ± 5 | 139 ± 36 | 169 ± 50 | 2 ± 2 | 0.4 ± 0.6 | 0.8 ± 0.7 | 10 |
| Heated soybeans (control tempeh) | 200 | 5 | 5 ± 1 | 18 ± 6 | 175 ± 68 | 205 ± 73 | 6 ± 4 | 2 ± 2 | 4 ± 3 | 16 |
| Oxygenated soybeans | 344 | 6 | 8 ± 2 | 24 ± 20 | 190 ± 115 | 245 ± 75 | 9 ± 9 | 2 ± 3 | 6 ± 8 | 22 |
| Nonoxygenated soybeans | 344 | 6 | 7 ± 1 | 28 ± 6 | 226 ± 62 | 217 ± 60 | 7 ± 4 | 4 ± 4 | 9 ± 14 | 18 |

[a] The hydrogen in the expired gas is generated by intestinal bacteria.

[b] The weight of each sample. Tests were conducted after the necessary preparations to ensure that the caloric values and compositions of the test food samples are about the same.

[c] The calculated area according to the measurements performed at 30-min intervals during the period 2.5 h to 10.5 h after intake.

[d] The total passage amount includes air (110 ± 27 ml).

*Source:* Calloway, D.H., Hickey, C.A., and Murrhy, E.L., *J. Food Sci.*, 36, 251–255, 1971. With permission.

**TABLE 15.4**
**Isoflavone Content in Tempeh[a]**

|                      | Daidzin | Genistin | Daidzein | Genistein |
|----------------------|---------|----------|----------|-----------|
| Soybean              | 1630    | 2130     | 92       | 178       |
| Tempeh               | 163     | 268      | 1063     | 2580      |
| Soybean paste (miso) | 480     | 362      | 483      | 1120      |
| Natto                | 1270    | 1185     | 183      | 127       |

[a] Content figured according to HPLC analysis (μg) per 1 g of dried soybeans.

*Source:* Sumi, H., Banba, T., and Yoshida, E., *Nippon Nogei Kagaku Kaishi* 71, 233, 1997 (in Japanese).

to be effective in lowering blood pressure, suppressing pain, inflammation, and allergies, and treating edemas.

Because, unlike natto, molds are mainly used for the production of tempeh, the modification activity for the isoflavones contained in soybeans is strong, resulting in an especially high concentration in tempeh of aglycon types including daidzein and genistein, which are easily absorbed by the human body (Table 15.4). With these aglycons functioning as female hormones, they account for why people can expect beauty care effects and effects against osteoporosis by eating tempeh.

### 15.3.3 Starters for Tempeh and High Nutritional Value

Traditional tempeh as it is consumed in Indonesia is rich in nutritional value, with the fermentation process increasing vitamins $B_{12}$, $B_2$, and $B_6$ and pantothenic acid, nicotinic acid, and folic acid. In particular, the amount of vitamin $B_{12}$ in 100 g of tempeh is enough to satisfy the daily requirement of an adult male. Because of this, tempeh drew attention some time ago as a food that is effective for the prevention of anemia. Subsequent research revealed that the vitamin $B_{12}$ is a product not of *Rhizopus* but of *Pseudomonas* molds, including *Klebsiella pneumoniae* bacteria.[47]

Laghi and usaruh, which are used as the starters for tempeh in Indonesia, contain many types of molds other than *Rhizopus*; the bacteria such as the *Lactobacillus;* and yeast fungi.[48] Thus, tempeh is the product of the combined fermentation of all these microorganisms. It is believed that more wide-ranging types of starters may be used from now on, leading to the development of tempeh with greater functional effects. It has also been reported that the tempeh bacteria (*Rhizopus oligosporus*) are effective in inhibiting the production of carcinogens (aflatoxin) produced by other molds such as *Aspergillus flavus*[49] (Figure 15.11).

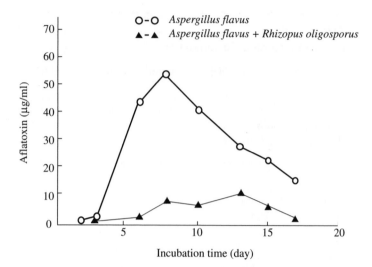

**FIGURE 15.11** The effects of the tempeh bacteria on aflatoxin-producing bacteria. (From Van Veen, A.G., Graham, D.C.W., and Steinkraus, K.H., *Cereal Sci. Today*, 13, 96, 1968. With permission.)

## 15.4 SHOYU (SOY SAUCE)

Shoyu (soy sauce) is a seasoning made from the fermentation of soybeans with malt (koji), which has a strong antibacterial activity used in the fermentation process. The existence and growth of other microbes and bacteria in general are not possible in soy sauce, which has a salt concentration of more than 16%, with the existence and growth of only the so-called shoyu yeast possible in this environment.

### 15.4.1 ANTIBACTERIAL, ANTIOXIDATION, AND DEPRESSOR EFFECTS

Akiba et al.[50] and Masuda et al.[51] showed that soy sauce has bacteriocidal activity against common intestinal pathogenic bacteria such as *E. coli* dysentery bacillus, *Vibrio cholerae, Salmonella typhi,* and the intestinal hemorrhagic *E. coli O-157*. Regarding the antioxidation activity of soy sauce as identified in the methanol extract liquid, Matsuda[52] found that daidzein and genistein, which are the aglycons of isoflavone, are involved in antioxidation activity. Yamaguchi et al.[53] found that the substances related to melanoidine in shoyu are involved in the antioxidation activity.

The most well-known physiological activities of shoyu in the human body are the lowering of blood pressure and gastric secretions. Regarding the depressor effects of shoyu, Kajimoto et al.[54] found that histamine absorbefacient substances are involved in the process, while Kinoshita et al.[55] showed the involvement of angiotensin-converting enzyme (ACE) inhibitor substances such as nicotinamine.

More recently, Nakamura et al.[56] conducted interference tests for 6 weeks for low-salt shoyu and miso, after which their effects on blood pressure were tested, confirming that, in particular, there was a significant lowering of blood pressure in the angiectatic phase.

Regarding the gastric secretion effects of shoyu, tests were conducted for 15 inpatients of the Internal Department of the College of Medicine of Gunma University. The intake of a clear soup (25 ml shoyu + 300 ml hot water) prepared with naturally brewed shoyu resulted in gastric secretions equivalent in amount to those from catsuchi calc caffeine liquid (0.07% caffeine), which was used as the control, but it was reported that the amount of gastric secretions was substantially lower with amino acid–based shoyu produced by chemical decomposition.[57]

### 15.4.2 ANTITUMOR EFFECTS

It has been confirmed that shoyu, along with miso (to be discussed later), is effective for the control of radiation-induced aberrations. Ito and Sato,[58] of the Research Institute for Radiation Biology and Medicine of Hiroshima University, conducted experiments in which radiation ($^{60}$Co) was irradiated on pregnant rats. In cases where shoyu was orally administered beforehand, it was possible to decrease the number of occurrences of abnormalities in the fetuses.

Shoyu has antitumor characteristics on its own, but 4-hydroxy-2-ethyl-5-methyl-3 (2$H$)-furanone (HEMF), which is an aromatic component of shoyu, has a very strong antitumor activity per unit weight, exceeding the level of activity in vitamin C (Table 15.5, Figure 15.12), and has strong inhibitor effects against

**TABLE 15.5**
**Antioxidation Activity of the Aromatic Components of Shoyu (Soy Sauce)[a]**

| Specimen | | Specimen Weight (mg/ml) | Antioxidation Activity per Unit Weight (neq/mg)[b] |
|---|---|---|---|
| Maltol | NA[c] | 0.25 | — |
| Cyclothene | 0.07 | 0.25 | 0.3 |
| HDMF | 3.2 | 0.25 | 12.8 |
| HMF | 2.3 | 0.25 | 9.3 |
| HEMF | 3.8 | 0.25 | 15.2 |
| Aqueous solution with 10,000 ppm of ascorbic acid | 101.0 | 10.0 | 10.1 |

[a] Each value is the average for the results of three tests.

[b] Nanoequivalents of antioxidation activity per 1 ml of specimen (neq/ml).

[c] Nanoequivalents of antioxidation activity per 1 ml of specimen (neq/ml).

*Source:* Nagahara, A. et al., *Cancer Res.*, 52, 1754–1756, 1992. With permission.

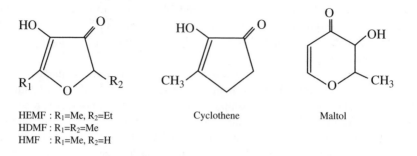

HEMF : R₁=Me, R₂=Et            Cyclothene            Maltol
HDMF : R₁=R₂=Me
HMF  : R₁=Me, R₂=H

**FIGURE 15.12** The aromatic components of shoyu (soy sauce).

carcinogenicity.[59,60] Figure 15.13 and Figure 15.14 show the effects of adding shoyu to mouse feed in relation to the proventriculus cancer of the mice induced by benzopyrene. There was a decrease in the tumor genesis rate for the group of mice fed shoyu; giving 25 ppm of HEMF led to a significant decrease in the

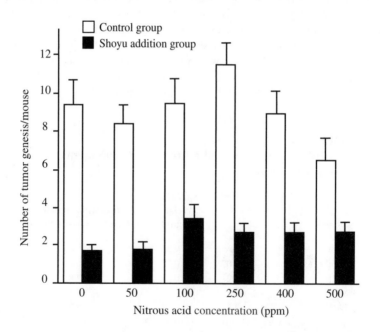

**FIGURE 15.13** Effects of the concentration of nitrous acid on the antitumor activity of shoyu (soy sauce). The figure shows the number of tumors generated per mouse for the group of mice given the feed containing 20% and the number of tumors generated per mouse for the group given feed containing no shoyu. Nitrous acid was added to drinking water, which was freely provided to the mice. The average values are shown as well as the standard deviations. (From Nagahara, A., *Nippon Jozo Kyokaishi*, 88, 859–863, 1993 [in Japanese]. With permission.)

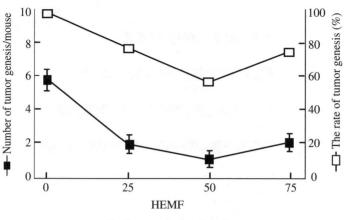

**FIGURE 15.14** The carcinogenesis inhibitor effects of HEMF against proventriculus tumors induced by benzo[a]pyrene. ■, Number of tumors generated/each mouse; □, rate of tumor genesis. The number of tumors generated is shown by M ± SE (*n* = 25 to 27 mice/ group). (From Nagahara, A., *Nippon Jozo Kyokaishi*, 88, 859–863, 1993 [in Japanese]. With permission.)

number and rate of tumor genesis; giving 50 ppm of HEMF inhibited carcinogenesis to a rate of about 60%.

## 15.5 MISO (SOYBEAN PASTE)

Miso (soybean paste) is a traditional fermented food in Japan, with a history going back about 1300 years. With soybeans as the main ingredient, yeast and salt are mixed in during the preparation phase, and then these ingredients are fermented for maturation. Different types of miso include rice miso, barley miso, and bean miso, which, respectively, use rice-derived yeast, barley-derived yeast, and bean-derived yeast. The most well-known functional activity of miso is probably its effectiveness against cancers.

### 15.5.1 Effectiveness of Soybean Paste for Cancer Prevention

At the Japanese Cancer Association convention in October 1981, Takeshi Hirayama, director of the Epidemiology Department of the National Cancer Center Research Institute, announced the results of an epidemiological survey of the relationship between the frequency of eating miso soup and mortality from stomach cancer.[61] In the survey, monitoring was carried out continuously for 13

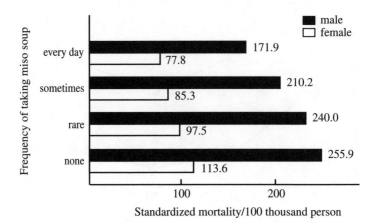

**FIGURE 15.15** Standardized mortality from stomach cancer relative to the level of frequency of eating miso soup. (From Hirayama, T., in *Diet Nutrition and Cancer*, Hayashi, Y., Ed., National Academy of Sciences, Washington, D.C., 1986, pp. 41–53. With permission.)

years from 1966, covering 265,119 adults (122,262 males and 142,857 females) who were 40 years or older and who were selected from among the residents in 29 districts under the jurisdiction of local public health centers in six prefectures across Japan. Their dietary habits along with whether they smoked or drank were investigated at first, and based on these results, the standard age-specific mortality caused by stomach cancer was calculated relevant to the level of frequency of eating miso soup, with the results shown in Figure 15.15. Research on mutagenicity based on the Ames test method using $N$-methyl-$N$-nitrosoguanidine (MNNG) and 3-amino-1,4-dimethyl-5$H$-pyrido[4,3-b]indole (Trip-P1) have shown that the methanol extract liquid from miso has a strong inhibitory activity and that the activity is especially strong in bean miso in comparison to barley miso or rice miso.[62]

Research has also been conducted on the antimutagen activity of miso. Okazaki et al.[63] conducted tests according to the Ames test method by using Trp-P1 and benzo[a]pyrene as the mutagens and identified antimutagen activity in the fatty acid ethyl ester, pyrazine, furfurals, and guaiacol contained in miso.

### 15.5.2 DEPRESSOR EFFECTS

Fermented soybeans generally have ACE inhibitor activity and depressor effects, but there is no correlation between the ACE activity as measured *in vitro* and the actual effects resulting from the intake of fermented soybeans. (ACE activity is again the strongest for bean miso, followed by rice miso and barley miso.) Iwashita et al.[64] orally administered 3.8 g/kg, relative to body weight, of the hydrothermal extracts of miso to SHRs and observed a lowering of their blood pressure by as

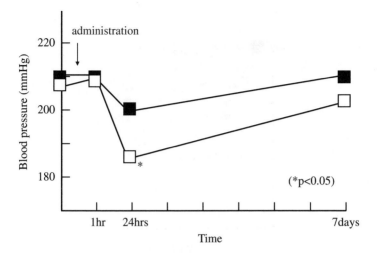

**FIGURE 15.16** Changes in blood pressure by oral administration of miso (soybean paste) extracts. ■, The group given distilled water; □, the group given miso extracts. (From Iwashita, A. et al., *Nippon Nogei Kagaku Kaishi*, 61, 84, 1993 [in Japanese]. With permission.)

much a 25 mmHg in 6 h to 24 h after the oral administration (Figure 15.16), Similar tendencies were also observed when hydrothermal extracts of miso were mixed into the feed to make up 10% of the feed, and the SHRs were allowed to freely eat the feed for 6 weeks.[65]

### 15.5.3 ANTIOXIDATION AND ANTIRADIOACTIVITY EFFECTS

Yoshiki and Okubo[66] found that partial fermentation of natural radical elimination substances occurs in the presence of active enzymes and acetaldehyde and by applying this method, revealed that the components of miso (isoflavone, saponin, etc.) have high levels of enzyme elimination activity. Kato[67] showed that the activity of capturing peroxy radicals is stronger for fully matured miso than for nonmatured miso. Santiago et al.[68] used electron spin resonance (ESR) to show that miso eliminates hydroxy radicals, superoxide radicals, and 1,1-dimethyl-2-picrylhydrazyl radicals. Regarding *in vivo* tests, Horii et al.[69] conducted tests in which desalted miso was added to make up 20% of the feed for rats, and observed a lowering of the serum cholesterol concentration in these rats. In relation to this study, Ide et al.[70] conducted research on the mechanism of the synthesis and decomposition of cholesterol in the liver microsome of rats, reporting that the phenomena are caused by the acceleration of the catabolism of cholesterol into bile acid.

The antiradioactivity effects of miso are also well-known worldwide. In 1986, a massive amount of radioactive material was discharged as a result of

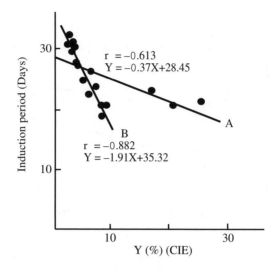

**FIGURE 15.17** Reaction between coloring degree of miso and its antioxidative activity. (A) All samples; (B) samples excluding white-miso. (From Yamaguchi, N., *Nippon Jozo Kyokaishi*, 87, 721–725, 1992 [in Japanese]. With permission.)

the nuclear reactor accident in Chernobyl, Ukraine, in the then-Soviet Union, and miso was distributed to the local residents who were exposed to the radiation. This action was based on testimonies that miso was effective for the aftereffects suffered from the atomic bombs in Hiroshima and Nagasaki.[71] Ito,[72] and Watanabe and Takahashi[73] administered [131]I and [134]Cs as feed to mice in their research on the effectiveness of miso-based feed and reported that, compared with the control group, the residual amount of radioactivity in the blood, kidneys, and muscles was relatively lower. Although the substances at work have not yet been identified, similar tests have been conducted regarding the mortality from X-radiation on the whole body, with reports on the effectiveness of miso for prolonging life.

Figure 15.17 shows the relationship between the depth of the coloring of miso and its antioxidation effects, as reported by Yamaguchi.[74] A correlation coefficient is identified between the depth of coloring and the induction period for all the samples ($r = -0.613$). When the three samples of shiro-miso (whitish miso) with light colors were excluded, there was a further rise in the value of the correlation coefficient. As this value shows, the miso with a deeper coloring has more antioxidation effects. The wide-ranging functional effects of melanoidine, which is the pigmentum nigrum for miso and shoyu, have recently attracted more attention; because the melanoidine content in shoyu, in particular, is very high at 700 to 2120 mg/100 ml, beneficial effects on health can likely be expected from normal daily intake of shoyu. Table 15.6 shows the data compiled from various reports.[75]

**TABLE 15.6**
**Functional Effects of Melanoidine Contained in Shoyu (Soy Sauce) and Miso (Soybean Paste)**

| Functional Effects | Melanoidine | Shoyu (Soy Sauce) | Miso (Soybean Paste) |
|---|---|---|---|
| Effects for preventing liver cancer | Yes | Yes | Yes |
| Effects for lowering cholesterol levels | Yes | — | Yes |
| Antimutagen effects | Yes | — | Yes |
| Antioxidation effects | Yes | Yes | Yes |
| Effects for radical elimination | Yes | Yes | Yes |
| Effects for inhibiting angiotensin conversion enzymes | Yes | Yes | Yes |
| Trypsin inhibition effects | Yes | Slightly yes | Slightly yes |
| Amylase inhibition effects | Yes | — | — |
| Lipase inhibition effects | Yes | — | — |
| Effects for improving glucose tolerance ability | Yes | — | — |
| Effects similar to simulating dietary fibers | Yes | — | — |
| Effects for increasing intestinal lactic acid bacteria | Yes | — | — |
| Effects for promoting the excretion of trace metal | Yes | — | — |

*Source:* Ariga, T., in *Maillard Reaction Products and Color*, Takahashi, K., Ed., Science Forum, Tokyo, 2004, pp. 298–300. With permission.

## 15.6 TOFUYO

Tofuyo is a unique fermented soybean food that has long been a tradition in Okinawa. Ordinary tofu is first produced from soybeans and after being dried at room temperature is pickled in a mixture containing yeast and awamori (a distilled liquor produced in Okinawa) for maturation. The *Aspergillus oryzae* including Monascus and Aspergillus bacteria are the microorganisms used in the fermentation process. Less salty than miso or shoyu, there is a certain sweetness to the taste of tofuyo, which has an elastic feel and a smooth texture like that of soft cheese.

The results of an analysis of tofuyo (matured for 3 months) produced by using *Monascus* bacteria showed the following composition in anhydride-converted values: crude protein: 29.2%, crude fat: 21.2%, crude ash content: 7.4%, crude fiber: 0%, reduced sugar: 24.2%, and salt: 3.2%. Tofuyo is not only a valuable protein source, but also helps improve blood circulation through the alcoholic effects of the awamori and is effective for stimulating the appetite. Yasuda et al.[76] conducted research on the antioxidation activity of tofuyo and found that the active component is probably a peptide-like substance observed in water extract fractions, with a ninhydrin positive reaction.

## REFERENCES

1. Yabe, K., On the vegetable cheese, *Bull. Coll. Agric. Tokyo Univ.*, 2, 68–72, 1894.
2. Hitomi, S., *Honcho Shokkan,* Shimada, I. Trans., Heibonsha, Tokyo, 1978, 334 pp. (in Japanese).
3. Oota, T., Natto ingestion for health, in *History of Natto,* Foods Pioneer Compilation, Eds., National Association of Natto Coop., Tokyo, 1975, 245 pp. (in Japanese).
4. Senbon, S., Bacillus natto as the anti-trichophytosis, *J. Formosan Med. Assoc. Taipei,* 39, 14–17, 1940.
5. Muramatsu, T., Experimental study concerning the treatment of carriers by the application of the antagonistic action of bacteria, *Kyoto Igakukaishi,* 12, 38–89, 1934 (in Japanese).
6. Arima, G., Experimental study on the antagonistic symptoms between *Bacillus subtilis natto* and dysentery bacillus, *Kaigun Igaku Zasshi,* 25, 509–527, 1936 (in Japanese).
7. Saito, T., Regarding the antagonistic action of *Bacillus subtilis natto* against *Salmonella typhi, Hokkai Igaku Zasshi,* 16, 82–92, 1938 (in Japanese).
8. Udo, S., Regarding the components of natto: the existence of dipicolinic acid in natto and its effects, *Nippon Nogei kagaku Kaishi,* 12, 386–394, 1936 (in Japanese).
9. Sumi, H. and Ohsugi, T., Anti-bacterial component dipicolic acid measured in Natto and Natto bacilli, *Nippon Nogei Kagaku Kaishi,* 73, 1289–1291, 1999 (in Japanese).
10. Sumi, H., Antibacterial activity of natto against pathogenic *E. coli* bacteria (*O-157*), *Bio Ind.,* 14, 47–50, 1997.
11. Sumi, H., The newly identified beneficial effects of natto, *Toyo Sinpo,* 1442, 5, 2002.
12. Sumi, H., Hamada, H., Tsushima, H., Mihara, H., and Muraki, H., A novel fibrinolytic enzyme nattokinase in the vegetable cheese natto: a typical and popular soybean food in the Japanese diet, *Experientia,* 43, 1110–1111, 1987.
13. Sumi, H., Taya, N., Nakajima, N., and Hiratani, H., Structure and fibrinolytic properties of nattokinase, *Fibrinolysis,* 6, 86, 1992.
14. Sumi, H., Nattokinase and human fibrinolytic system, *Kagaku to Seibutsu,* 29, 119–123, 1991 (in Japanese).
15. Fujita, M., Ito, Y., Hong, K., and Nishimoto, S., Characterization of nattokinase-degraded products from human fibrinogen or cross-linked fibrin, *Fibrinolysis,* 9, 157–164, 1995.
16. Sumi, H., Hamada, H., Nakanishi, H., and Hiratani, H., Enhancement of the fibrinolytic activity in plasma by oral administration of nattokinase, *Acta Haematol.,* 84, 139–143, 1990.
17. Fujita, M., Hong, K., Ito, Y., Misawa, S., Takeuchi, N., Kariya, K., and Nishimuro, S., Transport of nattokinase across the rat intestinal tract, *Biol. Pharm. Bull.,* 18, 1194–1196, 1995.

18.  Sumi, H., Yatagai, C., and Kishimoto, N., A very strong activity of pro-urokinase activator in natto, the traditional fermented soybean in Japan, *Fibrinolysis,* 10, 31, 1996.

19.  Urano, T., Ihara, H., Umemura, K., Suzuki, Y., Oike, M., Akita, S., Tsukamoto, Y., and Suzuki, T., The profibrinolytic enzyme subtilisin NAT purified from *Bacillus subtilis* cleaves and inactivates plasminogen activator inhibitor type I, *J. Biol. Chem.,* 276, 24690–24696, 2001.

20.  Nishimura, K., Hamamoto, J., Adachi, K., Yamazaki, A., Takagi, S., and Tamai, T., Examples of urgent-phase retinal embolism for which the intake of natto is believed to have been effective, *Ganka Rinsho Iho,* 88, 1381, 1994 (in Japanese).

21.  Cesarone, M.R., Belcaro, G., Nicolaides, A.N., Ricci, A., Geroulakos, G., Ippolito, E., Brandolini, R., Vinciguerra, G., Dugall, M., Griffin, M., Ruffini, I., Acerbi, G., Corsi, M., Riordan, N., Stuard, S., Barera, P., Dugall, M., Direnzo, A., Kenyon, J., and Errichi, B.M., Prevention of venous thrombosis in long-haul flights with flite tabs: The LONFLIT-FLITE randomized, controlled trial, *Antiology,* 54, 2003.

22.  Hayashi, U., Nagao, K., Tosa, S., and Yoshioka, S., Experimental study on the nutritional aspects of natto: regarding the relationships between natto-added diet and the blood pressures of SHR, 2, 9–17, 1979.

23.  Maruyama, M. and Sumi, H., Effect of natto diet on blood pressure, in *Basic and Clinical Aspects of Japanese Traditional Food Natto,* Vol. 2, Japan Technology Transfer Association, Tokyo, 1998, pp. 1–3 (in Japanese).

24.  Sumi, H., Yatagai, C., and Kishimoto, N., Fibrinolytic and anti-platelet aggregation activities in the Japanese fermented soybean natto, *Int. J. Hematol.,* S51, 1996.

25.  Kameda, Y., Kanamoto, S., Kameda, Y., and Saito, Y., A contact antitumor activity of *Bacillus natto* on solid type Ehrlich carcinoma cells, *Chem. Pharm. Bull.,* 16, 186–187, 1968.

26.  Suzuki, K., Analysis of protective effects of pretreatment with "*Bacillus natto*" on mice to lethal challenge with *Staphylococcus aureus, Tokyo Igaku Zasshi,* 33, 311–327, 1975 (in Japanese).

27.  Sumi, H., Yatagai, C., Wada, H., Yoshida, E., and Maruyama, M., Effect of *Bacillus natto*-fermented product (biozyme) on blood alcohol, aldehyde concentrations after whisky drinking in human volunteers, and acute toxicity of acetaldehyde in mice, *Jpn. J. Alcohol Drug Dependence,* 30, 69–79, 1995.

28.  Kaneki, M., Hedges, S.J., Hosoi, T., Fujiwara, S., Lyons, A., Crean, J., Ishida, N., Nakagawa, M., Takeshi, M., Sano, Y., Mizuno, Y., Hoshino, S., Miyano, M., Inoue, S., Horiki, K., Shiraki, M., Ouchi, Y., and Orimo, H., Japanese fermented soybean food as the major determinant of the large geographic difference in circulating levels of vitamin K2: possible implications for hip-fracture risk, *Nutrition,* 17, 315–321, 2001.

29.  Sumi, H., Determination of the vitamin K (menaquinone-7) content in fermented soybean natto and in the plasma of natto-ingested subjects, *J. Home Econ. Jpn.,* 50, 309–312, 1999 (in Japanese).

30.  Yatagai, C., Yanagisawa, Y., Ohsugi, T., and Sumi, H., Prolonged increase of plasma vitamin K2 concentration by natto (*Bacillus subtilis natto*) ingestion, *Pathophysiol. Haemost. Thromb.,* 89, 2003.

31.  Sumi, H. and Yatagai, C., Probiotics (natto bacillus) for anti-thrombosis and anti-osteoporosis, *Abstract of XVIIth International Congress on Fibrinolysis and Proteolysis,* 2004, p. 111.

32.  Orimo, H., The latest information on osteoporosis, *Nippon Iji Shinpo,* 3967, 1–11, 1976 (in Japanese).

33. Iwai, K., Nakaya, N., Kwasaki, Y., and Matsue, H., Inhibitory effect of natto, a kind of fermented soybeans, on LDL oxidation *in vitro*, *J. Agric. Food Chem.*, 50, 3592–3596, 2002.
34. Sumi, H., The mechanism of fermented soybeans for eliminating active oxygen: in particular, natto as an SOD agent, *Shokuhin Kogaku*, 41, 49–55, 1998 (in Japanese).
35. Iwai, K., Nakaya, N., Kawasaki, Y., and Matsue, H., Antioxidative functions of natto, a kind of fermented soybeans: effect on LDL oxidation and lipid metabolism in cholesterol-fed rats, *J. Agric. Food Chem.*, 50, 3597–3601, 2002.
36. Sumi, H., Sasaki, T., Yatagai, C., and Kozaki, Y., Determination and properties of the fibrinolysis accelerating substance (FAS) in Japanese fermented soybean "Natto," *Nippon Nogeikagaku Kaishi*, 74, 1259–1264, 2000 (in Japanese).
37. Winaro, F.G., *Proceedings of the IPB-JICA International Symposium on Agricultural Product Processing and Technology, IPB-JICA*, 1985.
38. Calloway, D.H., Hickey, C.A., and Murrhy, E.L., Reduction of intestinal gas-forming properties of legumes by traditional and experimental food processing methods, *J. Food Sci.* 36, 251–255, 1971.
39. Wang, H.L., Ellis, J.J., and Hesseltin, C.W., Antibacterial activity produced by molds commonly used in oriental food preparations, *Microgia*, 64, 218–221, 1972.
40. Karyadi, D., Salt-free fermented soybean foods in Asia, in STEP, Soda, H., Ueda, S., Murata, M., and Watanabe, T., Eds., Tokyo, 1986, pp. 112.
41. Sumi, H., Banba, T., and Yoshida, E., Bioactive substances in tempeh that are related to the circulatory system, *Nippon Nogei Kagaku Kaishi* 71, 233, 1997 (in Japanese).
42. Rilantono, L.I., Yuwono, H.S., and Nugrahadi, T., Dietary antioxidative potential in arteries, *Clin. Hemorheol. Microcirc.*, 23, 113–117, 2000.
43. Sumi, H., Okamoto, T., and Yatagai, C., *Abstract of 17th International Fibrinogen Workshop of the International Fibrinogen Research Society*, TH-02-10-0140, 2002.
44. Sumi, H. and Okamoto, T., Thrombolytic activity of an aqueous extract of Tempeh, *J. Home Econ. Jpn.*, 54, 337–342, 2003 (in Japanese).
45. Hasegawa, N., Ishida, K., and Yamada, N., Inhibitory effect of an aqueous extract of tempeh on compound 48/80-induced histamine release, *J. Home Econ. Jpn.*, 54, 1041–1043, 2003.
46. György, P., Murata, K., and Ikehata, H., Antioxidants isolated from fermented soybeans (tempeh), *Nature*, 203, 870–872, 1964.
47. Okada, N., Role of microorganism in tempeh manufacture, *Nippon Jozo Kyokaishi*, 81, 464–526, 1986 (in Japanese).
48. Imano, H., Regarding the starters for tempeh, *Daizu Geppo*, 8/9, 13–22, 1995 (in Japanese).
49. Van Veen, A.G., Graham, D.C.W., and Steinkraus, K.H., Fermented peanut press cake, *Cereal Sci. Today*, 13, 96, 1968.
50. Akiba, A., Ujiie, F., and Yokoyama, S., Anti bacterial activity of shoyu and sauce, *Choumi Kagaku*, 4, 1, 1957 (in Japanese).
51. Masuda, S., Kudo, Y., and Kumaya, S., The changes in intestinal hemorrhagic *E.coli* O-157: H7 in shoyu (soy sauce) and the components of shoyu (soy sauce), *Nippon Jozo Kyokaishi*, 94, 688–695, 1999 (in Japanese).
52. Matsuda, S., Regarding the anti-oxidant substances contained in shoyu (soy sauce), *Nippon Jozo Kyokaishi*, 93, 263–269, 1998 (in Japanese).

53. Yamaguchi, N., Yakoo, Y., and Fuimaki, M., Antioxidative activities of miso and soybean sauce on linoleic acid, *Nippon Shokuhin Kogyo Gakkaishi,* 26, 71–75, 1979 (in Japanese).

54. Kajimoto, Y., Depressor effect of soy-sauce, *Nippon Syokuhin Eisei Gakkaishi,* 4, 123–129, 1963 (in Japanese).

55. Kinoshita, E., Yamakoshi, J., Kikuchi, M., Regarding the depressor substances contained in shoyu (soy sauce), *Nippon Jozo Kyokaishi* 89, 126–130, 1994 (in Japanese).

56. Nakamura, M., Aoki, N., Yamada, T., and Kubo, N., Feasibility and effect on blood pressure of 6-week trail of low sodium soy sauce and Miso (fermented soybean paste), *Circ. J.,* 67, 530–534, 2003.

57. Kojima, T., Effect of soysauce on gastric juice secretion, *Rinsho Syoukabyou,* 2, 728–732, 1954 (in Japanese).

58. Ito, A. and Sato, Y., The effects of shoyu (soy sauce) regarding the occurrence of mutations induced by radiation, *Shoyu Kyoukai News,* 1990.

59. Nagahara, A., Benjamin, H., Storkson, J., Krewson, J., Sheng, K., Liu, W., and Pariza, M.W., Inhibition of benzo[a]pyrene-induced mouse forestomach neoplasia by a principal flavor component of Japanese-style fermented soy sauce, *Cancer Res.,* 52, 1754–1756, 1992.

60. Nagahara, A., Regarding the antitumor effects of shoyu (soy sauce), *Nippon Jozo Kyokaishi,* 88, 859–863, 1993 (in Japanese).

61. Hirayama, T., A large scale short study on cancer risks by diet with special reference to the risk reducing effects of green yellow vegetable consumption, in *Diet Nutrition and Cancer,* Hayashi, Y., Ed., National Academy of Sciences, Washington, D.C., 1986, pp. 41–53.

62. Okamoto, A., Hamagata, H., Matsumoto, E., Kawamura, Y., Koizumi, Y., and Yanagida, F., Angiotensin I converting enzyme inhibitory activities of various fermented foods, *Biosci. Biotechnol. Biochem.,* 59, 1147–1149, 1995.

63. Okazaki, S., Akiba, M., and Kimura, S., Regarding the research on anti-mutagen substances in the lipid of miso (soybean paste), *Nippon Nogei Kagaku Kaishi,* 58, 636, 1984 (in Japanese).

64. Iwashita, A., Okano, T., Takahama, A., Nakatsuka, M., and Kawamura, Y., Oral administration of miso extract on SHR, *Nippon Nogei Kagaku Kaishi,* 61, 84, 1993 (in Japanese).

65. Iwashita, A., Takahashi, Y., and Kawamura, Y., Physiological functions of miso, *Nippon Jozo Kyokaishi,* 89, 869–872, 1994 (in Japanese).

66. Yoshiki, Y. and Okubo, R., Reactive oxygen radical scavenging activity of soybean fermented foods: miso, *Nippon Jozo Kyokaishi,* 93, 702–708, 1998 (in Japanese).

67. Kato, H., Aging of cells prevented by miso (soybean paste) components, *Nippon Shokuhin Kogyo Gakkaishi,* 40, 82–86, 1994 (in Japanese).

68. Santiago, L.A., Mori, A., and Hiramatsu, M., Japanese soybean paste miso scavenges free radicals and inhibits lipid peroxidation, *J. Nutr. Sci. Vitaminol.,* 38, 297–304, 1992.

69. Horii, M., Ide, T., and Kawashima, K., Hypocholesterolemic activity of desalted miso in rats fed on atherogenic diet, *Nippon Shokuhin Kogyo Gakkaishi,* 37, 148–153, 1990.

70. Ide, T., Kano, S., and Moriuchi, H., Activities of hepatic rate-limiting enzymes in cholesterol biosynthesis and degradation in rats fed desalted miso, *Nippon Shokuhin Kogyo Gakkaishi,* 38, 435–440, 1991.

71. Akitsuki, T., *The Way To Health and Well-Being: Physical Constitution and Foods,* Kurieishuppannbu, Tokyo, 1980, 61 pp. (in Japanese).
72. Itoh, A., The effects of miso (soybean paste) for the elimination of radioactive substances, *Sci. Miso,* 1–6, 1993.
73. Watanabe, A. and Takahasi, T., The effects of miso (soybean paste) on small intestinal disorders of mice caused by X-radiation, *Miso no Kagaku to Gijyutsu,* 39, 29–32, 1991.
74. Yamaguchi, N., Antioxidative of miso, *Nippon Jozo Kyokaishi,* 87, 721–725, 1992 (in Japanese).
75. Ariga, T., The science of foods as seen through miso (soybean paste), shoyu (soy sauce), in *Maillard Reaction Products and Color,* Takahashi, K., Ed., Science Forum, Tokyo, 2004, pp. 298–300.
76. Yasuda, M., The fermented food from soybean protein (tofuyo) and its functional effects, *Abstract of 52th Japanese society of Nutrition and Food Science,* 1998, pp. 22.

# 16 Soybean Components and Food for Specified Health Uses (FOSHU)

*Takashi Yamamoto*

## CONTENTS

## 16.1 THE EFFECTIVENESS OF THE SOYBEAN

The soybean is an important food resource. It contains abundant protein, carbohydrate, and fat (Figure 16.1). It is a high-protein food and a good source of nitrogen for humans because the amino acid composition of protein in the soybean has the equivalent nutritional value as animal protein. Polysaccharides (dietary fiber) and oligosaccharides such as sucrose, raffinose, and stachyose are contained in the soybean as carbohydrates. Soybean fat contains abundant essential fatty acids such as linoleic acid and linolenic acid.

Furthermore, the soybean contains some useful minor components such as isoflavone, saponin, lecithin, and phytosterol. These minor components, as well as the major components, have some functions that are physiologically effective. The major physiological actions of soybean components are shown in Table 16.1.

The soy protein known as the "meat in the field" not only excels as a source of protein but also has many physiological functions. The effect of soy protein, as one of its effective physiological functions, on the plasma lipids and especially on plasma cholesterol concentration has been proved by many researchers, such as Carrol, Kritchevsky, Sirtori, Sugano, and their working groups, through clinical studies in human and animal tests. Extensive research on soy protein, which

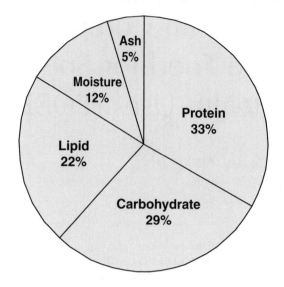

**FIGURE 16.1** Composition of soybean.

possibly reduces cholesterol concentration in the blood, has been conducted. The protein was the first soybean component recognized to have specified health uses. In addition, the effectiveness of soy protein control of plasma cholesterol concentration in fewer amounts is being studied in Japan (see Table 16.2).

**TABLE 16.1**
**Physiological Functions of Soybean Components**

| Component | Action |
| --- | --- |
| Protein | Cholesterol lowering, antiobesity, antiaging |
| Protein hydrolysate | Highly absorbent, antiobesity, antihypertensive |
| Lectin | Immune response |
| Trypsin inhibitor | Anticancer |
| Dietary fiber | Lipid lowering, anticolon cancer |
| Oligosaccharide | Substrate for bifidobacteria |
| Linoleic acid | Essential fatty acid, cholesterol lowering |
| Linolenic acid | Antiallergenic, reduction of coronary heart disease (CHD) risk |
| Lecithin | Lipid lowering, memory function |
| Sterol | Cholesterol lowering |
| Tocopherol | Antioxidant, reduction of CHD risk |
| Vitamin K | Anticoagulant, antiosteoporosis |
| Vitamin $B_1$ | Antiberiberi |
| Phytate | Mineral absorption, anticancer |
| Saponin | Lipid lowering, antioxidant |
| Isoflavone | Phytoestrogen, anticancer, antiosteoporosis |

**TABLE 16.2**
**Clinical Trials in Japan on Effects on Cholesterol Lowering**

| SPI (g/d) | Duration | Food | T Chol (mg/dl) | | HDL-Chol (mg/dl) | | References |
|---|---|---|---|---|---|---|---|
| | | | Before | After | Before | After | |
| 7 | 2–6 weeks | Nugget | 250 ± 24 | 238 ± 26[a] | 53.8 ± 15.1 | 52.2 ± 13.1 | Kambara, 1993 |
| 14 | 1 week | Nugget | 186 ± 16 | 175 ± 17[a] | 60 ± 9 | 59 ± 11 | Kito, 1993 |
| 5.8 | 4 months | Beverage | 255 ± 9 | 217 ± 8[a] | 55 ± 6 | 58 ± 7 | Imura, 1996 |
| 9.9 | 2 weeks | Sausage | 225 ± 8 | 208 ± 9[a] | 45.3 ± 3.1 | 50.2 ± 3.6 | Katsuta, 1997 |
| 9 | 2 weeks | Soup and cookies | 259 ± 8 | 244 ± 10[a] | 53.6 ± 3.3 | 53.1 ± 3.1 | Akioka, 1999 |
| 11 | 2 weeks | Hamburger | 223 ± 27 | 215 ± 23[a] | 55 ± 14 | 53 ± 14 | Ichinomiy, 1998 |
| 9 or 6 | 4 weeks | Yogurt | 243 ± 18 | 241 ± 31 | LDL 166 ± 24 | 160 ± 28 | Waki, 1999 |
| 7 | 2 weeks | Soup | 218 ± 21 | 206 ± 19[a] | 59.3 ± 19.0 | 60.8 ± 20.6 | Hirata, 2000 |
| 6 | 4 weeks | Milk | 257 ± 26 | 243 ± 25[a] | 61 ± 11 | 58 ± 9 | Akioka, 2000 |
| 6 | 13 weeks | Beverage | 244 ± 4 | 228 ± 5[a] | 56 ± 5 | 55 ± 3 | Ishikawa, 2002 |

[a] Significant difference ($p < 0.01 \sim 0.05$)

## 16.2  FOOD FOR SPECIFIED HEALTH USES (FOSHU)

Food labeling in Japan is regulated by health promotion law and food sanitation law announced by the Ministry of Health, Labor, and Welfare. FOSHU, defined by the Nutrition Improvement Law, which was succeeded by the Health Promotion Law, is the system to approve specific health claims on food labels. It took effect in 1991, and the first food based on this standard was produced in 1993. The market scale of FOSHU products exceeded 398 items and 566.9 billion yen by the end of 2003. The number of items approved by September 27, 2004 was 454 (Figure 16.2).

The Food Sanitation Law was established in April 2001 for food with health claims. Food with health claims is positioned between pharmaceutical products and general foods in the classification of substances to be taken by mouth (Table 16.3).

Foods with health claims are classified in two types. One is food with nutrient function claims, and the other is FOSHU. The former is the food labeling system based on the standard. Food can be labeled if it meets the standard by containing active ingredients specified by the standard. FOSHU is the labeling system that approves foods individually. Foods are individually examined for active ingredients, intake amount, safety, and contents of the label. Therefore, FOSHU is defined and contained in the category of food with health claims. Table 16.4 summarizes major health uses and components of FOSHU products approved to date. Previously, only food products could be approved as FOSHU products, but now tablets and capsules can also be approved. The food labeling system in Japan approves nutrition and health claims but not claims of reduction of disease risk.

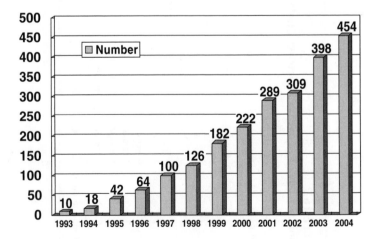

**FIGURE 16.2** Articles on food for specified health uses. (Courtesy of Japan Health Food and Nutrition Food Association.)

## TABLE 16.3
## Classification of Japanese Health Function Foods (Effective April 2001)

| | Health Function Foods (Foods with Health Claims) | | |
|---|---|---|---|
| Medicine | Food for Specified Health Uses (FOSHU) | Nutritional Functional Foods (Foods with Nutrient Function Claims) | Common Foods |
| Includes Quasi-drugs | Individual permission based | Standard based | Includes health foods and supplements |

*Source:* Ministry of Health, Labor, and Welfare.

## TABLE 16.4
## Specific Health Uses and Major Food Components with Health Claims

| Specific Health Uses | Related Properties |
|---|---|
| Foods that control bowel conditions | Oligosaccharides: xylo-oligosaccharide, fructo-oligosaccharide, galacto-oligosaccharide, isomalto-oligosaccharide, soy oligosaccharide, lact oligosaccharide, lactulose |
| | Lactic acid bacteria: *Lactbacillus* GG, *Bifidobacterium longum, L. acidophillus longum, Yakult bacillus, B. blebe, Yakult bacillus* |
| | Dietary fiber: polydextrose, cyalume (plantain seed coat), resistant dextrin, low polymer sodium alginate |
| Foods that control high blood cholesterol levels | Soybean protein, chitosan, low polymer sodium alginate, phytosterol |
| Foods that control high blood pressure | Lact tripeptide, casein dodecapeptide, sardine peptide, tuna oligopeptide |
| Foods that control high blood glucose level | Resistant dextrin, wheat albumin, guava polyphenol, L-arabinose |
| Foods for weak bones | Vitamin $K_2$, soy isoflavones |
| Foods that help the absorption of minerals | Calcium citrate malate (CCM), casein phospho peptide (CPP), hemoferrum, fructo-oligosaccharide |
| Foods that suppress the occurrence of triglyceride in the blood after food intake | Diacylglycerol, globin hydrolysate |
| Foods that suppress the causes of dental caries | Paratinose, maltitol, xylitol, erythritol, tea polyphenol |
| Foods that help maintain healthy teeth | Xylitol, reduced paratinose, second calcium phosphate, colpomenia sinuosa extract, casein phospho peptide noncrystallized calcium phosphate complex (CPP-ACP) |
| Food that may prevent body fat accumulation | Diacylglycerol |

## 16.3  FOSHU PRODUCTS WITH SOYBEAN COMPONENTS

There is no denying that soybeans contribute a great deal to the health of Japanese people. The soybean contains many protein components, which have many physical and physiological functions. Therefore, it is used to make food with new functions that use its functional ingredients. Four kinds of active ingredients are known to have been used for FOSHU products as of September 2004. These are soy protein, soy isoflavone, soy oligosaccharides, and phytosterol.

There are two more components contained in the soybean. One of them is the bound substance of soy protein hydrolysate and lecithin, and the other is vitamin $K_2$, which is formed abundantly by the action of bacillus natto, which makes natto, a Japanese traditional fermented food.

### 16.3.1  CHOLESTEROL LOWERING

Cholesterol is one of the essential components of the body. It is also one of the components that comprise the cell membrane; bile acids and hormones are also made from cholesterol. Though cholesterol is an important component of the body, it can become an issue because increased blood cholesterol may increase the risk of vascular events such as coronary disease due to changes of life-style, including diet. It has been long known that soybean or its components affect blood lipid and especially blood cholesterol level. Research on soy protein has been ongoing since the 1960s. Food made from soy protein was first approved as a FOSHU product in 1994.

The content of approved food labeling is "Helpful to improve dietary life for those who care for cholesterol because this product was made so that soy protein, which has the action to lower the blood cholesterol level, can be taken easily." Foods that contain soy protein as an active ingredient flooded the market as food for people who are concerned about plasma cholesterol concentration. There are many types of these foods such as soybean milk, soybean milk yogurt, soup, fried foods, hamburger steak, meatballs, Vienna sausages, and high protein drinks. The diversity of foods enables diversity of dietary life. The amount of soy protein contained in these foods is approximately 6 g per serving. The major FOSHU products that contain soybean components are shown in Table 16.5.

Furthermore, there is a food made by combining phospholipids and polypeptides with abundant hydrophobic components, which are considered to be very effective soy proteins for lowering cholesterol. The effective amount depends on the product but on average is 1.5 g per serving in 10 g powder and it is taken mixed with water. Two servings per day are recommended to reduce cholesterol.

Phytosterol is another soybean component used for lowering cholesterol. Phytosterol enters the micelle and competes with cholesterol when it is digested and absorbed. The absorbability of phytosterol is extremely low and cholesterol absorption is reduced because the cholesterol that cannot enter the micelle is passed out of the body without being absorbed. Therefore, foods made using phytosterol or sterol esters from soybeans have been approved as FOSHU products

## TABLE 16.5
## Selected FOSHU Products Containing Soybean Components

| Related Properties (Valid Properties) | Food | Company | Date of Permission |
|---|---|---|---|
| Soybean protein | Soybean Fry (fried food) | FUJI OIL CO., LTD | April 24, 1998 |
| | Balance Meatball (chilled meatball) | Nippon Meat Packers, Inc. | May 23, 2001 |
| | Balance Hamburger (chilled hamburger) | Nippon Meat Packers, Inc. | May 23, 2001 |
| | G–9 (soft drinks) | KANESA Co., Ltd. | August 27, 2001 |
| | Balance Winner | Nippon Meat Packers, Inc. | October 21, 1997 |
| | Balance Frankfurter | Nippon Meat Packers, Inc. | October 21, 1997 |
| | Healthy Burger | Marudai Food Co., Ltd. | December 24, 1999 |
| | Healthy Ball (meatball) | Marudai Food Co., Ltd. | August 30, 2001 |
| | Soybean Milk (controlled soybean milk) | TORAKU CO., LTD. | March 23, 2001 |
| | Soybean Yogurt | TORAKU CO., LTD. | March 28, 2000 |
| | Soybean Yogurt giving fruit taste | TORAKU CO., LTD. | December 6, 2002 |
| | Soybean Milk Yogurt Drink (fermented soybean milk) | TORAKU CO., LTD. | January 18, 2001 |
| | Soybean Soup (dry soup) | Meiji Seika Co., Ltd. | December 28, 2000 |
| | Body Support Soft Drink (soybean protein soft drink) | Nestle Japan Group | December 6, 2002 |
| | Kensei Soybean (soybean protein soft drink) | Nestle Japan Group | June 11, 2003 |
| | Soymilk from SOYA FARM (controlled soymilk) | TORAKU CO., LTD. | June 11, 2003 |
| | Yeah (controlled soybean milk) | FUJI OIL CO., LTD. | June 11, 2003 |
| Phosphatide | Soybean Peptid Remake (powdered soft drink) | KYOWA HAKKO KOGYO Co., Ltd. | December 12, 2002 |
| Vegetable sterol | Econa Healthy Oil | Kao Corporation | June 4, 1999 |
| | Kenkosarara (soybean oil) | AJINOMOTO CO., INC. | December 26, 2001 |
| | Healthy Coleste (soybean oil) | Nisshin OilliO, Ltd. | September 25, 2003 |
| Vegetable sterol estel | Ramapro (margarine) | Nipponlever | April 9, 2001 |
| Soy oligosaccharide | Oligo CC (carbonated drink) | CALPIS CO., Ltd. | October 25, 2001 |
| | Soybean Oligosugar Syrup (table sugar) | CALPIS CO., Ltd. | October 25, 2001 |
| | Soybean Oligosugar Syrup (lactic acid drink) | CALPIS CO., Ltd. | December 12, 2000 |

(*continued*)

**TABLE 16.5 (Continued)**
**Selected FOSHU Products Containing Soybean Components**

| Related Properties (Valid Properties) | Food | Company | Date of Permission |
|---|---|---|---|
| | ELTOS Syrup (table sugar) | Taisho Pharmaceutical Co., Ltd. | April 22, 2002 |
| | Sutto (soft drink) | Tokiwa Pharmaceutical Co., Ltd. | October 23, 1997 |
| | Pises (soft drink) | Tokiwa Pharmaceutical Co., Ltd. | October 23, 1997 |
| | Pises (table sugar) | Taisho Pharmaceutical Co., Ltd. | April 22, 2002 |
| Soy isoflavone | Soybean Fermented Tea (soft drink) | Fujicco Co., Ltd. | March 23, 2001 |
| | Black Soybean Tea (soft drink) | Fujicco Co., Ltd. | September 9, 2001 |
| | Black Soybean Drink (soybean drink) | Fujicco Co., Ltd. | October 18, 2001 |
| | Black Bean Tea Gold (soft drink) | Fujicco Co., Ltd. | May 27, 2002 |
| | Kotsukotsu Kenkotsu Healthy Life (soft drink) | SSP Co., Ltd. | April 30, 2001 |
| | Kotsukotsu Kenkotsu Healthy Life (soft drink) | SSP Co., Ltd. | January 8, 2004 |
| | Active Life B K (soft drink) | Maruwa Co., Ltd. | January 8, 2004 |
| | Kaikotsubijin Iron (soft drink) | Maruwa Co., Ltd. | June 8, 2004 |
| | Bisset (soft drink) | Maruwa Co., Ltd. | June 8, 2004 |
| | Flavonamin (soft drink) | Maruwa Co., Ltd. | June 8, 2004 |
| Vitamin $K_2$ | Honegenki Gold Soybean (natto) | Mizkan Group Co., Ltd. | December 27, 2002 |
| | Honegenki Organic Growing (natto) | Mizkan Group Co., Ltd. | December 27, 2004 |
| | Honegenki Hikiwari (natto) | Mizkan Group Co., Ltd. | December 27, 2002 |

as "food for those who care for cholesterol." These foods included blended oils containing 1.79 to 3.2 g of phytosterol 100 g of blended oil. The recommended daily dose is 109 to 14 g of the oil.

An example of the content of approved labeling for FOSHU products is as follows: This food made from soy germ has features to lower the blood total cholesterol and low-density lipoprotein (LDL)-cholesterol levels because it abundantly contains natural phytosterol that has an action to block the absorption of cholesterol, and is recommended for people with high cholesterol levels to take everyday.

### 16.3.2 REGULATING INTESTINAL FUNCTION

The category that includes the richest variety of FOSHU products is the regulation of bowel function. Many kinds of active ingredients are used for these products and are mainly classified into three categories for FOSHU, namely, oligosaccharides, lactic acid bacteria, and dietary fiber.

Carbohydrates account for about 28% of soybean. Soybean contains very few starches, unlike other legumes. Dietary fiber accounts for about 16% of soy carbohydrates. Insoluble components such as cellulose, hemicellulose, and pectinic substances account for the most of the fiber. Oligosaccharides such as sucrose, stachyose, and raffinose account for the remaining parts.

Oligosaccharide that can be broken down neither by amylase nor by disaccharidase in the human body is a good substrate for bifidobacteria. Raffinose and stachyose in soybean cannot be digested by human digestive enzymes but can be broken down by intestinal bacteria. They can easily be substrates, especially for bifidobacteria. That is why soybean oligosaccharide is used as "food suitable for those who want to regulate the bowels." The content of approved labeling is as follows: This product is suitable for those who care for the bowel condition because it maintains good intestinal environment by increasing bifidobacteria.

Oligosaccharide is used for table sugar, soft drinks, and carbonated drinks. An adequate intake of the drink per day is estimated to be one 100 ml bottle that contains about 4 g of soybean oligosaccharide. Soybean oligosaccharide accounts for 20% to 30% of the syrup, so intake of two or three spoons (15 to 25 g) per day is appropriate when used as table sugar. The caloric value of soybean oligosaccharide is less than that of sucrose by two thirds and it is less sweet than normal sugar by three fourths. A small decrease in energy intake can be expected.

### 16.3.3 BONE HEALTH

The soybean also contains isoflavone, a kind of polyphenol, mainly in the germ. Soy isoflavone is effective at maintaining bone density. That is why foods made using soy isoflavone have been developed as FOSHU products for people who are concerned about bone health. The contents of approved labeling for these products are as follows: "This drink is suitable for those who care for bone health because it contains soy isoflavone that intervenes in the process of calcium loss from bone." "This drink is suitable for those who care for bone health because it contains soy isoflavone helpful to maintain the amount of calcium in the bone." "This product is suitable for those who care for bone health because it was made from soy isoflavone helpful to maintain the amount of calcium in the bone and made easy to take."

Soy germ tea and soft drinks containing isoflavone have been made as FOSHU products. The product (soybean tea) contains 40 mg of isoflavone per can, and the above-mentioned effect is expected from drinking a can per day.

Soybean originally contains approximately 18 μg of vitamin $K_2$ per 100 g and is a valuable source of vitamin $K_2$ by itself, but natto bacillus can significantly increase the amount of vitamin $K_2$. For example, natto, a traditional Japanese soybean food, is rich in vitamin $K_2$ and considered to be effective for increasing calcium deposits in the bones. Bone protein (osteocalcin) made in the osteoblast is very important for bone formation because it absorbs calcium into the bone by combining with it. γ-Carboxylation (conversion to Gla) of the glutamic acid residue is required for osteocalcin to function, and vitamin K is a coenzyme indispensable for that action. The abundant vitamin $K_2$ in natto has the same effect. For these reasons, *Bacillus subtilis* OUV23481 strain, natto bacillus, which produces vitamin $K_2$, was approved as an active ingredient for FOSHU products.

The content of approved labeling is as follows: This product contains abundant vitamin $K_2$ by the action of natto bacillus, *Bacillus subtilis* OUV23481 strain, and was made to enhance function of bone protein (osteocalcin) which helps calcium to deposit into the bone. Natto contains over 700 μg of vitamin $K_2$ per pack (50 g), and the recommended intake is one pack per day.

## 16.4  CONCLUSIONS

There is nothing comparable to soybean for having various functional components in a single food item in addition to being used widely as active ingredients for FOSHU products. The soybean greatly contributes to human nutrition and health.

# 17 Soy in Health and Disease: Perspectives

*David Kritchevsky*

## CONTENTS

## 17.1  BACKGROUND

At the beginning of the twentieth century, pathologists were already acquainted with the idea that lipids were deposited in the human aorta. They tried to duplicate this observation in rabbits using a combination of diet and physical trauma, and a few were successful. The first demonstration that diet alone was sufficient to induce atherosclerosis in rabbits was made by Ignatowski in 1908.[1] Working from the hypothesis that a diet rich in animal protein was the cause of atherosclerosis, he induced atherosclerotic lesions in weanling rabbits by feeding them milk and eggs and in adult rabbits by feeding them horse meat.[1,2] Several other investigators were able to confirm Ignatowski's findings. Stuckey[3] observed aortic lesions in rabbits fed either ox brain or egg yolk and concluded that a nonprotein common to egg yolk and ox brain was the atherogenic agent. Stuckey's findings stimulated studies by Chalatow[4] and Wesselkin[5] that pointed to cholesterol as the putative atherogenic agent. Feeding studies conducted by Anitschkow and Chalatow[6] and Wacker and Heuck[7] confirmed the atherogenicity of dietary cholesterol. Subsequent research, indeed until today, focused primarily on the roles of cholesterol in atherogenesis and virtually ignored all other dietary components. However, some investigators continued to seek dietary factors other than cholesterol that could be atherogenic per se or might enhance the observed cholesterol effects. The early history of proteins in atherosclerosis has been described.[8] An exhaustive study of protein effects in atherosclerosis has recently been published.[9]

Interest in the possible atherogenic effects of vegetable protein was evinced by Freyberg in 1937,[10] who found no effect. The first direct comparison of the atherogenic properties of animal protein (casein) and vegetable protein (soy) was made by Meeker and Kesten.[11,12] They found a casein-based diet to be significantly more atherogenic for rabbits than one based on soy protein. Although proteins of origin other than casein or soy have been used to study protein effects in atherosclerosis, most published studies use casein and soy as the examples of animal and vegetable protein, respectively. In 1959, casein was reported to be more cholesterolemic than soy protein in both conventional and germ-free chickens,[13] and a few years later, soy flour and soy protein were shown to be less cholesterolemic and atherogenic for rabbits than casein.[14] One human study, published in the 1960, merits comment. Hodges et al.[15] studied a group of six human subjects ingesting a mixed protein diet and switched them to a series of diets of varying carbohydrate (simple complex) composition in which the protein was vegetable protein. Regardless of carbohydrate mix, serum cholesterol levels were significantly lower than they had been at the start of the study. Going from the mixed protein to the vegetable protein diet decreased cholesterol levels by 28% ($p < 0.01$), and, in the final stage, going back to the mixed protein from the vegetable protein diet increased cholesterol levels by 34% ($p < 0.01$).

## 17.2   PRESENT STATUS

In the 1960s, Carroll and colleagues[16] initiated a concentrated program of research into the lipidemic and atherogenic effects of proteins. Rabbits were fed semipurified diets containing a variety of proteins, and, in general, animal proteins were found to be more cholesterolemic than proteins of plant origin.[16]

Feeding of amino acid mixtures approximating the composition of casein or soy protein gave surprising results. Cholesterol levels in rabbits fed the casein amino acid mixture approximate those of rabbits fed casein. However, the soy amino acid mixture raised cholesterol levels by 80%. When partial enzymic hydrolysates of the proteins were fed serum cholesterol, levels were reduced by 16% in rabbits fed the casein hydrolyzate. This study suggests that the changes in cholesterol level might be evoked by small peptides.[17] Sugano et al.[18] found that an undigested fraction of soy protein was hypocholesterolemic for rats. They later prepared an undigested high-molecular-weight fraction of soybean protein by exposing the intact protein to exhaustive digestion by microbial proteinases. This washed protein fraction reduced the serum cholesterol levels of rats fed cholesterol and cholic acid by 55%.[19] In other studies of protein hydrolysis products, it has been shown that soy β-conglycinin (7S globulin) inhibits atherosclerosis in mice.[20] Sirtori and colleagues have contributed greatly to our knowledge of the mechanisms of action of soy protein peptides. They have reported that β-conglycinin subunits regulate liver low-density lipoprotein receptors.[21,22] Variation in only one amino acid is sufficient to cause differences. As an example, cow's milk containing β-casein A[1] is significantly more cholesterolemic and atherogenic for rabbits than is milk containing β-casein A[2]. The difference is between the presence of a histidine (A[1]) or proline (A[2]) residue at codon 67.[23]

Examination of the published data and of the composition of casein and soy protein raised the possibility that the lysine to arginine (L:A) ratio (which is

**TABLE 17.1**
**Influence of Fish Protein, Casein, or Whole Milk Protein
on Atherosclerosis in Rabbits (Effect of Lysine to Arginine Ratio)**

| | Protein | | |
|---|---|---|---|
| **No.** | **Fish**<br>**10/12** | **Casein**<br>**10/12** | **Whole Milk**<br>**9/12** |
| Lysine/arginine | 1.44 | 1.89 | 2.44 |
| Serum lipids (mg/dl) | | | |
|   Cholesterol (C) | $283 \pm 46^{ab}$ | $530 \pm 76^{a}$ | $462 \pm 62^{b}$ |
|   % HDL-C | $15.7 \pm 1.4^{c}$ | $11.8 \pm 1.1^{c}$ | $11.9 \pm 1.5$ |
|   Triglycerides | $122 \pm 26^{d}$ | $177 \pm 47$ | $251 \pm 56^{d}$ |
| Atherosclerosis (0–4) | | | |
|   Arch | $1.55 \pm 0.23^{e}$ | $2.05 \pm 0.25$ | $2.61 \pm 0.16^{e}$ |
|   Thoracic | $0.95 \pm 0.17^{f}$ | $1.10 \pm 0.25$ | $1.56 \pm 0.19^{f}$ |

Diet contains 40% sucrose, 25% protein, 14% coconut oil, 15% fiber. Fed for 8 months.
Atherosclerosis graded on a 0 to 4 scale.
Values in horizontal row bearing same superscript letter are significantly different ($P < 0.05$).
All values ± standard error of mean (SEM).

*Source:* After Kritchevsky, D. et al., *Atherosclerosis* 41:429–431, 1982.

higher in animal protein) may, in part, determine the atherogenic potential of a protein.[24] In several studies, we showed that the L:A ratios of casein and soy protein did indeed determine atherogenicity and that a 1:1 mix of beef protein and textured vegetable protein (TVP) was more cholesterolemic than textured beef protein but not more atherogenic.[25] Comparison of the atherogenic effects of fish protein (L:A, 1.44), casein (L:A, 1.89), and whole milk protein (L:A, 2.44) showed a statistically significant relationship, with severity of atherosclerosis being directly related to the L:A ratio[26] (Table 17.1).

Finally, we conducted a study[27] in which rabbits were fed one of four proteins: casein (C), casein plus arginine to give an L:A equal to that of soy protein (CA), soy protein (S), or soy protein plus lysine to give the L:A of casein (SL) (Table 17.2). Serum cholesterol levels in group SL were significantly elevated when compared to serum cholesterol levels in group S. Average severity of atherosclerosis (arch plus thoracic/2) in group C was 2.45 times that of group C. In group CA, atherogenicity was reduced by 17% compared to group C and in group SL, it was raised by 64% compared to group S. Addition of the specific amino acids changed the plasma lipoprotein spectra as well. The rabbits fed soy protein (in a semipurified diet) excreted 42% less feces (grams/day) than those fed a commercial diet but more than those fed casein (by 109%). On diet CA, fecal output was not increased compared to diet C, but the ratio of acidic to neutral steroids rose by 47%. On diet SL, fecal output fell by 43% compared to diet C, and the ratio of fecal acidic and neutral steroids fell by 48% (Table 17.3).

## TABLE 17.2
### Influence of Addition of a Single Amino Acid on Experimental Atherosclerosis in Rabbits (Average of Three Experiments)

| No. | Casein (C) 20/31 | Soy (S) 25/31 | C + Arginine 20/31 | S + Lysine 25/31 |
|---|---|---|---|---|
| | | Group | | |
| % Protein | 23.9 | 23.5 | 23.9 | 23.5 |
| % Amino acid | 1.9 | 1.3 | 1.9 | 1.3 |
| Serum lipids (mg/dl) | | | | |
| Cholesterol | $241 \pm 28^a$ | $130 \pm 13^{abc}$ | $232 \pm 36^b$ | $189 \pm 20^c$ |
| Triglycerides | $102 \pm 11^{de}$ | $63 \pm 7^{df}$ | $105 \pm 15^f$ | $74 \pm 6^e$ |
| Atherosclerosis (0–4) | | | | |
| Arch | $1.63 \pm 0.22^g$ | $0.71 \pm 0.15^{gh}$ | $1.30 \pm 18^h$ | $1.10 \pm 0.16$ |
| Thoracic | $1.05 \pm 0.20^i$ | $0.44 \pm 11^i$ | $0.73 \pm 0.15$ | $0.79 \pm 0.11$ |

Values in horizontal row bearing same superscript letter are significantly different ($P < 0.05$). All values $\pm$ SEM.

*Source:* After Kritchevsky, D. et al., in *Current Topics in Nutrition and Disease*, Vol. 8, Alan R. Liss, New York, 1983, pp. 85–100.

A review of the possible mechanisms of cholesterolemic action of dietary casein and soy protein suggests increased cholesterol absorption in casein-fed animals and enhancement of fecal output of sterols and bile acids under the influence of soy protein.[28] We reasoned that the effect was due to the finding that lysine feeding inhibited arginase,[29,30] resulting in less available arginine. With the

## TABLE 17.3
### Fecal Steroid Excretion in Rabbits Fed Casein, Soy, Casein + Arginine, or Soy + Lysine (1 Week Collection)

| | Chow | Casein (C) | Soy (S) | C + Arginine | S + Lysine |
|---|---|---|---|---|---|
| | | | Group | | |
| Feces (g/d) | 20.0 | 5.6 | 11.7 | 5.3 | 6.7 |
| Steroids (mg/d) | | | | | |
| Acidic (A) | $31.6 \pm 10.0$ | $9.4 \pm 2.2$ | $33.0 \pm 10.3$ | $12.9 \pm 2.6$ | $12.1 \pm 2.5$ |
| Neutral (N) | $19.3 \pm 2.9$ | $8.5 \pm 2.6$ | $15.4 \pm 4.2$ | $7.9 \pm 3.0$ | $10.9 \pm 0.6$ |
| A/N | 1.64 | 1.11 | 2.14 | 1.63 | 1.11 |

Diet contains 40% sucrose, 25% protein, 14% coconut oil, 15% fiber. Fed for 8 months. All values $\pm$ SEM.

*Source:* After Kritchevsky, D. et al., in *Current Topics in Nutrition and Disease*, Vol. 8, Alan R. Liss, New York, 1983, pp. 85–100.

emergence of knowledge about the cardiovascular benefits of nitric oxides, comes the possibility that lysine may influence NO production. The antiatherogenic effects of dietary arginine have been reported,[31] and an attempt has been made to relate them to antioxidant effects.

In addition to its influence on arginine metabolism, lysine may exert other, as yet unstudied, effects on atherosclerosis. Moore et al.[32–36] have published a study on diet and atherosclerosis involving 253 subjects for whom they had exhaustive data on diet and eating patterns. They found a significant positive trend for increased percentage of raised coronary lesions and lysine intake[35] Positive trends were also found for myristic and oleic acids, fructose, niacin, riboflavin, calcium, and iodine.

Interaction of dietary proteins with other dietary components can influence cholesterolemia and atherogenesis in rabbits. The standard semipurified diet contains casein as the protein, sucrose as the carbohydrate, and cellulose as the fiber source. Substitution of soy protein for casein reduces cholesterol levels by 38% and average atherosclerosis by 17%. When the fiber is alfalfa, serum cholesterol levels and atherosclerosis are significantly lower than levels in the cellulose group. The difference in cholesterol level is only 18% higher in the casein group, and average atherosclerosis is 17% lower.[37] These observations show that changes in dietary components other than protein also affect cholesterolemia and atherosclerosis (Table 17.4).

The interaction of soy protein with other dietary components has rarely been studied because the thrust of the experiments has been comparison of proteins. Examining other aspects of the diet may indicate new ingredient combinations that could affect cholesterolemia and atherogenesis.

**TABLE 17.4**
**Interaction of Protein and Fiber in Rabbits Fed Semipurified Diets**

| Protein | Fiber | No. | Serum Cholesterol (mg/dl) | Atherosclerosis | |
| | | | | Arch | Thoracic |
|---|---|---|---|---|---|
| Casein | Cellulose | 8 | 402 ± 40 | 1.81 ± 0.20 | 1.19 ± 0.29 |
| Soy | Cellulose | 5 | 248 ± 44 | 1.50 ± 0.39 | 1.00 ± 0.52 |
| Casein | Wheat straw | 12 | 375 ± 42 | 1.17 ± 0.22 | 0.88 ± 0.18 |
| Soy | Wheat straw | 13 | 254 ± 35 | 1.04 ± 0.28 | 0.77 ± 0.24 |
| Casein | Alfalfa | 10 | 193 ± 34 | 0.70 ± 0.11 | 0.55 ± 0.20 |
| Soy | Alfalfa | 13 | 159 ± 20 | 0.88 ± 0.22 | 0.58 ± 0.17 |

Diet contains 40% sucrose, 25% protein, 14% coconut oil, 15% fiber. Fed for 8 months.
Atherosclerosis graded on a 0 to 4 scale.
All values ± SEM.

*Source:* After Kritchevsky, D. et al., *Atherosclerosis*, 26, 397–403, 1977.

Because of the critical involvement of cholesterol and dietary fat in the atherogenic process, the influences of other dietary components have not been exploited thoroughly. In 1953, Keys[38] postulated that increased levels of dietary fat were correlated with increased mortality from heart disease. Keys used his own data on fat intake derived from the Seven Countries Study and World Health Organization (WHO) data on heart disease incidence. Yerushalmy and Hilleboe[39] used the same WHO data to point out that protein intake correlated with heart disease mortality as well (or better) as did fat intake.

## 17.3  FUTURE STUDIES

The influences of dietary protein on atherosclerosis have only recently become a subject for research. The emphasis has been on comparisons of animal and vegetable protein. The demonstrations that soy protein peptides can affect cholesterolemia have led to efforts to isolate active peptides and eventually to develop synthetic peptides that would become the basis of treatment. The thrust here has been on the most widely used protein, soy protein, but vigorous investigation into the effects of other vegetable proteins might be instructive. Exploration of the possible effects of the L:A ratio has led to important findings, but these, like most studies, have involved major substitutions of one protein for the other. However, small changes may suffice. In rabbits, it has been shown that a 1:1 mix of animal and vegetable protein will reduce serum cholesterol levels and severity of atherosclerosis.[22] Sirtori et al.[40] showed that a small addition of soymilk to the diet of hypercholesterolemic subjects was enough to lower cholesterol levels. These observations are important because most subjects will readily accept small changes in diet but may resist large substitutions.

Investigations into the physiological effects of soy protein have shown that it can exert beneficial effects on cholesterolemia and atherosclerosis. Much has been learned about mechanisms of action of soy protein.

It would be useful to extend these studies to include other commonly eaten vegetable proteins. Large changes in diet may be resisted, but if positive effects of small changes in diet composition can be reproduced, they would probably be acceptable and would enable us to enjoy the positive benefits of ingestion of animal protein (trace minerals, $B_{12}$, etc.) while leading to reduction in risk. Most dietary advice promotes ingestion of a varied diet taken in moderation. Increasing soy (or other plant) protein intake rather than wholesale replacement may be the most acceptable advice.

In the area of research, there remains much to be learned such as mechanisms of action of soy protein, influence of soy peptides on health and disease, and roles of apolipoprotein E isoforms, to list a few. In the public health area, we know that relatively minor substitution or addition of soy protein to the conventional diet can have healthful consequences.

# REFERENCES

1. Ignatowski, A., Influence de la nourriture animale sur l'organisme des lapins, *Arch. Med. Exp. Anat. Pathol.*, 20, 1–20, 1908.
2. Ignatowski, A., Über die wirkung des tierischen eiweisses auf die aorta und die parenchymatisen organe der kaninchen, *Virchows Arch. Pathol. Anat. Physiol. Klinische Med.*, 198, 248–270, 1909.
3. Stuckey, H.W.I., Über die veranderungen der Kaninchen aorta bei der reichlichen tierschen Kost, *Central Allgemeine Pathol. Patholog. Anat.*, 22, 379–380, 1911.
4. Chalatow, S.S., Über das verhaltender Leber gegenüber den verschnederen Arten von Speisefett, *Virchows Arch. Pathol. Anat. Physiol. Klinische. Med.*, 207, 452–469, 1912.
5. Wesselkin, N.W., Über die Ablagerung von fettartigen Stoffen in den Organen, *Virchows Arch. Pathol. Anat. Physiol. Klinische. Med.*, 212, 225–235, 1913.
6. Anitschkow, N. and Chalatow, S., Über experimentelle cholesterinsteatose und ihre bedeutung für die entstehung einiger pathologische prozesse, *Centralbl. Allg. Path. Path. Anat.*, 24, 1–9, 1913.
7. Wacker, L. and Hueck, W., Über experimentelle atherosklerose und cholesterinanie, *Münch. Med. Wochenschr.*, 60, 2097–2106, 1913.
8. Kritchevsky, D., Dietary protein, cholesterol and atherosclerosis: a review of the early history, *J. Nutr.*, 125, 589S–593S, 1995.
9. Debry, G., *Dietary Proteins and Atherosclerosis*, CRC Press: Boca Raton, FL, 2004, 340 pp.
10. Freyberg, R.H., Relation of experimental atherosclerosis to diets rich in vegetable protein, *Arch. Int. Med.*, 59, 660–666, 1937.
11. Meeker, D.R. and Kesten, H.D., Experimental atherosclerosis and high protein diets, *Proc. Soc. Exp. Biol. Med.*, 45, 543–545, 1940.
12. Meeker, D.R. and Kesten, H.D., Effect of high protein diets on experimental atherosclerosis of rabbits, *Arch. Pathol.*, 31, 147–162, 1941.
13. Kritchevsky, D., Kolman, R.R., Guttmacher, R.M., and Forbes, M., Influence of dietary carbohydrate and protein on serum and liver cholesterol in germ-free chickens, *Arch. Biochem. Biophys.*, 85, 444–451, 1959.
14. Howard, A.N., Gresham, G.A., Jones, D., and Jennings, I.W., The prevention of rabbit atherosclerosis by soya bean meal, *J. Atheroscler. Res.*, 5, 330–337, 1965.
15. Hodges, R.E., Krehl, W.A., Stone, D.B., and Lopez, A., Dietary carbohydrates and low cholesterol diets: effects on serum lipids on man, *Am. J. Clin. Nutr.*, 20, 198–208, 1967.
16. Carroll, K.K. and Hamilton, R.M.G., Effects of dietary protein and carbohydrate on plasma cholesterol levels in relation to atherosclerosis, *J. Food Sci.*, 40, 18–23, 1975.
17. Huff, M.W., Hamilton, R.M., and Carroll, K.K., Plasma cholesterol levels in rabbits fed low fat, cholesterol-free, semipurified diets: effects of dietary proteins, protein hydrolysates and amino acid mixtures, *Atherosclerosis*, 28, 187–195, 1977.
18. Sugano, M., Yamada, Y., Yoshida, K., Hashimoto, Y., Matsuo, T. et al. The hypocholesterolemic action of the undigested fraction of soybean protein in rats, *Atherosclerosis*, 72, 115–122, 1988.
19. Sugano, M., Goto, S., Yamada, Y., Yoshida, K., Hashimoto, Y. et al., Cholesterol-lowering activity of various undigested fractions of soybean protein in rats, *J. Nutr.*, 120, 977–985, 1990.

20. Adams, M.R., Golden, D.L., Franke, A.A., Potter, S.M., Smith, H.S. et al., Dietary soy beta-conglycinin (7S globulin) inhibits atherosclerosis in mice, *J. Nutr.*, 134, 511–516, 2004.
21. Kritchevsky, D., Vegetable protein and atherosclerosis, *J. Am. Oil Chem. Soc.*, 56, 135–140, 1979.
22. Lovati, M.R., Manzoni, C., Gianazza, E., and Sirtori, C.R., Soybean protein products as regulators of liver low-density lipoprotein receptors. I. Identification of active β-conglycinin subunits, *J. Agri. Food Chem.*, 46, 2474–2480, 1998.
23. Manzoni, C., Lovati, M.R., Gianazza, E., Morita, Y., and Sirtori, C., Soybean protein products as regulators of liver low-density lipoprotein receptors. II. α-α′ rich commercial soy concentrate and α′ deficient mutant differently affect low-density lipoprotein receptor activation, *J. Agri. Food Chem.*, 46, 2481–2484, 1998.
24. Tailford, K.A., Berry, C.L., Thomas, A.C., and Campbell, J.H., A casein variant in cow's milk is atherogenic, *Atherosclerosis*, 170, 13–19, 2003.
25. Kritchevsky, D., Tepper, S.A., Czarnecki, S.K., Klurfeld, D.M., and Story, J.A., Experimental atherosclerosis in rabbits fed cholesterol-free diets. Part 9. Beef protein and textured vegetable protein, *Atherosclerosis*, 39, 169–175, 1981.
26. Kritchevsky, D., Tepper, S.A., Czarnecki, S.K., and Klurfeld, D.M., Atherogenicity of animal and vegetable protein. Influence of the lysine to arginine ratio, *Atherosclerosis*, 41, 429–431, 1982.
27. Kritchevsky, D., Tepper, S.A., Czarnecki, S.K., Klurfeld, D.M., and Story, J.A., Animal and vegetable proteins in lipid metabolism and atherosclerosis, in *Current Topics in Nutrition and Disease*, Vol. 8, Alan R. Liss, New York, 1983, pp. 85–100.
28. Beynen, A.C., van der Meer, R., West, C.E., Sugano, M., and Kritchevsky, D., Possible mechanisms underlying the differential cholesterolemic effects of dietary casein and soy protein, in *Nutrition Effects on Cholesterol Metabolism*, Transmondial, Voortheuzen, The Netherlands, 1986, pp. 29–45.
29. Hunter, A. and Downs, C.E., *The inhibition of arginase by amino acids, J. Biol. Chem.*, 157, 427–446, 1945.
30. Cittadini, D., Pietropaolo, C., Decristofaro, D., and D'Ayjello-Caracciolo, M., *In vivo* effect of L-lysine on rat liver arginase, *Nature*, 203, 643–644, 1964.
31. Cooke, J.P., Singer, A.H., Tsao, P., Zera, P., Rowan, R.A. et al., Antiatherogenic effects of L-arginine in the hypercholesterolemic rabbit, *J. Clin. Invest.*, 90, 1168–1172, 1992.
32. Moore, M.C., Moore, E.M., Beasley, C.D., Hankins, G.J., and Judlin, B.C., Dietary-atherosclerosis study on deceased persons, *J. Am. Diet. Assoc.*, 56, 13–22, 1970.
33. Moore, M.C., Moore, E.M., and Beasley, C.D., Dietary-atherosclerosis study on deceased persons, *J. Am. Diet. Assoc.*, 56, 23–28, 1970.
34. Moore, M.C., Guzman, M.A., Schilling, P.E., and Strong, J.P., Dietary-atherosclerosis study on deceased persons. Relation of eating pattern to raised coronary lesions, *J. Am. Diet. Assoc.*, 67, 22–28, 1975.
35. Moore, M.C., Guzman, M.A., Schilling, P.E., and Strong, J.P., Dietary-atherosclerosis study on deceased persons. Relation of selected dietary components to raised coronary lesions, *J. Am. Diet. Assoc.*, 68, 216–223, 1976.
36. Moore, M.C., Guzman, M.A., Schilling, P.E., and Strong, J.P., Dietary-atherosclerosis study on deceased persons. Further data on the relation of selected nutrients to raised coronary lesions, *J. Am. Diet. Assoc.*, 70, 602–606, 1977.

37. Kritchevsky, D., Tepper, S.A., Williams, D.E., and Story, J.A., Experimental atherosclerosis in rabbits fed cholesterol-free diets. Part 7. Interaction of animal or vegetable protein with fiber, *Atherosclerosis,* 26, 397–403, 1977.
38. Keys, A., Atherosclerosis: a problem in newer public health, *J. Mt. Sinai Hosp. NY,* 20, 118–139, 1953.
39. Yerushalmy, J. and Hilleboe, H.E., Fat in the diet and mortality from heart disease: a methodologic note, *NY State J. Med.,* 57, 2343–2354, 1957.
40. Sirtori, C.R., Pazzucconi, F., Colombo, L., Battistin, P., Bondioli, A. et al., Double-blind study of the addition of high-protein soya milk v. cows' milk to the diet of patients with severe hypercholesterolaemia and resistance to or intolerance of statins, *Br. J. Nutr.,* 82, 91–96, 1999.

# Index